T0259525

Women's Mental Health

Guest Editors

SUSAN G. KORNSTEIN, MD
ANITA H. CLAYTON, MD

PSYCHIATRIC CLINICS OF NORTH AMERICA

www.psych.theclinics.com

June 2010 • Volume 33 • Number 2

SAUNDERS an imprint of ELSEVIER, Inc.

W.B. SAUNDERS COMPANY
A Division of Elsevier Inc.

1600 John F. Kennedy Boulevard • Suite 1800 • Philadelphia, PA 19103-2899

http://www.theclinics.com

PSYCHIATRIC CLINICS OF NORTH AMERICA Volume 33, Number 2
June 2010 ISSN 0193-953X, ISBN-13: 978-1-4377-1868-3

Editor: Sarah E. Barth
Developmental Editor: Donald Mumford

Psychiatric Clinics of North America (ISSN 0193-953X) is published quarterly by Elsevier Inc., 360 Park Avenue South, New York, NY 10010-1710. Months of issue are March, June, September, and December. Business and Editorial Offices: 1600 John F. Kennedy Blvd., Suite 1800, Philadelphia, PA 19103-2899. Periodicals postage paid at New York, NY and additional mailing offices. Subscription prices are $248.00 per year (US individuals), $430.00 per year (US institutions), $125.00 per year (US students/residents), $297.00 per year (Canadian individuals), $535.00 per year (Canadian Institutions), $369.00 per year (foreign individuals), $535.00 per year (foreign institutions), and $185.00 per year (international & Canadian students/residents). Foreign air speed delivery is included in all *Clinics'* subscription prices. All prices are subject to change without notice. **POSTMASTER:** Send address changes to *Psychiatric Clinics of North America*, Elsevier Health Sciences Division, Subscription Customer Service, 3251 Riverport Lane, Maryland Heights, MO 63043. Customer Service: 1-800-654-2452 (US). From outside the United States, call 1-314-447-8871. Fax: 1-314-447-8029. E-mail: journalscustomerservice-usa@elsevier.com (for print support) and journalsonlinesupport-usa@elsevier.com (for online support).

Reprints. For copies of 100 or more, of articles in this publication, please contact the Commercial Reprints Department, Elsevier Inc., 360 Park Avenue South, New York, New York 10010-1710. Tel.: (212) 633-3813, Fax: (212) 462-1935, E-mail: reprints@elsevier.com.

Psychiatric Clinics of North America is covered in *MEDLINE/PubMed (Index Medicus), Current Contents/Social and Behavioral Sciences, Social Science Citation Index, Embase/Excerpta Medica,* and PsycINFO.

Printed and bound by CPI Group (UK) Ltd, Croydon, CR0 4YY

Transferred to Digital Print 2011

Contributors

GUEST EDITORS

SUSAN G. KORNSTEIN, MD
Professor of Psychiatry and Obstetrics-Gynecology; Executive Director, Institute for Women's Health; Executive Director, Mood Disorders Institute; Medical Director, Clinical Trials Office, Virginia Commonwealth University, Richmond, Virginia

ANITA H. CLAYTON, MD
David C. Wilson Professor, Department of Psychiatry and Neurobehavioral Sciences; Professor of Clinical Obstetrics and Gynecology, University of Virginia, Charlottesville, Virginia

AUTHORS

LESLEY M. ARNOLD, MD
Professor of Psychiatry; Director, Women's Health Research Program, Department of Psychiatry, University of Cincinnati College of Medicine, Cincinnati, Ohio

LEILA AZARBAD, PhD
Assistant Professor, Department of Behavioral Sciences, Rush University Medical Center, Chicago, Illinois

SUDIE E. BACK, PhD
Associate Professor, Associate Director, Drug Abuse Research Track, Clinical Neuroscience Division, Department of Psychiatry, Medical University of South Carolina, Charleston, South Carolina

MUDHASIR BASHIR, MD
Assistant Professor, Department of Psychiatry and Neurobehavioral Sciences, University of Virginia Health System, Charlottesville, Virginia

KATHLEEN T. BRADY, MD, PhD
Distinguished University Professor; Director, Clinical Neuroscience Division, Department of Psychiatry, Medical University of South Carolina; Research Director, South Carolina Clinical and Translational Research Institute, Charleston, South Carolina

KEIRA CHISM, MD
Instructor; Associate Director, Consultation-Liaison Psychiatry, Methodist Hospital; Department of Psychiatry and Human Behavior, Thomas Jefferson University, Philadelphia, Pennsylvania

ANITA H. CLAYTON, MD
David C. Wilson Professor, Department of Psychiatry and Neurobehavioral Sciences; Professor of Clinical Obstetrics and Gynecology, University of Virginia, Charlottesville, Virginia

LEE S. COHEN, MD
Perinatal and Reproductive Psychiatry Clinical Research Program; Department of Psychiatry, Massachusetts General Hospital, Harvard Medical School, Boston, Massachusetts

KRISTINA M. DELIGIANNIDIS, MD
Assistant Professor of Psychiatry; Director, Depression Specialty Clinic; Psychiatrist, Women's Mental Health Specialty Clinic, UMass Memorial Medical Center; Center for Psychopharmacologic Research and Treatment, University of Massachusetts Medical School, Worcester, Massachusetts

ANIQUE FORRESTER, MD
Resident PGY 3, Department of Psychiatry and Human Behavior, Thomas Jefferson University, Philadelphia, Pennsylvania

MARLENE P. FREEMAN, MD
Perinatal and Reproductive Psychiatry Clinical Research Program; Department of Psychiatry, Massachusetts General Hospital, Harvard Medical School, Boston, Massachusetts

BENICIO N. FREY, MD, PhD
Department of Psychiatry and Behavioural Neurosciences; Department of Obstetrics and Gynecology, McMaster University; Women's Health Concerns Clinic, St Joseph's Healthcare, Hamilton, Ontario, Canada

LINDA GONDER-FREDERICK, PhD
Associate Professor, Department of Psychiatry and Neurobehavioral Sciences; Clinical Director, Behavioral Medicine Center, Department of Psychiatric Medicine, University of Virginia Health System, Charlottesville, Virginia

SHELLY F. GREENFIELD, MD, MPH
Chief Academic Officer; Director, Clinical Research and Education, Alcohol and Drug Abuse Treatment Program, McLean Hospital, Belmont; Associate Professor of Psychiatry, Harvard Medical School, Boston, Massachusetts

DAVID V. HAMILTON, MD, MA
Fellow, Department of Psychiatry and Neurobehavioral Sciences, Institute for Law, Psychiatry, and Public Policy, University of Virginia, Charlottesville, Virginia

SUZANNE HOLROYD, MD
Professor, Department of Psychiatry and Neurobehavioral Sciences, University of Virginia Health System, Charlottesville, Virginia

ELISABETH J.S. KUNKEL, MD
Professor of Psychiatry and Human Behavior; Vice Chair for Clinical Affairs; Director, Consultation-Liaison Psychiatry, Thomas Jefferson University, Philadelphia, Pennsylvania

KATIE LAWSON, MA
Study Coordinator, Clinical Neuroscience Division, Department of Psychiatry, Medical University of South Carolina, Charleston, South Carolina

ELIZABETH L. LEMON, MA
Perinatal and Reproductive Psychiatry Clinical Research Program; Department
of Psychiatry, Massachusetts General Hospital, Harvard Medical School,
Boston, Massachusetts

DIMITRI MARKOV, MD
Assistant Professor, Department of Psychiatry and Human Behavior; Department of
Medicine, Thomas Jefferson University, Philadelphia, Pennsylvania

RUTA NONACS, MD, PhD
Perinatal and Reproductive Psychiatry Clinical Research Program; Department
of Psychiatry, Massachusetts General Hospital, Harvard Medical School,
Boston, Massachusetts

MICHELLE R. PELCOVITZ, BA
Clinical Research Coordinator, Mount Sinai School of Medicine; James J. Peters Veterans
Affairs Medical Center, Bronx, New York, New York

LAURA C. PRATCHETT, PsyD
Psychology Post-Doctoral Fellow, Mount Sinai School of Medicine; James J. Peters
Veterans Affairs Medical Center, Bronx, New York, New York

JULIA J. RUCKLIDGE, PhD
Associate Professor of Psychology, Department of Psychology, University of Canterbury,
Christchurch, New Zealand

ELKA SERRANO, MD
Staff Psychiatrist, Family and Children's Services, Tulsa, Oklahoma

CLAUDIO N. SOARES, MD, PhD, FRCPC
Associate Professor, Departments of Psychiatry and Behavioural Neurosciences and
Obstetrics and Gynecology; Academic Head, Mood Disorders Division, McMaster
University; Director, Women's Health Concerns Clinic, St Joseph's Healthcare, Hamilton,
Ontario, Canada

MEIR STEINER, MD, PhD, FRCPC
Department of Psychiatry and Behavioural Neurosciences; Department of Obstetrics
and Gynecology, McMaster University; Women's Health Concerns Clinic, St Joseph's
Healthcare, Hamilton, Ontario, Canada

SIMONE N. VIGOD, MD, FRCPC
Lecturer, Department of Psychiatry, University of Toronto, Women's College Hospital,
Women's College Research Institute, Toronto, Ontario, Canada

ADELE C. VIGUERA, MD
Perinatal and Reproductive Psychiatry Clinical Research Program; Department
of Psychiatry, Massachusetts General Hospital, Harvard Medical School,
Boston, Massachusetts

BETTY WANG, MD
Perinatal and Reproductive Psychiatry Clinical Research Program; Department
of Psychiatry, Massachusetts General Hospital, Harvard Medical School,
Boston, Massachusetts

JULIA K. WARNOCK, MD, PhD
Professor of Psychiatry, Department of Psychiatry, The University of Oklahoma College
of Medicine-Tulsa, Tulsa, Oklahoma

TAL WEINBERGER, MD
Clinical Instructor, Consultation-Liaison Psychiatry; Department of Psychiatry
and Human Behavior, Thomas Jefferson University, Philadelphia, Pennsylvania

KIRSTEN M. WILKINS, MD
Assistant Professor of Psychiatry, Department of Psychiatry, The University
of Oklahoma College of Medicine-Tulsa, Tulsa, Oklahoma

RACHEL YEHUDA, PhD
Mental Health Patient Care Center Director, James J. Peters Veterans Affairs Medical
Center, Bronx; Professor of Psychiatry and Neurobiology, Director of Traumatic Stress
Studies Division, Mount Sinai School of Medicine, New York, New York

Contents

> As many as 7% of women experience significant social or occupational dysfunction as a result of severe premenstrual mood disturbance. Biological, psychological, and sociocultural factors are implicated in the cause of premenstrual dysphoric disorder, but the interaction between these factors remains to be elucidated. Mental health practitioners can aid women by providing diagnostic clarity and by initiating an integrated step-wise management approach.

> Studies suggest that pregnancy does not protect women from the emergence or persistence of mood disorders. Mood and anxiety disorders are prevalent in women during the childbearing years and, for many women, these mood disorders are chronic or recurrent. Maintenance antidepressant therapy is often indicated during the reproductive years and women face difficult treatment decisions regarding psychotropic medications and pregnancy. Treatment of psychiatric disorders during pregnancy involves a thoughtful weighing of the risks and benefits of proposed interventions and the documented and theoretical risks associated with untreated psychiatric disorders such as depression. Collaborative decision-making that incorporates patient treatment preferences is optimal for women trying to conceive or who are pregnant. This article reviews the diagnosis and treatment guidelines of mood disorders during pregnancy and postpartum, with specific reference to the use of psychotropic medications during this critical time.

> Women are at a higher risk than men of developing depression and anxiety and such increased risk might be particularly associated with reproductive cycle events. Recent evidence suggests that the transition to menopause may constitute a window of vulnerability for some women for the development of new onset and recurrent depression. Several biological and environmental factors seem to be independent predictors or modulating factors for the occurrence of depression in menopausal women; they include the presence and severity of hot flushes, sleep disturbances, history of severe premenstrual syndrome or postpartum blues, stressful life

events, history of depression, socioeconomic status, and use of hormones and psychotropic agents. The regulation of monoaminergic systems by ovarian hormones might explain, at least in part, the emergence of depressive symptoms and/or anxiety in biologically predisposed subpopulations. The use of transdermal estradiol, as well as serotonergic and noradrenergic antidepressants, is an efficacious strategy in the treatment of depression and vasomotor symptoms in symptomatic women in midlife. In this review, the authors discuss the existing evidence of a greater risk for the development of depression during the menopausal transition and the putative underlying mechanisms contributing to this window of vulnerability. Hormonal and nonhormonal treatment strategies for depression and anxiety in this particular population are critically examined, although more tailored treatment options are still needed.

This article reviews depressive symptoms in women as they relate to infertility and infertility treatments. Common causes of infertility in women are discussed and the literature on depressive symptoms before and during various infertility treatments is presented. Recommendations are made from a psychiatric perspective regarding how to manage depressive symptoms in women in the context of infertility.

Sexual dysfunctions diminish the quality of life for many women, frequently causing enough distress to warrant the diagnosis of a sexual disorder. Problems with sexual function can occur in any stage of the sexual response cycle. Dysfunction is further influenced by a variety of factors: medical, psychiatric, cultural, and stage of life. A variety of treatment modalities exist, though current research has not yet provided Food and Drug Administration-approved therapies for sexual disorders in women.

Gender differences in substance use disorders (SUDs) and treatment outcomes for women with SUDs have been a focus of research in the last 15 years. This article reviews gender differences in the epidemiology of SUDs, highlighting the convergence of male/female prevalence ratios of SUDs in the last 20 years. The telescoping course of SUDs, recent research on the role of neuroactive gonadal steroid hormones in craving and relapse, and sex differences in stress reactivity and relapse to substance abuse are described. The role of co-occurring mood and anxiety, eating, and posttraumatic stress disorders is considered in the epidemiology, natural history, and treatment of women with SUDs. Women's use of alcohol, stimulants, opioids, cannabis, and nicotine are examined in terms of recent epidemiology, biologic and psychosocial effects, and treatment. Although women may be less likely to enter substance abuse treatment than men over the course of the lifetime, once they enter treatment, gender itself is not a predictor of treatment retention, completion, or outcome. Research on gender-specific treatments for women with SUDs and behavioral couples treatment has yielded promising results for substance abuse treatment outcomes in women.

Attention-deficit hyperactivity disorder (ADHD) is recognized to exist in males and females although the literature supports a higher prevalence in males. However, when girls are diagnosed with ADHD, they are more often diagnosed as predominantly inattentive than boys with ADHD. This article provides a review of gender differences noted across the lifespan. Males and females with ADHD are more similar than different, and generally ADHD profiles are not sex specific. Small gender differences have been found: adolescent girls with ADHD have lower self-efficacy and poorer coping strategies than adolescent boys with ADHD; rates of depression and anxiety may be higher, and physical aggression and other externalizing behaviors lower in girls and women with ADHD. Men with ADHD seem to be incarcerated more often than women with ADHD. However, many studies suffer from small sample sizes, referral biases, differences in diagnostic procedures, and possible rater influences. Treatments are reviewed and discussed with reference to the reported gender differences in functioning and the global deficits noted in all samples. The data available so far suggest that treatments are likely to be equally effective in males and females. However, referral bias is a problem, in that females with ADHD are less likely to be referred for treatment than males with ADHD. Future research should include equal representation of both sexes in samples such that sex by treatment analyses can be routinely conducted.

Research in fibromyalgia has increased understanding of the possible genetic and environmental factors that could be involved in the etiology of fibromyalgia. There is now substantial evidence for augmentation of central pain processing in fibromyalgia. Because the clinical presentation of fibromyalgia is heterogeneous, treatment recommendations must be individualized for each patient. The rapid growth of trials in fibromyalgia in recent years has resulted in new evidence-based approaches to pharmacological and nonpharmacological treatment.

Breast cancer is a relatively common diagnosis for American women and depressive symptoms occur in many women with breast cancer. Identification of women with breast cancer and concomitant depressive symptoms and mood disorders requires particular attention by heath care providers, and may be aided by the administration of a variety of diagnostic and/or screening tools. Insomnia is also a significant problem for women with breast cancer at various stages of diagnosis and treatment, including after remission. Although many studies on the treatment of depression in women with breast cancer have been done, and the data do point to the efficacy of several antidepressants in this population, there are no data to support the widely held hypothesis that treatment of depression in patients with breast cancer may positively affect morbidity and mortality. Breast cancer treatments may give rise to depressive symptoms and this should be considered in the approach to pharmacotherapy. Several psychotherapeutic modalities offer relief of the symptoms and syndromes of depression in breast cancer. Future research can answer the question of which approach is most appropriate for which patients, and whether therapy can improve a variety of health outcomes and survival for women with breast cancer.

Obesity carries a unique disease burden on women and is influenced by a variety of biological, hormonal, environmental, and cultural factors. Reproductive transitions, such as pregnancy and menopause, increase the risk for obesity. Psychologically, obese women experience greater weight-related stigma and discrimination and are at increased risk for depression than obese men. Women are also particularly susceptible to psychological stress, sleep debt, and lack of physical activity, all of which are risk factors for the development of excess weight. Obesity risk is increased among women with psychiatric disorders and those who use certain psychotropic medications. Obesity treatment should take into consideration degree of obesity, health risks, past weight loss attempts, and individual differences in motivation and readiness for treatment.

Complementary and alternative medicine (CAM) therapies are commonly practiced in the United States and are used more frequently among women than men. This article reviews several CAM treatments for depressive disorders in women, with a focus on major depressive disorder across the reproductive life cycle. The CAM therapies selected for this review (ie, S-adenosylmethionine, omega-3 fatty acids, St John's wort, bright light therapy, acupuncture, and exercise) were based on their prevalence of use and the availability of randomized, placebo-controlled data. Further study is necessary to delineate the role of specific CAM therapies in premenstrual syndrome, premenstrual dysphoric disorder, antepartum and postpartum depression, lactation, and the menopausal transition.

Posttraumatic stress disorder (PTSD) as a response to trauma is repeatedly found to be more common among women than men. This article explores prevalence rates and gender differences. Explanations for this gender bias and examined and the literature on trauma types and resulting PTSD is reviewed. Other disorders that may result from trauma that also have gender biases are considered as a potential way to understand this difference. Risk and resilience can perhaps more appropriately be considered specific to symptom picture rather than merely development of pathology.

Mudhasir Bashir and Suzanne Holroyd

With the growth of the elderly population, and the female elderly population in particular, healthcare providers will see increasing numbers of elderly women with psychiatric disorders. To properly care for this group of patients, better understanding is needed not only of group differences in this patient population but also of the differences in each individual, as they age, given their unique life experiences, cohort effects, medical comorbidity, social situation, and personality traits. Understandably, these characteristics will interact with psychiatric disorders in ways that may increase the challenge to correctly diagnose and treat these patients. In addition, understanding late life changes, the prevalence of various mental disorders and the sometimes unique presentation of mental disorders in this age group is required to better diagnose and treat this population.

THE CLINICS ARE NOW AVAILABLE ONLINE!

Access your subscription at:
www.theclinics.com

Preface

Advances in Women's Mental Health

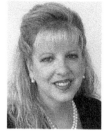 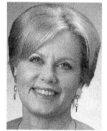

Susan G. Kornstein, MD   Anita H. Clayton, MD
Guest Editors

Women's health is escalating in importance in the national health care agenda with new data about gender differences being acquired quickly, an increasing percentage of the population being female, and health insurance reform under intense debate. Since the requirement that women be included in clinical research studies, with subsequent analysis of gender differences when appropriate, the knowledge base has increased dramatically with regard to the prevalence, etiology, presentation, and treatment response of disorders in women. Women's health has increasingly become an area of specialty, with residency tracks, fellowships, conferences, and organizations dedicated to this important clinical and research focus.

This volume updates some topics covered in the 2003 issue of *Psychiatric Clinics of North America* that was devoted to women's health, and introduces new topic areas. The effect of reproductive status on psychiatric symptoms is examined in several articles, including a review of premenstrual dysphoria by Simone Vigod and colleagues, identification and management of depression during pregnancy and the postpartum period by Lee Cohen and colleagues, presentation on the interrelationship between mood and climacteric symptoms in the menopausal transition by Claudio Soares and Benicio Frey, and discussion of the influence of infertility and its treatment on women's mental health presented by Kirsten Wilkins and colleagues.

Gender differences in psychiatric diagnoses are addressed by Shelly Greenfield and colleagues with regard to substance abuse problems and by Julia Rucklidge related to attention-deficit/hyperactivity disorder. In addition, the effects of gender are considered in sexual functioning and dysfunction by Anita Clayton and David Hamilton and in the elderly psychiatric patient by Mudhasir Bashir and Suzanne Holroyd.

Psychiatr Clin N Am 33 (2010) xiii–xiv
doi:10.1016/j.psc.2010.02.002
0193-953X/10/$ – see front matter
psych.theclinics.com

Medical conditions with comorbid psychiatric symptoms that occur more frequently in women are also presented. Fibromyalgia is reviewed by Lesley Arnold; Tal Weinberger and colleagues discuss breast cancer; and Leila Azarbad and Linda Gonder-Frederick speak to obesity in women. Additionally, Kristina Deligiannidis and Marlene Freeman provide a detailed analysis of complementary and alternative medicine interventions for psychiatric disorders. In contrast trauma and violence toward women is addressed by Laura Pratchett and coworkers.

These comprehensive reviews provide new insights into caring for women with psychiatric conditions. Application of the wealth of information in these articles will improve the care of women and should stimulate further research into this important clinical area.

Susan G. Kornstein, MD
Department of Psychiatry, Institute for Women's Health,
Mood Disorders Institute, and Clinical Trials Office
Virginia Commonwealth University
PO Box 980710
Richmond, VA 23298-0710, USA

Anita H. Clayton, MD
Department of Psychiatry and Neurobehavioral Sciences
University of Virginia
PO Box 801210
Charlottesville, VA 22908-1210, USA

E-mail addresses:
skornste@vcu.edu (S.G. Kornstein)
AHC8V@hscmail.mcc.virginia.edu (A.H. Clayton)

Approach to Premenstrual Dysphoria for the Mental Health Practitioner

Simone N. Vigod, MD, FRCPC[a], Benicio N. Frey, MD, PhD[b,c],
Claudio N. Soares, MD, PhD, FRCPC[b,c,d,e],
Meir Steiner, MD, PhD, FRCPC[b,c,d,*]

KEYWORDS

• PMDD • PMS • Dysphoria • Mental Health • Mood disorder

For many centuries, the menstrual cycle has held negative connotations for women. It has been held as evidence for a generalized sense that women were incompetent or unstable, with their resultant exclusion from opportunities in education, employment, and positions of influence.[1,2] Such views are no longer in the mainstream.

Dr Vigod is supported by a Fellowship from the Ontario Mental Health Foundation and by the Department of Psychiatry, Women's College Hospital, Toronto, Ontario, Canada.

Dr Frey is has received grant/research support from Canadian Institutes of Health Research, Eli Lilly, Father Sean O'Sullivan Research Centre, Stanley Medical Research Institute, and Wyeth Pharmaceuticals. He has participated as a member of the speakers' bureau of AstraZeneca and Wyeth Pharmaceuticals and as a member of advisory boards for AstraZeneca and Wyeth Pharmaceuticals.

Dr Claudio N. Soares has received grant/research support from Eli Lilly, AstraZeneca, Physicians Services Incorporated (PSI) Foundation, Allergen National Centre of Excellence, Hamilton Community Foundation, Lundbeck, Wyeth, and Canadian institute of Health Research (CIHR). He has worked as a research consultant for Wyeth, Lundbeck, Bayer Healthcare Pharmaceuticals; he has participated as a member of the speakers' bureau of AstraZeneca, Wyeth, Bayer Healthcare Pharmaceuticals, and is a member of the advisory boards for AstraZeneca, Wyeth, and Bayer Healthcare Pharmaceuticals.

Dr Steiner is a consultant for Wyeth Pharmaceuticals, Bayer Shering Pharmaceuticals, AstraZeneca, Azevan Pharmaceuticals, and Servier; has received grant and research support from Canadian Institutes of Health Research, Physicians Services Inc., Wyeth Pharmaceuticals, AstraZeneca, and Lundbeck and received honoraria from Azevan Pharmaceuticals, Bayer, Canada, and Ortho-McNeil.

[a] Department of Psychiatry, University of Toronto, Women's College Hospital, Women's College Research Institute, Room 944C, Toronto, ON M5S 1B2, Canada

[b] Department of Psychiatry and Behavioural Neurosciences, McMaster University, Hamilton, ON, Canada

[c] Women's Health Concerns Clinic, St Joseph's Healthcare, Fontbonne Building, 6th Floor, 301 James Street South, Hamilton, ON L8P 3B6, Canada

[d] Department of Obstetrics and Gynecology, McMaster University, Hamilton, ON, Canada

[e] Mood Disorders Division, McMaster University, Hamilton, ON, Canada

* Corresponding author. Department of Psychiatry and Behavioural Neurosciences, McMaster University, Hamilton, ON, Canada.
E-mail address: mst@mcmaster.ca

There has been clear advancement of knowledge with the advent of understanding that female sex hormones underlie the menstrual cycle and that mood disorders related to menstruation are a significant problem for some women. Women commonly present to health care practitioners complaining of premenstrual mood disturbance, warranting diagnosis and treatment. However, it can be challenging for providers to feel confident about managing these complaints because of the wide array of symptoms that women report, the multiple physical and psychiatric conditions on the differential diagnosis, and the psychosocial connotations of the disorder. This review presents an approach to the diagnosis and management of premenstrual mood disturbance and specifically reviews a biopsychosocial approach to the management of premenstrual dysphoric disorder (PMDD) for the mental health practitioner.

SCOPE OF THE PROBLEM
Prevalence

Varying reports in the literature on the prevalence of premenstrual mood disturbance depend in part on the definitions used. The American Psychiatric Association (APA) explicitly acknowledges in the Diagnostic and Statistical Manual for Mental Disorders (DSM-IV-TR) that up to 70% of women are affected by at least mild symptoms of premenstrual syndrome (PMS).[3] The American College of Obstetricians and Gynecologists (ACOG) reports that up to 85% of women experience PMS as defined by at least 1 emotional and 1 physical symptom, present in 3 consecutive menstrual cycles, and severe enough to interfere in daily life.[4] The APA has defined, and ACOG acknowledges, PMDD as a more severe and pervasive form of premenstrual mood disturbance that affects a much smaller, albeit significant, proportion of women.[3,4]

Studying the prevalence of PMDD in community samples has been challenging because the strict DSM-IV-TR diagnostic criteria for PMDD include prospective symptom measurement, exclusion of other psychiatric and physical disorders, and evaluation of functional impairment. Most community prevalence estimates have been based on retrospective symptom reports and have contained variable definitions of severe symptoms. Prevalence estimates based on DSM-IV-TR diagnostic criteria, but without the requirement for prospective symptom ratings, seem to be in the range of 5% to 6% in samples from North America and Europe.[5,6] However, there may be cultural variability in prevalence or symptom reporting as shown by a reported prevalence of only 1.2% in a Japanese study of 1152 women aged from 15 to 49 years in a cancer screening clinic.[7] Studies that measure symptoms prospectively reveal slightly lower estimates in some cases, with prevalence estimates ranging from 1.6% to 6.4%. Studies of clinical or volunteered populations tend to report prevalence estimates on the higher end of that range.[8–11] For example, in older premenopausal women recruited into the Harvard Study for Moods and Cycles (women aged 36–44 years), 6.4% of those who completed 1 menstrual cycle of prospective ratings met criteria for PMDD.[8] Estimates from 2 community-based prospective studies in which participants were sampled with the intent of generalizing the information to the general population revealed slightly lower estimates. Using the National Registry of Iceland, Sveindottir and Backstrom[12] reported a prevalence of PMDD between 2% and 6%. In the United States, Gehlert and colleagues[13] interviewed 1246 women (ages 13–55 years) in their homes, and the participants completed prospective daily symptom checklists over 2 menstrual cycles. In this study, only 1.6% of the women were diagnosed with PMDD using strict DSM-IV-TR criteria.

Clinical Correlates

Discerning correlates of PMS and PMDD can aid practitioners in identifying women at risk for the disorder and in need of treatment. However, although these variables may be associated with premenstrual mood disturbance, and therefore can help with identifying who is at risk, they do not necessarily lie along the causal pathway to PMS or PMDD. Potential etiological variables that may help guide treatment are discussed further in this article.

Few demographic variables are associated with increased risk for PMS or PMDD. Although younger age was associated with increased severity of symptoms in 1 study, clinical experience suggests that older women, particularly those with multiple children, may be more likely to report severe symptoms.[14] It is possible that this observation is confounded by the higher likelihood that younger women (before starting their families) are more likely to be using concomitant hormonal treatments for birth control, thereby reducing the severity of their premenstrual symptoms. The relationship between education level and PMDD has been studied, with conflicting results. Although women with higher levels of education tend to report more premenstrual symptoms,[15] in older premenopausal women from the Harvard Study of Moods and Cycles, PMDD was associated with lower levels of education.[8] Additional evidence from the same sample suggests that this effect may have been the result of high comorbidity of PMDD with major depressive disorder.[16]

Another important clinical correlate of premenstrual mood dysphoria is life stress. Several studies have shown an association between PMS/PMDD and stressful life events, including past sexual abuse in up to 40% of women,[17–21] a substantially higher rate of sexual abuse than has been reported in the female general population.[22] Premenstrual mood disturbance has also been associated with high levels of day-to-day stress.[23]

Family history of PMDD increases a woman's risk of having the disorder herself, with twin studies suggesting heritability in the range of 44% to 56%.[24,25] Personal history of major depressive disorder, particularly when related to other reproductive life stages such as depression in pregnancy or the postpartum period, may also be associated with an increased risk of PMDD.[26]

Effects

It has been difficult to specify the distinction between PMS and PMDD regarding the effects of these problems on social and occupational dysfunction. Steiner and colleagues[27] found that preexisting beliefs about work may affect the findings in studies that use self-reports. However, significant evidence of the negative effects of PMDD has been documented. For example, a large study of randomly selected members of a health maintenance organization found that women with PMDD reported decreased work productivity compared with women with milder premenstrual symptoms.[28] More recently, Yang and colleagues[29] attempted to compare the health-related quality of life in women with PMDD with that of women in the general population and women with other chronic health conditions in a community sample based in the United States. They found that the mental health–related quality of life burden for women with PMDD was greater than for women in the general population. It was also greater than for women with chronic back pain, and comparable with women with type II diabetes mellitus, hypertension, osteoporosis, and rheumatoid arthritis.

DIAGNOSTIC CONSIDERATIONS
PMS Versus PMDD

Premenstrual psychiatric symptoms are currently conceptualized and treated as part of the mood disorder spectrum. As outlined earlier, the DSM-IV-TR contains a definition of PMS as a syndrome that may include mild psychological discomfort or physical discomfort such as bloating and breast tenderness.[3] However, these symptoms do not result in significant functional impairment, and PMS symptoms are not considered to be disordered. However, PMDD is listed in DSM-IV-TR[3] as an example of a depressive disorder not otherwise specified and is described as follows:

> In most menstrual cycles during the past year, five (or more) of the following symptoms were present for most of the time during the last week of the luteal phase, began to remit within a few days after the onset of the follicular phase, and were absent in the week post-menses .... The disturbance markedly interferes with work or school or with usual social activities and relationships with others (p. 774).

In appendix B, the DSM-IV-TR specifies research criteria for PMDD whereby a diagnosis must include a least 1 of the essential symptoms of marked and persistent anger/irritability, depressed mood, anxiety, or affective lability with a total of 5 (out of a possible 11) symptoms. The other 7 symptoms are anhedonia, lack of energy, change in appetite, change in sleep, sense of feeling overwhelmed or out of control, and other physical symptoms (eg, breast tenderness or swelling, headaches, joint or muscle pain, a sensation of bloating or weight gain). The diagnosis of PMDD also requires a minimum of 2 consecutive months of prospectively daily symptom ratings.[3] These prospective ratings are considered essential because of concern that retrospective reports of premenstrual symptoms might not be reliable,[30] and because, due to mood and cognitive changes, there may be differential symptom reporting depending on the phase of the menstrual cycle in which women are queried.[31,32] Prospective daily symptom ratings are usually made using Likert or visual analog scales. Validated tools were described in a recent comprehensive review by Pearlstein and Steiner.[33] Many women do report some premenstrual symptoms during the follicular phase. A change score for symptom severity between the luteal and follicular phases may therefore be a more meaningful outcome, with a change of 30% to 50% having been recommended as an indication that a diagnosis of PMDD is appropriate.[34]

Other Conditions as Differential Diagnoses

Physical disorders that may mimic PMDD can usually be readily differentiated from PMDD by careful history, physical examination, and other relevant investigations. These disorders include systemic diseases such as autoimmune disorders, diabetes mellitus, anemia and hypothyroidism, and gynecologic conditions such as dysmenorrhea and endometriosis in which premenstrual exacerbations are commonly seen.[35]

Distinguishing PMDD from premenstrual exacerbations or magnification of psychiatric disorders is important because, with successful treatment of the primary condition, premenstrual symptoms will often remit.[36] Women who report premenstrual depressive symptoms should be screened for psychiatric symptoms across all phases of the cycle (and be treated accordingly). Premenstrual exacerbations of depressive disorders are commonly reported. For example, Hartlage and colleagues[37] found that 44% of nondepressed women taking antidepressants reported premenstrual mood symptoms in a community sample in the United States. Results from the National Institutes of Mental Health's Sequenced Treatment Alternatives to Relieve Depression

(STAR-D) trial found that, of 433 female participants with major depression, 64% reported a worsening of their depressive symptoms 5 to 10 days before menses.[38] Bipolar disorder must also be considered in the differential diagnosis of PMDD. Women with underlying bipolar disorder may experience premenstrual exacerbations of depressed mood or irritability.[39] Women with personality disorders may also experience increased irritability and interpersonal difficulties in the premenstrual period.[40]

PROPOSED ETIOLOGICAL FACTORS

It has been argued that PMS is a culture-bound syndrome in which women in Western cultures have been socialized to have negative expectations about menstruation.[41] It has been put forward that North American culture and the media further perpetuate the idea that the premenstrual period is associated with negative affect and mood instability,[2] with the result that women negatively interpret normal physiological changes that are essentially neutral in nature.[42–44] However, there is also clear evidence that sociocultural expectations do not form the complete picture of the cause of PMS, and certainly not of PMDD. As is the case with other psychiatric disorders, evidence is mounting that the cause of PMDD is likely complex, involving multiple biological, psychological, and sociocultural determinants. It is difficult to study how such factors might interact to produce the clinical picture of PMDD. This section highlights factors known to be important in the cause of this disorder, and that may be useful in guiding management and future development of treatment options.

Female Sex Hormones

Although symptoms of PMDD and phases of the menstrual cycle are temporally related, not all women suffer severe premenstrual mood symptoms. It is now being hypothesized that women with PMDD are more vulnerable than women without PMDD to the normal physiological changes associated with the menstrual cycle. This theory has been supported in 2 studies, in which women with and without PMDD responded differently to challenges with physiological levels of estrogen and progesterone.[45,46] In the first study, women with PMDD responded with more depressive mood than controls,[45] and, in the second study, the 2 groups had differential gonadotropin hormone level responses.[46] The centrally active progesterone metabolite allopregnanolone has also been investigated for its potential role in the pathogenesis of PMDD. In women with PMS and PMDD, there seems to be a relationship between allopregnanolone serum concentrations and the severity of premenstrual symptoms,[47,48] although some investigators have hypothesized that women with PMDD have differential sensitivity to allopregnanolone, and not to absolute levels of the neurosteroid.[49] Imaging studies show that women with PMDD have differential sensitivity at their γ-aminobutyric acid A (GABA-A) receptors (ie, where allopregnanolone acts in the central nervous system),[50] and that the severity of symptoms in women with PMDD seems to be related to their sensitivity to GABA steroids.[51] In addition, women with PMDD show differential sensitivity to other compounds with GABA-A activity, such as the benzodiazepine antagonist flumazenil[52] and several benzodiazepines compared with controls.[53,54] Possibly because of drug modulating effects on allopregnanolone levels, via GABA-A receptors, this sensitivity seems to normalize during treatment with serotonin reuptake inhibitors.[55]

Other Hormones and Endocrine Factors

Because of the prominence of irritability as a symptom of PMDD, androgens have also been investigated. Increased testosterone levels have been observed in women who report severe premenstrual irritability,[56,57] although one study revealed significantly lower total and free plasma testosterone levels in PMS patients compared with healthy controls.[58] There is little consistent evidence for the involvement of other endocrine factors, including cortisol, thyroid hormone, prolactin, melatonin, aldosterone, and endorphins in the cause of PMS/PMDD.[33]

Serotonin

Research has revealed that there is a relationship between serotonin function and ovarian hormone secretion, contributing to the plausibility of a complex interaction between hormone secretion and serotonin fluctuation.[59] In support of this hypothesis, a role for serotonin in the pathophysiology of PMDD has been consistently shown in research investigations using several experimental models. During the premenstrual phase, patients with PMDD have lower whole blood serotonin levels[60] and lower platelet serotonin uptake[61] than controls without PMDD, and Melke and colleagues[62] found that women with premenstrual dysphoria had fewer platelet paroxetine binding sites (ie, fewer serotonin transporters) compared with controls. Positron emission technology has revealed differences between women with PMDD and controls in brain serotonergic function across the menstrual cycle.[63] Challenges with serotonergic agents, such as L-tryptophan, fenfluramine, and buspirone, have also provided evidence of serotonin dysfunction in women with PMDD.[64–68] In addition, serotonergic drugs, and selective serotonin reuptake inhibitors (SSRIs) in particular, can treat PMDD rapidly (see later discussion), strongly supporting the hypothesis that serotonin is involved in the cause of PMDD. Only approximately 60% of patients with PMDD respond to treatment with SSRIs,[69] therefore isolated premenstrual serotonin deficiency is not likely to be the only etiological variable in all PMDD patients.

Genetic Factors

As mentioned earlier, there is evidence that PMDD is a heritable disorder. This has led to a search for genes that may be important in the pathophysiology of PMDD. From the evidence outlined earlier, most of the focus on genetic factors has been on genes related to serotonin and estrogen, as these are believed to be of primary importance in PMDD. Praschak-Rieder and colleagues[70] found an association between PMDD and 5HTLLPR heterozygosity in women with seasonal affective disorder, and Steiner and colleagues[57] identified a relationship between polymorphism in the serotonin transporter gene and severity of PMDD symptoms. More recently, Huo and colleagues[71] identified allelic variation in ESR1, the estrogen-α receptor gene in women with PMDD. This work forms an important basis for future research into the pathophysiology of PMDD.

Psychosocial Factors

There is little literature investigating how biological and sociocultural variables may interact in the development of severe PMS and PMDD. However, sexual abuse (and childhood sexual abuse in particular) has lasting effects on psychological and physiological responses to stress.[72] It has been hypothesized that past abuse could predispose women to psychiatric disorders, including PMDD through psychological and biological mechanisms.[73] For example, from a psychological perspective, some evidence suggests that women with premenstrual symptoms tend to rely more than other women on less effective strategies for coping with stress, such as avoidance or wishful thinking, than on strategies such as problem-focused coping or direct action.[2,74] From a biological perspective, preliminary evidence suggests that the high prevalence of sexual abuse among women seeking treatment of premenstrual symptoms may account for findings of dysregulated cardiovascular and neuroendocrine responses to laboratory stress in PMDD patients.[75] In fact, Bunevicius and colleagues[76] found that women with PMDD with and without histories of sexual abuse had differential autonomic nervous system responses to a challenge with the α-adrenergic receptor agonist clonidine. There is potential in this field for further development of the understanding of how biological and psychosocial factors interact to produce psychiatric illness.

MANAGEMENT

Although the precise pathophysiology of premenstrual mood dysphoria has yet to be elucidated, treatment strategies for PMDD have been informed by the findings to date. As PMDD has multiple biological and sociocultural etiological determinants, its treatment should involve an integrated approach. Treatment should appropriately reflect the severity and functional impairment associated with the symptoms, with a step-wise approach beginning with the least invasive treatments. An outline of the approach to treatment of PMDD is given in **Box 1**. For all women, treatment of comorbid psychiatric or medical disorders and issues related to any persistent life stressors, or any past or current physical or sexual abuse, is essential.

Lifestyle Factors

Education about the condition, supportive counseling, and general healthy lifestyle measures, such as regular exercise and healthy diet, may be sufficient to result in symptom improvement in women with mild symptoms. These recommendations can be made and patients can attempt to follow them during a 2-month trial while the patient completes the prospective daily ratings necessary to confirm the diagnosis of PMDD.[77] Increased consumption of fruits, vegetables, legumes, whole grains, and water is recommended, and women can be encouraged to reduce or eliminate intake of salty foods, sugar, caffeine (especially coffee), red meat, and alcohol. Eating smaller, more frequent meals that are high in carbohydrates may specifically improve symptoms of tension and depression.[77] Recommendations for regular exercise include 20- to 30-minute periods of aerobic exercise 3 to 4 times per week.[78] Reduction of body weight to within 20% of ideal, if possible, is an appropriate goal.[36] Because sleep irregularities are present in many women with PMDD, education about sleep hygiene is important.[79] Women can be encouraged to adopt a regular

---

Box 1
Step-wise approach to management of PMDD

A. Psychoeducation

B. Lifestyle modification: healthy eating, regular exercise, good sleep hygiene, limit setting and stress management, moderate alcohol use

C. Dietary supplementation: calcium, vitamin B6

D. Behavioral treatments

E. Psychotherapy

F. Psychopharmacology

G. Hormonal treatments

H. Complementary and alternative therapies (at any time during the course of treatment)

sleep-wake pattern by adhering to consistent bedtimes and waking times throughout their menstrual cycle. Another helpful component of a treatment program is to ensure that women monitor their symptoms and begin to identify triggers of symptom exacerbation. This approach can help women to set appropriate limits and avoid scheduling highly stressful activities during the premenstrual period.

Dietary Supplementation

There is some evidence for calcium supplementation in treating PMS/PMDD with one large trial finding that 1200 mg of calcium daily reduced symptoms of PMS, including depression, by the second or third treatment cycle.[80] Calcium is not known to be associated with any adverse effects so long as doses do not exceed 1500 mg daily.[78] Evidence for vitamin B6 (pyridoxine) in the treatment of depressive symptoms in premenopausal women[81] led to investigation into pyridoxine as a treatment of premenstrual mood symptomatology, although no trials have been done in women with strictly diagnosed PMDD. A recent double-blind placebo-controlled trial of 94 women with premenstrual mood and somatic symptoms revealed a greater decrease in psychiatric symptoms with 80 mg of vitamin B6 compared with placebo.[82] Vitamin B6 supplementation does have risks; higher doses have been associated with peripheral neuropathy.[83] With the rationale that increased tryptophan availability might increase serotonin synthesis, the effects of complex carbohydrate supplementation have been studied, and 2 studies have reported positive effects of a carbohydrate-rich beverage on affective symptoms in women with PMS.[84,85] Although other dietary supplements are recommended in the lay press for treatment of PMS/PMDD symptoms, little scientific evidence is available to support these recommendations.[86,87]

Psychoeducation and Behavioral Treatments

There is some evidence for group psychoeducation and support in treating women with PMS and PMDD.[88–91] Specifically, women with PMDD who received a psychoeducational group intervention that focused on positive reframing of women's perceptions of their menstrual cycles had reduced premenstrual symptoms and premenstrual impairment compared with women in a control group. However, the intervention did not result in differences in posttreatment depression or anxiety scores.[88] Relaxation therapy can also be added to the treatment regimen, particularly for women who report high daily stress levels.[92,93]

Psychotherapy

A systematic review by Lustyk and colleagues[94] identified 7 published peer-reviewed studies (3 randomized controlled trials) evaluating the efficacy of cognitive-behavioral therapy (CBT) for PMS and PMDD. The reviewers concluded that, although CBT may provide some benefit, the magnitude of the effect is likely to be smaller than for pharmacotherapy and even relaxation treatments. However, CBT remains an option for women who prefer not to attempt pharmacotherapeutic treatment.

Psychopharmacology

Some women will not respond to the nonpharmacological strategies mentioned earlier. Other women will have severe symptoms of PMDD in need of immediate treatment. Serotonergic medications, specifically SSRIs, have become the mainstay of pharmacological treatment with established safety and efficacy.[33,95,96] The US Federal Drug Administration (FDA) has approved the use of fluoxetine, sertraline, and paroxetine for PMDD. A Cochrane Database meta-analysis also reveals good evidence of effectiveness for fluvoxamine, citalopram, and the serotonergic tricyclic antidepressant clomipramine.[96] There is also evidence in randomized controlled trials for efficacy of the selective serotonin and norepinephrine reuptake inhibitor class of medications (ie, venlafaxine and duloxetine).[97,98]

In the treatment of major depressive disorder, SSRIs generally require at least 2 weeks for onset of therapeutic efficacy. However, used for PMDD, SSRIs have shown efficacy when used continuously or only in the luteal (premenstrual) phases of each cycle. One advantage of luteal-phase dosing is that SSRI discontinuation effects are rarely seen, perhaps because of the lack of sustained use. Regardless of dosing method, symptoms can recur rapidly when treatment is discontinued, and women with the most severe symptoms at baseline are most at risk.[99]

Hormone Manipulation

The next step in the treatment algorithm involves manipulating female sex hormones to avoid the periodic fluctuations associated with menstruation (and hence avoid associated mood fluctuations). Although there is a strong theoretical basis to this treatment, few ovulation-suppression treatments have been effective for PMDD, and some come with significant risk for adverse effects. These include deep vein thrombosis and pulmonary embolus from oral contraceptives, androgenization and osteoporosis from gonadotropin-releasing hormone (GnRH) agonists, permanent sterilization from oophorectomy.

Because oral contraceptives do provide a reasonably safe means of inhibiting ovulation (and may be most appropriate if women also desire oral contraceptives as a form of birth control), the efficacy of traditional oral contraceptives in treatment of PMDD has not been well established. However, a recent Cochrane Database systematic review supports the efficacy of a combination of ethinyl estradiol and drospirenone for the treatment of PMDD.[100] The FDA has approved this treatment of PMDD; however, indication has been limited to women who also wish to use the medication for contraception, likely because the potential for adverse effects is greater than for SSRIs.

GnRH agonists, such as leuprolide acetate, have shown efficacy in PMS/PMDD, but the effect seems to be greater for physical than for emotional symptoms.[69,101,102] As described, long-term use (ie, greater than 6 months) of GnRH agonists has been associated with several unfavorable side effects such as risk for hypoestrogenism and osteoporosis.[69] The synthetic steroid danazol can reduce emotional and physical symptoms of PMS/PMDD[103]; however, at low doses (200 mg/d), ovulation, and thus conception, are still possible, and danazol can cause virilization of the fetus. Undesirable side effects, including weight gain, mood changes, and acne, have been observed with higher doses sufficient to inhibit ovulation (600–800 mg/d).[69] Suppression of ovulation through bilateral ovariectomy with hysterectomy has been reported to be highly effective in permanently eliminating symptoms of PMS. However, because of the extreme nature of this treatment method, it is not usually recommended, even in severe cases of PMDD.[104]

Complementary and Alternative Strategies

Many patients and practitioners are turning to herbal, complementary, and other treatment options for management of PMS and PMDD. Some of these treatments have been supported by research. At present, the strongest evidence seems to be for *Vitex agnus castus* (chasteberry), although it may be more beneficial for physical rather than psychological symptoms of PMDD.[33] Chasteberry may act as a dopamine agonist to reduce follicle-stimulating hormone or prolactin levels. Small randomized controlled trials also support saffron, Qi therapy, massage, reflexology, chiropractic manipulation, and biofeedback.[105,106] There is some evidence provided in open trials for the efficacy of yoga, guided imagery, photic stimulation, and acupuncture.[33] With the rationale that it may induce rapid increase in serotonin (without the side effects of psychotropic medication), bright-light therapy has been studied as a treatment of PMDD, and a systematic review of 4 trials suggests that bright-light therapy may be an effective option for women with PMDD.[107]

SUMMARY

Premenstrual mood symptoms are common and a small but significant proportion of women experience recurrent premenstrual mood symptoms that are severe enough to cause substantial social and occupational dysfunction. There is convincing evidence for important roles for biological and sociocultural variables in the development of premenstrual mood symptoms. There are several effective treatments, used alone or in combination, that have been found to ameliorate psychological symptoms associated with the menstrual cycle. Further interdisciplinary research into risk factors for PMDD, and the interaction between them, will provide a more complete understanding of the cause of this disorder, and ultimately guide future developments in treatment.

REFERENCES

1. Delaney J, Lupton MJ, Toth E. The curse: a cultural history of menstruation. New York: E.P. Dutton; 1976.
2. Chrisler JC, Johnston-Robledo I. Raging hormones? Feminist perspectives on premenstrual syndrome and postpartum depression. In: Ballou M, Brown LS, editors. Rethinking mental health and disorder: feminist perspectives. New York: Guilford Press; 2002. p. 174–97.
3. American Psychiatric Association. Diagnostic and statistical manual of mental disorders. Text revision (DSM-IV-TR). Fourth edition. Washington, DC: American Psychiatric Association; 2000. p. 771–4.
4. American College of Obstetricians and Gynecologists. Premenstrual syndrome. Patient Education Pamphlet, by the American College of Obstetricians and Gynecologists; 2003. Available at: www.acog.org/publications/patient_education/bp057.cfm. Accessed February 16, 2010.
5. Wittchen HU, Becker E, Lieb R, et al. Prevalence, incidence and stability of premenstrual dysphoric disorder in the community. Psychol Med 2002;32: 119–32.
6. Steiner M, Macdougall M, Brown E. The premenstrual symptoms screening tool (PSST) for clinicians. Arch Womens Ment Health 2003;6(3):203–9.
7. Takeda T, Tasaka K, Sakata M, et al. Prevalence of premenstrual syndrome and premenstrual dysphoric disorder in Japanese women. Arch Womens Ment Health 2006;9(4):209–12.
8. Cohen LS, Soares CN, Otto MW, et al. Prevalence and predictors of premenstrual dysphoric disorder (PMDD) in older premenopausal women. The Harvard Study of Moods and Cycles. J Affect Disord 2002;70:125–32.
9. Rivera-Tovar AD, Frank E. Late luteal phase dysphoric disorder in young women. Am J Psychiatry 1990;147:1634–6.
10. Banerjee N, Roy KK, Takkar D. Premenstrual dysphoric disorder—a study from India. Int J Fertil Womens Med 2000;45:342–4.

11. Rojnic Kuzman M, Hotujac L. Premenstrual dysphoric disorder–a neglected diagnosis? Preliminary study on a sample of Croatian students. Coll Antropol 2007;31(1):131–7.
12. Sveindottir H, Backstrom T. Prevalence of menstrual cycle symptom cyclicity and premenstrual dysphoric disorder in a random sample of women using and not using oral contraceptives. Acta Obstet Gynecol Scand 2000;79(5):405–13.
13. Gehlert S, Song IH, Chang CH, et al. The prevalence of premenstrual dysphoric disorder in a randomly selected group of urban and rural women. Psychol Med 2009;39(1):129–36.
14. Freeman EW, Rickels K, Schweizer E, et al. Relationships between age and symptom severity among women seeking medical treatment for premenstrual symptoms. Psychol Med 1995;25:309–15.
15. Marvan ML, Diaz-Erosa M, Montesinos A. Premenstrual symptoms in Mexican women with different educational levels. J Psychol 1998;132:517–26.
16. Soares CN, Cohen LS, Otto MW, et al. Characteristics of women with premenstrual dysphoric disorder (PMDD) who did or did not report history of depression: a preliminary report from the Harvard Study of Moods and Cycles. J Womens Health Gend Based Med 2001;10:873–8.
17. Beck LE, Gevirtz R, Mortola JF. The predictive role of psychosocial stress on symptom severity in premenstrual syndrome. Psychosom Med 1990;52:536–43.
18. Warner P, Bancroft J. Factors related to self-reporting of the pre-menstrual syndrome. Br J Psychiatry 1990;157:249–60.
19. Fontana AM, Palfai TG. Psychosocial factors in premenstrual dysphoria: stressors, appraisal, and coping processes. J Psychosom Res 1994;38:557–67.
20. Paddison PL, Gise LH, Lebovits A, et al. Sexual abuse and premenstrual syndrome: comparison between a lower and higher socioeconomic group. Psychosomatics 1990;3:265–72.
21. Friedman RC, Hurt SW, Clarkin J, et al. Sexual histories and premenstrual affective syndrome in psychiatric inpatients. Am J Psychiatry 1982;139:1484–6.
22. MacMillan HL, Fleming JE, Streiner DL, et al. Childhood abuse and lifetime psychopathology in a community sample. Am J Psychiatry 2001;158:1878–83.
23. Woods NF, Most A, Longenecker GD. Major life events, daily stressors, and perimenstrual symptoms. Nurse Res 1985;34:263–7.
24. Kendler KS, Karkowski LM, Corey LA, et al. Longitudinal population-based twin study of retrospectively reported premenstrual symptoms and lifetime major depression. Am J Psychiatry 1998;155:1234–40.
25. Treloar SA, Heath AC, Martin NG. Genetic and environmental influences on premenstrual symptoms in an Australian twin sample. Psychol Med 2002; 32(1):25–38.
26. Payne JL, Palmer JT, Joffe H. A reproductive subtype of depression: conceptualizing models and moving toward etiology. Harv Rev Psychiatry 2009;17(2):72–86.
27. Steiner M, Brown E, Trzepacz P, et al. Fluoxetine improves functional work capacity in women with premenstrual dysphoric disorder. Arch Womens Ment Health 2003;6:71–7.
28. Chawla A, Swindle R, Long S, et al. Premenstrual dysphoric disorder: is there an economic burden of illness? Med Care 2002;40:1101–12.
29. Yang M, Wallenstein G, Hagan M, et al. Burden of premenstrual dysphoric disorder on health-related quality of life. J Womens Health (Larchmt) 2008; 17(1):113–21.
30. Rubinow DR, Roy-Byrne P, Hoban MC, et al. Prospective assessment of menstrually related mood disorders. Am J Psychiatry 1984;141:684–6.

31. Meaden PM, Hartlage SA, Cook-Karr J. Timing and severity of symptoms associated with the menstrual cycle in a community-based sample in the Midwestern United States. Psychiatry Res 2005;134(1):27–36.

32. Lane T, Francis A. Premenstrual symptomatology, locus of control, anxiety and depression in women with normal menstrual cycles. Arch Womens Ment Health 2003;6(2):127–38.

33. Pearlstein T, Steiner M. Premenstrual dysphoric disorder: burden of illness and treatment update. J Psychiatry Neurosci 2008;33(4):291–301.

34. Smith MJ, Schmidt PJ, Rubinow DR. Operationalizing DSM-IV criteria for PMDD: selecting symptomatic and asymptomatic cycles for research. J Psychiatr Res 2003;37:75–83.

35. Steiner M, Peer M, Soares CN. Comorbidity and premenstrual syndrome: recognition and treatment approaches. Gynaecology Forum 2006;11:13–6.

36. Steiner M, Born L. Psychiatric aspects of the menstrual cycle. In: Kornstein SG, Clayton AH, editors. Women's mental health: a comprehensive textbook. New York: Guilford Press; 2002. p. 48–69.

37. Hartlage SA, Brandenburg DL, Kravitz HM. Premenstrual exacerbation of depressive disorders in a community-based sample in the United States. Psychosom Med 2004;66(5):698–706.

38. Kornstein SG, Harvey AT, Rush AJ, et al. Self-reported premenstrual exacerbation of depressive symptoms in patients seeking treatment for major depression. Psychol Med 2005;35(5):683–92.

39. Kim DR, Gyulai L, Freeman EW, et al. Premenstrual dysphoric disorder and psychiatric co-morbidity. Arch Womens Ment Health 2004;7(1):37–47.

40. Critchlow DG, Bond AJ, Wingrove J. Mood disorder history and personality assessment in premenstrual dysphoric disorder. J Clin Psychiatry 2001;62(9): 688–93.

41. Johnson TM. Premenstrual syndrome as a Western culture-specific disorder. Cult Med Psychiatry 1987;11:337–56.

42. Anson O. Exploring the bio-psycho–social approach to premenstrual experiences. Soc Sci Med 1999;49:67–80.

43. Marvan ML, Escobedo C. Premenstrual symptomatology: role of prior knowledge about premenstrual syndrome. Psychosom Med 1999;61:163–7.

44. Ruble DN. Premenstrual symptoms: a reinterpretation. Science 1977;197: 291–2.

45. Schmidt PJ, Nieman LK, Danaceau MA, et al. Differential behavioral effects of gonadal steroids in women with and in those without premenstrual syndrome. N Engl J Med 1998;338:209–16.

46. Eriksson O, Backstrom T, Stridsberg M, et al. Differential response to estrogen challenge test in women with and without premenstrual dysphoria. Psychoneuroendocrinology 2006;31(4):415–27.

47. Freeman EW, Frye CA, Rickels K, et al. Allopregnanolone levels and symptom improvement in severe premenstrual syndrome. J Clin Psychopharmacol 2002;22:516–20.

48. Nyberg S, Backstrom T, Zingmark E, et al. Allopregnanolone decrease with symptom improvement during placebo and gonadotropin-releasing hormone agonist treatment in women with severe premenstrual syndrome. Gynecol Endocrinol 2007;23(5):257–66.

49. Andreen L, Nyberg S, Turkmen S, et al. Sex steroid induced negative mood may be explained by the paradoxical effect mediated by GABAA modulators. Psychoneuroendocrinology 2009;34(8):1121–32.

50. Epperson CN, Haga K, Mason GF, et al. Cortical gamma-aminobutyric acid levels across the menstrual cycle in healthy women and those with premenstrual dysphoric disorder: a proton magnetic resonance spectroscopy study. Arch Gen Psychiatry 2002;59:851–8.
51. Sundstrom I, Andersson A, Nyberg S, et al. Patients with premenstrual syndrome have a different sensitivity to a neuroactive steroid during the menstrual cycle compared to control subjects. Neuroendocrinology 1998;67(2):126–38.
52. Le Melledo JM, Van Driel M, Coupland NJ, et al. Response to flumazenil in women with premenstrual dysphoric disorder. Am J Psychiatry 2000;157: 821–3.
53. Sundstrom I, Ashbrook D, Backstrom T. Reduced benzodiazepine sensitivity in patients with premenstrual syndrome: a pilot study. Psychoneuroendocrinology 1997;22:25–38.
54. Sundstrom I, Nyberg S, Backstrom T. Patients with premenstrual syndrome have reduced sensitivity to midazolam compared to control subjects. Neuropsychopharmacology 1997;17:370–81.
55. Sundstrom I, Backstrom T. Citalopram increases pregnanolone sensitivity in patients with premenstrual syndrome: an open trial. Psychoneuroendocrinology 1998;23(1):73–88.
56. Eriksson E, Sundblad C, Landen M, et al. Behavioural effects of androgens in women. In: Steiner M, Yonkers KA, Eriksson E, editors. Mood disorders in women. London: Martin Dunitz; 2000. p. 233–46.
57. Steiner M, Dunn EJ, MacDougall M, et al. Serotonin transporter gene polymorphism, free testosterone, and symptoms associated with premenstrual dysphoric disorder. Biol Psychiatry 2002;51:91S.
58. Bloch M, Schmidt PJ, Su TP, et al. Pituitary-adrenal hormones and testosterone across the menstrual cycle in women with premenstrual syndrome and controls. Biol Psychiatry 1998;43:897–903.
59. Steiner M, Pearlstein T. Premenstrual dysphoria and the serotonin system: pathophysiology and treatment. J Clin Psychiatry 2000;61(Suppl 12):17–21.
60. Rapkin AJ, Edelmuth E, Chang LC, et al. Whole-blood serotonin in premenstrual syndrome. Obstet Gynecol 1987;70:533–7.
61. Taylor DL, Mathew RJ, Ho BT, et al. Serotonin levels and platelet uptake during premenstrual tension. Neuropsychobiology 1984;12:16–8.
62. Melke J, Westberg L, Landen M, et al. Serotonin transporter gene polymorphisms and platelet [3H] paroxetine binding in premenstrual dysphoria. Psychoneuroendocrinology 2003;28(3):446–58.
63. Jovanovic H, Cerin A, Karlsson P, et al. A PET study of 5-HT1A receptors at different phases of the menstrual cycle in women with premenstrual dysphoria. Psychiatry Res 2006;148(2–3):185–93.
64. Bancroft J, Cook A, Davidson D, et al. Blunting of neuroendocrine responses to infusion of L-tryptophan in women with perimenstrual mood change. Psychol Med 1991;21:305–12.
65. Yatham LN. Is 5HT1α receptor subsensitivity a trait marker for late luteal phase dysphoric disorder? A pilot study. Can J Psychiatry 1993;38:662–4.
66. FitzGerald M, Malone KM, Li S, et al. Blunted serotonin response to fenfluramine challenge in premenstrual dysphoric disorder. Am J Psychiatry 1997; 154:556–8.
67. Steiner M, Yatham LN, Coote M, et al. Serotonergic dysfunction in women with pure premenstrual dysphoric disorder: is the fenfluramine challenge test still relevant? Psychiatry Res 1999;87:107–15.

68. Rasgon N, Serra M, Biggio G, et al. Neuroactive steroid-serotonergic interaction: responses to an intravenous L-tryptophan challenge in women with premenstrual syndrome. Eur J Endocrinol 2001;145:25–33.
69. Mitwally MF, Kahn LS, Halbreich U. Pharmacotherapy of premenstrual syndromes and premenstrual dysphoric disorder: current practices. Expert Opin Pharmacother 2002;3:1577–90.
70. Praschak-Rieder N, Willeit M, Winkler D, et al. Role of family history and 5-HTTLPR polymorphism in female seasonal affective disorder patients with and without premenstrual dysphoric disorder. Eur Neuropsychopharmacol 2002; 12(2):129–34.
71. Huo L, Straub RE, Roca C, et al. Risk for premenstrual dysphoric disorder is associated with genetic variation in ESR1, the estrogen receptor alpha gene. Biol Psychiatry 2007;62(8):925–33.
72. Heim C, Newport DJ, Heit S, et al. Pituitary-adrenal and autonomic responses to stress in women after sexual and physical abuse in childhood. JAMA 2000;284: 592–7.
73. Kendler KS, Gardner CO, Prescott CA. Toward a comprehensive developmental model for major depression in women. Am J Psychiatry 2002;159:1133–45.
74. Ornitz AW, Brown MA. Family coping and premenstrual symptomatology. J Obstet Gynecol Neonatal Nurs 1993;22:49–55.
75. Matsumoto T, Ushiroyama T, Kimura T, et al. Altered autonomic nervous system activity as a potential etiological factor of premenstrual syndrome and premenstrual dysphoric disorder. Biopsychosoc Med 2007;1:24.
76. Bunevicius R, Hinderliter AL, Light KC, et al. Histories of sexual abuse are associated with differential effects of clonidine on autonomic function in women with premenstrual dysphoric disorder. Biol Psychol 2005;69(3):281–96.
77. Jarvis CI, Lynch AM, Morin AK. Management strategies for premenstrual syndrome/premenstrual dysphoric disorder. Ann Pharmacother 2008;42(7): 967–78.
78. Frackiewicz EJ, Shiovitz TM. Evaluation and management of premenstrual syndrome and premenstrual dysphoric disorder. J Am Pharm Assoc 2001;41: 437–47.
79. Baker FC, Kahan TL, Trinder J, et al. Sleep quality and the sleep electroencephalogram in women with severe premenstrual syndrome. Sleep 2007;30(10): 1283–91.
80. Thys-Jacobs S, Starkey P, Bernstein D, et al. Calcium carbonate and the premenstrual syndrome: effects on premenstrual and menstrual symptoms. Am J Obstet Gynecol 1998;179:444–52.
81. Williams AL, Cotter A, Sabina A, et al. The role for vitamin B-6 as treatment for depression: a systematic review. Fam Pract 2005;22(5):532–7.
82. Kashanian M, Mazinani R, Jalalmanesh S. Pyridoxine (vitamin B6) therapy for premenstrual syndrome. Int J Gynaecol Obstet 2007;96(1):43–4.
83. Wyatt KM, Dimmock PW, Jones PW, et al. Efficacy of vitamin B-6 in the treatment of premenstrual syndrome: systematic review. BMJ 1999;318:1375–81.
84. Sayegh R, Schiff I, Wurtman J, et al. The effect of a carbohydrate-rich beverage on mood, appetite, and cognitive function in women with premenstrual syndrome. Obstet Gynecol 1995;86:520–8.
85. Freeman EW, Stout AL, Endicott J, et al. Treatment of premenstrual syndrome with a carbohydrate-rich beverage. Int J Gynaecol Obstet 2002; 77(3):253–4.

86. Khine K, Rosenstein DL, Elin RJ, et al. Magnesium (Mg) retention and mood effects after intravenous Mg infusion in premenstrual dysphoric disorder. Biol Psychiatry 2006;59(4):327–33.
87. Bendich A. The potential for dietary supplements to reduce premenstrual syndrome (PMS) symptoms. J Am Coll Nutr 2000;19:3–12.
88. Morse G. Positively reframing perceptions of the menstrual cycle among women with premenstrual syndrome. J Obstet Gynecol Neonatal Nurs 1999;28:165–74.
89. Walton J, Youngkin E. The effect of a support group on self-esteem of women with premenstrual syndrome. J Obstet Gynecol Neonatal Nurs 1987;16:174–8.
90. Seideman RY. Effects of a premenstrual syndrome education program on premenstrual symptomatology. Health Care Women Int 1990;11:491–501.
91. Taylor D. Effectiveness of professional–peer group treatment: symptom management for women with PMS. Res Nurs Health 1999;22:496–511.
92. Goodale IL, Domar AD, Benson H. Alleviation of premenstrual syndrome symptoms with the relaxation response. Obstet Gynecol 1990;75:649–55.
93. Morse CA, Dennerstein L, Farrell E, et al. A comparison of hormone therapy, coping skills training, and relaxation for the relief of premenstrual syndrome. J Behav Med 1991;14:469–89.
94. Lustyk MK, Gerrish WG, Shaver S, et al. Cognitive-behavioral therapy for premenstrual syndrome and premenstrual dysphoric disorder: a systematic review. Arch Womens Ment Health 2009;12(2):85–96.
95. Steiner M, Pearlstein T, Cohen LS, et al. Expert guidelines for the treatment of severe PMS, PMDD, and comorbidities: the role of SSRIs. J Womens Health (Larchmt) 2006;15(1):57–69.
96. Brown J, O'Brien PM, Marjoribanks J, et al. Selective serotonin reuptake inhibitors for premenstrual syndrome. Cochrane Database Syst Rev 2009;(2): CD001396.
97. Freeman EW, Rickels K, Yonkers KA, et al. Venlafaxine in the treatment of premenstrual dysphoric disorder. Obstet Gynecol 2001;98(5):737–44.
98. Ramos MG, Hara C, Rocha FL. Duloxetine treatment for women with premenstrual dysphoric disorder: a single-blind trial. Int J Neuropsychopharmacol 2009;12(8):1081–8.
99. Freeman EW, Rickels K, Sammel MD, et al. Time to relapse after short- or long-term treatment of severe premenstrual syndrome with sertraline. Arch Gen Psychiatry 2009;66(5):537–44.
100. Lopez LM, Kaptein AA, Helmerhorst FM. Oral contraceptives containing drospirenone for premenstrual syndrome. Cochrane Database Syst Rev 2009;(2): CD006586.
101. Muse KN, Cetel NS, Futterman LA, et al. The premenstrual syndrome: effects of "medical ovariectomy". N Engl J Med 1984;311:1345–9.
102. Freeman EW, Sondheimer SJ, Rickels K. Gonadotropin-releasing hormone agonist in the treatment of premenstrual symptoms with and without ongoing dysphoria: a controlled study. Psychopharmacol Bull 1997;33:303–9.
103. O'Brien PMS, Abukhalil I. Randomised controlled trial of the management of premenstrual mastalgia using luteal phase only Danazol. Am J Obstet Gynecol 1999;180:18–23.
104. Cronje WH, Vashisht A, Studd JWW. Hysterectomy and bilateral oophorectomy for severe premenstrual syndrome. Humanit Rep 2004;19(9):2152–5.

105. Agha-Hosseini M, Kashani L, Aleyaseen A, et al. *Crocus sativus* L. (saffron) in the treatment of premenstrual syndrome: a double-blind, randomised and placebo-controlled trial. BJOG 2008;115(4):515–9.
106. Jang HS, Lee MS. Effects of qi therapy (external qigong) on premenstrual syndrome: a randomized placebo-controlled study. J Altern Complement Med 2004;10(3):456–62.
107. Krasnik C, Montori VM, Guyatt GH, et al. Medically Unexplained Syndromes Study Group. The effect of bright light therapy on depression associated with premenstrual dysphoric disorder. Am J Obstet Gynecol 2005;193(3 Pt 1): 658–61.

Treatment of Mood Disorders During Pregnancy and Postpartum

Lee S. Cohen, MD*, Betty Wang, MD,
Ruta Nonacs, MD, PhD, Adele C. Viguera, MD,
Elizabeth L. Lemon, MA, Marlene P. Freeman, MD

KEYWORDS

• Mood disorders • Pregnancy • Postpartum

Although pregnancy was once believed to be a time of emotional well-being for women,[1] studies now suggest that pregnancy does not protect women from the emergence or persistence of mood disorders.[2–7] Mood and anxiety disorders are prevalent in women during the childbearing years[8,9] and, for many women, these mood disorders are chronic or recurrent. Maintenance antidepressant therapy is often indicated during the reproductive years and women face difficult treatment decisions regarding psychotropic medications and pregnancy. Treatment of psychiatric disorders during pregnancy involves a thoughtful weighing of the risks and benefits of proposed interventions (eg, pharmacological treatment) and the documented[10–12] and theoretical risks associated with untreated psychiatric disorders such as depression. Collaborative decision making that incorporates patient treatment preferences is optimal for women trying to conceive or who are pregnant.

With increasing evidence of high rates of relapse following discontinuation of psychotropic medications (eg, antidepressants,[13] mood stabilizers,[14] antipsychotics,[15] and benzodiazepines[16]) and other data that describe new-onset psychiatric illness during pregnancy,[2,6,17] the value of psychiatric consultation during pregnancy and after delivery is intuitive. The risks of untreated mood disorders during pregnancy to the mother and the baby (eg, preterm delivery, poor nutrition, inadequate weight gain, poor prenatal care, inability to care for oneself, substance use, termination of the pregnancy, and postpartum depression[12,18]) also deserve attention. Depression

Perinatal and Reproductive Psychiatry, Department of Psychiatry, Massachusetts General Hospital, Harvard Medical School, 185 Cambridge Street, Boston, MA 02114, USA
* Corresponding author.
E-mail address: lcohen2@partners.org

Psychiatr Clin N Am 33 (2010) 273–293
doi:10.1016/j.psc.2010.02.001
0193-953X/10/$ – see front matter © 2010 Elsevier Inc. All rights reserved.

during pregnancy is a strong predictor of postpartum depression, a condition that can have dire consequences for the mother, the baby, and the entire family. Therefore, it could be argued that nothing is more critical than sustaining maternal emotional well-being during pregnancy.

Because of the substantial unknowns of long-term effects of medication exposure during pregnancy and those of untreated mood disorders, women with similar illness histories often make different decisions about their care in collaboration with their physicians during pregnancy. Because rapid discontinuation of medication seems to increase the risk of relapse of mood episodes,[19,20] women should be educated about the risks and benefits of medications during pregnancy so that medications are not abruptly stopped (out of fear of exposing the fetus to medication). Furthermore, medications with benign reproductive safety profiles across classes of molecules should be used as first-line agents in women of reproductive age being treated for psychiatric illness.

Acute major depressive episodes are often untreated or undertreated during pregnancy.[21,22] Screening for, and successful treatment of, depression during pregnancy can minimize maternal suffering, as well as the potential negative consequences of untreated maternal depression on infant development and family functioning.[12]

This article reviews the diagnosis and treatment guidelines of mood disorders during pregnancy and post partum, as well as the use of psychotropic medications during this time.

PERINATAL PSYCHIATRY: FROM SCREENING TO TREATMENT

Clinicians who manage the care of female psychiatric patients before, during, and after pregnancy may be called to evaluate women who experience a broad spectrum of difficulties. Symptoms may be mild, although the consultant is typically requested when symptoms become severe. It is not uncommon for women to present weeks or even months after the onset of psychiatric symptoms. Many women and their health care providers mistakenly believe that even serious mood symptoms are normal postpartum reactions, and many women may be afraid or embarrassed to disclose that they are suffering from depression. Psychiatric disorders may emerge anew during pregnancy, although more often clinical presentations represent persistence or exacerbation of an existing illness. Physicians, therefore, should screen more aggressively for psychiatric disorders either before conception or during pregnancy, integrating questions about psychiatric symptoms and treatment into the obstetric history. Identification of at-risk women allows the most thoughtful, acute treatment before, during, and after pregnancy.

One recent report has described the finding that even among women with identified psychiatric illness during pregnancy, definitive treatment is frequently lacking or incomplete.[21] The extent to which women suffering from postpartum psychiatric illness are under treated as a group is also well described. One of the reasons for failure to treat women with psychiatric disorders during pregnancy is the concern regarding potential risks associated with fetal exposure to psychotropics. Many clinicians can conceptualize the need to weigh relative risks of fetal exposure on the one hand versus the risk of withholding treatment on the other. However, given the inability to quantify these risks absolutely, clinicians often defer treatment entirely and consequently put patients at risk for the sequelae of untreated maternal psychiatric illness. Clinicians should realize that the process of managing psychiatric illness during pregnancy and the puerperium is not a process like threading a needle; it is not clear-cut and much treatment described in the literature is not evidence based. Despite the growing number of reviews on the subject, management of antenatal depression is still largely guided by experience, with few definitive data and no controlled treatment studies to inform treatment. The best treatment algorithms depend on the severity of the disorder, on a patient's psychiatric history, her current symptoms, and her attitude toward the use of psychiatric medications during pregnancy, and, ultimately, the patient's wishes. However, thoughtful collaborative decisions can still be made with these patients as clinicians review the best available evidence with them and as clinician and patient realize that no decision is risk free and no decision is perfect. Thoughtful treatment decisions can be made nonetheless, taking into account available information regarding relative risks of treatment and the patient's wishes.

PHARMACOLOGICAL TREATMENT OF DEPRESSION DURING PREGNANCY
Clinical Guidelines

Making the diagnosis of depression during pregnancy can be difficult because disturbances in sleep and appetite, symptoms of fatigue, and changes in libido can be normal during pregnancy. Clinical symptoms that may support the diagnosis of major depressive disorder (MDD) include anhedonia, feelings of guilt and hopelessness, poor self-esteem, and thoughts of suicide. In addition, symptoms that interfere with function signal a psychiatric condition that warrants treatment. Suicidal ideation is not uncommon[23–25]; however, risk of frank self-injurious or suicidal behaviors seems to be low in women who develop depression during pregnancy.[24,25]

Multiple reviews have been published in the last decade[26–31] regarding the risks associated with fetal exposure to antidepressants. Although data accumulated in the last 30 years have suggested that some antidepressants have favorable risk/benefit profiles during pregnancy,[32–34] information regarding the full spectrum and relative severity of risks of prenatal exposure to psychotropic medications is still incomplete. Moreover, the risks of medication use must be balanced against the risks associated with untreated psychiatric disorders that may adversely affect the mother and the fetus.

As with other medications, 4 types of risk are typically cited with respect to potential use of antidepressants during pregnancy: (1) risk of pregnancy loss or miscarriage, (2) risk of organ malformation or teratogenesis, (3) risk of neonatal toxicity or withdrawal syndromes during the acute neonatal period, and (4) risk of long-term neurobehavioral sequelae.[33] To guide physicians about the reproductive safety of various prescription medications, the US Food and Drug Administration (FDA) has established a system that classifies medications into 5 risk categories (A, B, C, D, and X) based on data derived from human and animal studies. Medications in category A are designated as safe for use during pregnancy, whereas category X drugs are contraindicated, as they are known to have risks to the fetus that outweigh any benefit to the patient. Most psychotropic medications are classified as category C agents, for which human studies are lacking and for which risk cannot be ruled out. No psychotropic drugs are classified as safe for use during pregnancy (ie, category A).

This system of classification has noteworthy limitations. First, categorization is often ambiguous and may lead to unwarranted conclusions. For example, certain tricyclic antidepressants (TCAs) have been labeled as category D agents, indicating positive evidence of risk, although the pooled available data do not support this assertion and suggest that these drugs are safe for use during pregnancy.[35,36] Second, the categorization is usually assigned when only a small amount of animal data is available, and when human data are sparse or absent. Third, when larger and more rigorous studies become available on the reproductive safety profile of a medication, the category is rarely altered. Fourth, the categorization system fails to take into account the risks of the untreated maternal psychiatric disorder for the woman and her fetus. Therefore, the physician must also rely on other sources of information when counseling patients about the potential use of psychotropics during pregnancy. Randomized, placebo-controlled studies that examine the effects of medication use on pregnant populations are lacking. Therefore, many of the data related to the profile of reproductive safety for a medication are derived from retrospective studies and case reports. More recently, studies that have evaluated the reproductive safety of antidepressants have used a more rigorous prospective design,[35–40] or have relied on large administrative databases or multicenter birth defect surveillance programs.[41,42] Given the lack of clarity of the FDA risk categories, this agency has recently proposed a modification of the classification system that incorporates a more individualized and sophisticated approach to the use of medications in pregnancy.[43]

As a general guiding principle, treatment of depression during pregnancy is determined by the severity of the underlying disorder, history of treatment responses, and individual patient preferences. For women who present with the new onset of depressive symptoms during pregnancy, or mild to moderate major depression, nonpharmacological treatment strategies should be explored first, consistent with recent recommendations by representatives of the American Psychiatric Association and the American College of Obstetrics and Gynecology.[44] Women with mild to moderate depressive symptoms may benefit from nonpharmacological treatments that include supportive psychotherapy, cognitive behavioral therapy (CBT), or interpersonal therapy (IPT).[45–48] These interventions may be beneficial for reducing the severity of depressive symptoms and may either limit or obviate medications. Given the importance of interpersonal relationships in couples who are expecting a child and the significant role transitions that take place during pregnancy and after delivery, IPT may be ideally suited for the treatment of depressed pregnant women.[48] In general, pharmacological treatment is pursued when nonpharmacological strategies have failed or when it is thought that the risks associated with psychiatric illness during pregnancy outweigh the risks of fetal exposure to a particular medication.

In patients with less severe major depression, discontinuation of ongoing pharmacological therapy during pregnancy should be considered. Although data on the use of IPT or CBT to facilitate antidepressant discontinuation before conception are not available, it makes sense to pursue such treatment of women on maintenance antidepressant therapy who are planning to become pregnant. These treatment modalities may reduce the risk of recurrent depressive symptoms during pregnancy; however, this has not been studied systematically. Close monitoring of affective status during pregnancy is essential throughout pregnancy for women with a history of a mood disorder, regardless of whether medication is continued or discontinued. Psychiatrically ill women are at high risk for relapse during pregnancy, and early detection and treatment of recurrent illness may significantly reduce morbidity associated with affective disorder.

Many women who discontinue antidepressants during pregnancy experience recurrent depressive symptoms.[49,50] In 1 recent study, women who discontinued their medications were 5 times more likely to relapse (with a rate of relapse of 68%)[5] compared with women who maintained their antidepressants across pregnancy. Thus, women with recurrent or refractory depressive illness may decide (in collaboration with their clinician) that the safest option is to continue pharmacologic treatment during pregnancy to minimize the risk for recurrent illness. In this setting, the clinician should attempt to select medications during pregnancy that have a well-characterized reproductive safety profile that may necessitate switching psychotropics (to one with a better reproductive safety profile). In an ideal world, modification of the treatment plan would occur before pregnancy, and allow time for confirming euthymia on a new medication. For example, one might switch from duloxetine, a medication for which there are sparse data on reproductive safety, to an agent such as fluoxetine or citalopram. In other situations, one may decide to use a medication for which information regarding reproductive safety is sparse (eg, a woman with refractory depression who has responded only to 1 particular antidepressant for which specific data on reproductive safety are limited [eg, venlafaxine]). The patient may choose to continue this medication during pregnancy rather than risk potential relapse associated with antidepressant discontinuation or switch to another antidepressant for which she has no history of response.

Even if a woman continues an antidepressant during pregnancy, relapse may occur. Cohen and colleagues[5] reported that 26% of women who continue antidepressants had a relapse of MDD during pregnancy. Therefore, careful monitoring is required even if maintenance medications are continued. Only a small amount of information is available on the pharmacokinetic profile of selective serotonin reuptake inhibitors (SSRIs) and newer antidepressants across pregnancy,[51–54] with some but not all women having lower plasma concentrations of medication in late pregnancy. Therefore, some women may require higher doses of medication as pregnancy progresses to maintain therapeutic benefits; this supports a need for frequent assessment.

Antidepressant Use During Pregnancy

In situations in which pharmacological treatment is more clearly indicated, the clinician should select medications with the safest reproductive profile. Fluoxetine and citalopram, with extensive data that support their reproductive safety, can be considered as first-line choices. Among the SSRIs, paroxetine is the most controversial, given reports regarding cardiovascular malformations with first-trimester exposure. However, more comprehensive studies and pooled teratovigilance data did not support this risk. Nevertheless, many women and their obstetrical health care providers may remain anxious about use of paroxetine in pregnancy. The TCAs and bupropion have also been well characterized and can be considered reasonable treatment options during pregnancy. Among the TCAs, desipramine and nortriptyline are frequently cited as preferred because they are less anticholinergic and less likely to exacerbate orthostatic hypotension during pregnancy. The amount of literature on the reproductive safety of the newer SSRIs is increasing, and these agents may be useful in certain settings, particularly if a woman has had a good response to 1 of them yet has poorer responses to better-characterized antidepressants.[9,39,55] When prescribing medications during pregnancy, an attempt should be made to simplify the medication regimen. For instance, a more sedating antidepressant may be selected for a woman who presents with depression and sleep disturbance instead of selecting a more activating antidepressant in combination with trazodone or a benzodiazepine.

Cumulative reports that describe the reproductive safety of SSRIs have been recently reviewed.[30,31] These reports provide some reassurance that as a group of medicines, SSRIs are not major teratogens. Initially, some[56,57] reports suggested that first-trimester exposure to paroxetine was associated with an increased risk of cardiac defects (including atrial and ventricular septal defects). Although these findings prompted the FDA to change the labeling of paroxetine from category C to D, 2 independent, peer-reviewed, comprehensive meta-analyses of studies assessing paroxetine exposure during the first trimester[41,42,58,59] failed to prove the increased teratogenicity of paroxetine. Therefore, although it is widely believed that paroxetine may confer an increased risk of congenital malformations with first-trimester exposure, the most comprehensive studies to date have not supported this; paroxetine should still be considered a treatment option for women who, before pregnancy, have had a positive response to the agent.

The data about the risk of major malformations after first-trimester use of SSRIs remain inconsistent. A large body of literature has failed to show a risk of major malformations with first-trimester exposure, but 1 study suggested that SSRI use during the first trimester of pregnancy was associated with increased risk of omphalocele, craniosynostosis, and anencephaly.[41] Another study suggested that first-trimester SSRI use was not associated with significantly increased rates of craniosynostosis, omphalocele, or cardiac defects, but did note an increase in malformations with particular SSRIs. In this analysis, sertraline was associated with omphalocele and septal defects, whereas paroxetine exposure was associated with right ventricular outflow tract obstruction defects.[42]

Bupropion may be an attractive option for women who have not responded well to fluoxetine or TCAs. Data thus far have not indicated an increased risk of malformations associated with bupropion use during pregnancy.[60–62] Bupropion deserves special consideration if a woman is attempting to abstain from smoking during pregnancy, as it is also approved by the FDA for smoking cessation, and tobacco use during pregnancy is associated with a spectrum of risks. Bupropion may be an attractive option for women with attention deficit disorder who are receiving stimulants, as reproductive safety data regarding this class of medicines are more sparse than those for bupropion, an antidepressant that has been used with benefit in some patients with attention-deficit/hyperactivity disorder.[63,64]

Limited data are available on the use of the serotonin-norepinephrine reuptake inhibitor (SNRI) venlafaxine[40] during pregnancy. Nonetheless, given the frequency of use of these medicines and the frequency of unplanned pregnancy,[65] the data supporting safety of venlafaxine are increasingly reassuring. There is little information available on the use of duloxetine in pregnancy. Mirtazapine is a novel piperazinoazepine antidepressant; although the data regarding the use of this medication during pregnancy are sparse, in 1 small study it did not seem to increase the rate of major malformations.[66] Although small studies of medication exposures may provide reassuring preliminary information, large definitive trials are necessary to assess risks that might be rare (and observable only with adequate sample sizes).

Although selection of the safest antidepressant based on teratogenic potential is critical if pharmacotherapy is to be pursued during pregnancy, other clinical considerations such as dosage of medication used across pregnancy also warrant comment. Clinicians must use an adequate dosage of medication to obtain and sustain euthymia. Frequently the dosage of a medication is reduced during pregnancy in an attempt to limit risk to the fetus. However, this type of modification in treatment may instead place the woman at greater risk for recurrent illness. During pregnancy, changes in plasma volume and increases in hepatic metabolism and renal clearance may significantly affect drug levels.[67,68] Several investigators have described a reduction (up to 65%) in serum levels of TCAs during pregnancy.[36,69] Subtherapeutic levels may be associated with depressive relapse[36]; therefore, an increase in daily TCA or SSRI dosage may be required to obtain sustain affective well-being.[52]

Perinatal Outcomes Following Antidepressant Exposure

Despite the growing literature that supports the relative safety of fetal exposure to SSRIs with respect to teratogenic risk, multiple reports[37,70,71] have described adverse perinatal outcomes (including decreased gestational age, low birth weight, and poor neonatal adaptation) following in utero exposure to these medicines. Nonetheless, other studies[35,72,73] have failed to note these associations. Particular concern has been raised regarding the potential effects of late-pregnancy exposure to SNRI; 1 recent report[74] noted jitteriness, tachypnea, and tremulousness. These effects have been described as transient (limited to several days following delivery). In general, most reports characterize a neonatal syndrome following maternal antidepressant use as mild and not requiring clinical intervention.

Conflicting reports have also raised a question about whether SSRI use in later pregnancy is associated with a serious but rare developmental lung condition, persistent pulmonary hypertension of the newborn (PPHN). Chambers and colleagues[75] raised this concern when they noted an association between PPHN and SSRI use in a nested case-controlled study. They reported the risk of PPHN with exposure to SSRIs after 20 weeks at about 1%. However, more recent studies have shown a lower or perhaps absent association. Källén and Otterblad[76] also found an association between late SSRI use in pregnancy and PPHN, albeit a substantially smaller risk than that found by Chambers and colleagues.[75] The most recent study, however, failed to show any association between SSRI use during pregnancy and PPHN.[77] PPHN is correlated with multiple established risk factors, including cesarean section, race, body mass index (calculated as weight in kilograms divided by the square of height in meters), and other factors not associated with SSRI use.[78]

Another concern about antidepressant use in late pregnancy is neonatal withdrawal or adaptation syndrome. Further investigation is warranted to clarify the association between SSRI use and neonatal risks, as symptoms reported to be associated with late-pregnancy antidepressant use have also been reported among neonates of mothers with untreated depression and anxiety. Most reports that have attempted to delineate the potential effects of peripartum exposure to SSRIs have been limited by small sample size, nonsystematic assessment of infant outcome, and frequent use of nonblinded raters.

With multiple studies supporting the finding of transient jitteriness, tremulousness, and tachypnea associated with peripartum use of SSRIs[74,79] some physicians (as well as labeling across the SSRIs mandated by the FDA) have suggested the discontinuation of antidepressants just before delivery to minimize the risk of neonatal toxicity. Another potential rationale for antidepressant discontinuation before delivery is derived from the assumption that this would attenuate the risk of PPHN that has been associated with late-trimester exposure to SSRIs.[75] The recommendation is not data driven and such a practice may carry significant risk as it withdraws treatment from a patient precisely as she is about to enter the postpartum period, a time of heightened risk for affective illness. In consideration of the well-characterized risks to mother, baby, and family associated with untreated maternal mood disorder, treatment goals should include having a woman enter the postpartum period in a depression euthymic state. The strategy of medication discontinuation before delivery, however, may increase the risk of recurrent depression on the cusp of the puerperal period and may be associated with significant morbidity, and recovery from recrudescing illness may also take considerable time.

Although a limited amount of data are available regarding the long-term effects of fetal exposure to antidepressants as a class, fluoxetine and TCAs are the best-characterized agents in this regard. In children exposed to fluoxetine, TCAs or no medication, no differences have been detected in behavioral or cognitive development (in terms of IQ, language, temperament, behavior, reactivity, mood, distractibility, and activity level[38,72]) among groups when followed through early childhood. Although the greatest emphasis of research regarding antidepressant use and pregnancy has addressed the effect of antidepressant drugs on risk for congenital malformation, more research is needed to assess the long-term effects of prenatal antidepressant exposure. Therefore, although these and other data[80] available are reassuring, they are still limited and further, more definitive, investigation into the long-term neurobehavioral effects of prenatal exposure to antidepressants is warranted.

Electroconvulsive Therapy

Consideration of the use of electroconvulsive therapy (ECT) during pregnancy typically generates anxiety among clinicians and patients. However, its safety record has been well documented in the last 50 years,[81–83] particularly when instituted in collaboration with a multidisciplinary treatment team, including an anesthesiologist, psychiatrist, and obstetrician.[83–86] Requests for psychiatric consultation for pregnant patients who require ECT tend to be emergent and dramatic. For example, expeditious treatment is imperative in instances of mania during pregnancy or psychotic depression with suicidal thoughts and disorganized thinking. Such clinical situations are associated with a danger from impulsivity or self-harm. A limited course of treatment may be sufficient followed by institution of treatment with 1 or a combination of agents (such as antidepressants, neuroleptics, benzodiazepines, or mood stabilizers).

ECT during pregnancy tends to be underused because of concerns that treatment will harm the fetus. Despite 1 report of placental abruption associated with the use of ECT during pregnancy,[87] considerable experience supports its safe use in severely ill gravid women. Reviews of ECT during pregnancy note the efficacy and safety of this procedure.[84,88,89] In a review of the 339 cases of ECT during pregnancy published in the past 65 years, only 11 of the 25 fetal or neonatal complications, including 2 deaths, were likely caused by ECT. Given its relative safety, ECT may also be considered an alternative to conventional pharmacotherapy for women who wish to avoid extended exposure to psychotropics during pregnancy or for women who fail to respond to standard antidepressants.

BIPOLAR DISORDER DURING PREGNANCY

Although the effect of pregnancy on the natural course of bipolar disorder (BPD) is not well described, studies suggest that any protective effects of pregnancy on risk for recurrence of mania or depression in women with BPD are limited[90] and the risk for relapse and chronicity following discontinuation of mood stabilizers is high.[19,91–94] Given these data, clinicians and women with BPD who are either pregnant or who wish to conceive find themselves between a "teratologic rock and a clinical hard place."[95]

Historically, women with BPD have been counseled to defer pregnancy (given an apparent need for pharmacological therapy with mood stabilizers) or to terminate pregnancies following prenatal exposure to drugs (such as lithium or valproic acid). However, more recent and comprehensive data suggest that women can select treatment strategies that allow for pregnancy with the mother and baby's safety in mind. The risk of lithium exposure during pregnancy has been reassessed and is considered safer than it was decades ago. Concerns regarding fetal exposure to lithium, for example, have typically been based on early reports of higher rates of cardiovascular malformations (eg, Ebstein anomaly) following prenatal exposure to this drug.[96,97] More recent data suggest the risk of cardiovascular malformations following prenatal exposure to lithium is smaller than previous estimates (1/2000 vs 1/1000).[98] Prenatal screening with high-resolution ultrasound and fetal echocardiography is recommended at or about 16 to 18 weeks of gestation to screen for cardiac anomalies. Nonetheless, the woman with BPD is faced with a decision regarding use of lithium during pregnancy; it is appropriate to counsel such a patient about the small risk of organ dysgenesis associated with prenatal exposure to this medicine.

Lamotrigine is another mood stabilizer that is an option for pregnant women with BPD who show a clear need for prophylaxis with mood stabilizer. Although previous reports failed to show an increased risk of malformations associated with lamotrigine exposure,[99–102] data from the North American Anti-Epileptic Drug registry indicate an increased risk of oral cleft in infants exposed to lamotrigine during the first trimester; the prevalence was approximately 9 per 1000 births.[103]

Compared with lithium and lamotrigine, prenatal exposure to some anticonvulsants is associated with a far greater risk for organ malformation. An association between prenatal exposure to mood stabilizers, including valproic acid and carbamazepine, and neural tube defects (3%–8%) and spina bifida (1%) also has been observed.[104–106] Fetal exposure to anticonvulsants has been associated not only with high rates of neural tube defects, such as spina bifida, but also with multiple anomalies (including midface hypoplasia [also known as the anticonvulsant face], congenital heart disease, cleft lip or palate, growth retardation, and microcephaly). Factors that may increase the risk for teratogenesis include high maternal serum anticonvulsant levels and exposure to more than 1 anticonvulsant. This finding of dose-dependent risk for teratogenesis is at variance with that for some other psychotropics (eg, antidepressants). Thus, when using anticonvulsants during pregnancy, the lowest effective dose should be used, anticonvulsant levels should be monitored closely, and the dosage adjusted appropriately. Ideally, women of reproductive age should avoid treatment with valproate, and it should not be considered a first-line therapy in women with reproductive potential.

Information about the reproductive safety of newer anticonvulsants sometimes used to treat BPD (including gabapentin, oxcarbazepine, and topiramate) remains sparse.[102] Other efforts are under way to accumulate data from prospective registries regarding teratogenic risks across a broad range of anticonvulsants. The North American Antiepileptic Drug Pregnancy Registry was established as a way of collecting such information rapidly and efficiently (http://www.aedpregnancyregistry.org).

Prenatal screening following anticonvulsant exposure for congenital malformations (including cardiac anomalies) with fetal ultrasound at 18 to 22 weeks of gestation is recommended. The possibility of fetal neural tube defects should be evaluated with maternal serum α fetoprotein and ultrasonography. In addition, 4 mg a day of folic acid before conception and in the first trimester for women receiving anticonvulsants is frequently recommended. However, supplemental use of folic acid to attenuate the risk of neural tube defects in the setting of anticonvulsant exposure has not been systematically evaluated.

Although use of mood stabilizers (including lithium and some anticonvulsants) has become the mainstay of treatment of the management of acute mania and the maintenance phase of BPD, most patients with BPD are not treated with monotherapy. Rather, use of adjunctive conventional and newer antipsychotics has become common clinical practice for many patients with BPD. Moreover, with increasing data supporting the use of atypical antipsychotics as monotherapy in the treatment of BPD, patients and clinicians will seek information regarding the reproductive safety of these newer agents. To date, some data exist that support the reproductive safety of typical antipsychotics; these data have been reviewed extensively elsewhere.[32] However, despite their expanding use in psychiatry, available reproductive safety data regarding the atypical antipsychotics are limited, but increasing. The National Pregnancy Registry for Atypical Antipsychotics (http://www.womensmentalhealth.org/pregnancyregistry) was established to systematically collect data on the maternal and fetal outcome of women who continue atypical antipsychotic medication during pregnancy. Some patients who benefit from treatment with antipsychotics may decide with their clinician to discontinue an atypical antipsychotic or switch to a typical antipsychotic with a better-characterized safety profile. Atypical antipsychotics are best avoided if possible, although they are not absolutely contraindicated during pregnancy. Atypical antipsychotics should be reserved for use in more challenging clinical situations in which treatment with more conventional agents has not been helpful. Given the limited data supporting the use of typical antipsychotics as monotherapy for BPD, that course of therapy should not be pursued.

Patients with a history of a single episode of mania and prompt full recovery, followed by sustained well-being, may tolerate discontinuation of a mood stabilizer before an attempt to conceive.[90,98] Even among women with a history of prolonged well-being and sustained euthymia, discontinuation of prophylaxis for mania may be associated with subsequent relapse. In 1 study, the risk of recurrence of a mood episode during pregnancy in women who discontinued their mood stabilizer during pregnancy was 71%.[20]

For women with BPD and a history of multiple and frequent recurrences of mania or bipolar depression, several options can be considered. Some patients may choose to discontinue a mood stabilizer before conception, as outlined earlier. An alternative strategy for this high-risk group is to continue treatment until pregnancy is verified and then taper off the mood stabilizer. Because the uteroplacental circulation is not established until approximately 2 weeks following conception, the risk of fetal exposure is minimal. Home pregnancy tests are reliable and can document pregnancy as early as 10 days following conception, and with a home ovulation predictor kit, a patient may be able to time her treatment discontinuation accurately. This strategy minimizes fetal exposure to drugs and extends the protective treatment up to the time of conception, which may be particularly prudent for older patients because the time required for them to conceive may be longer than for younger patients. However, a potential problem with this strategy is that it may lead to abrupt discontinuation of treatment, thereby potentially placing the patient at increased risk for relapse. With close clinical follow-up, however, patients can be monitored for early signs of relapse, and medications may be reintroduced as needed. Another problem with the strategy of discontinuation of mood stabilizers emerges when the patient is being treated with valproic acid. The teratogenic effect of valproic acid occurs early in gestation (between weeks 4 and 5), often before the patient even knows she is pregnant. In such a scenario, any potential teratogenic insult from valproic acid may already have occurred by the time the patient discovers the pregnancy.

For women who tolerate discontinuation of maintenance treatment, the decision of when to resume treatment is a matter for clinical judgment. Some patients and clinicians prefer to await the initial appearance of symptoms before restarting medication; others prefer to limit their risk of a major recurrence by restarting treatment after the first trimester of pregnancy. Preliminary data suggest that pregnant women with BPD who remain well throughout pregnancy may have a lower risk for postpartum relapse than those who become ill during pregnancy.[90]

For women with particularly severe forms of BPD, such as with multiple severe episodes, and especially with psychosis and prominent thoughts of suicide, maintenance treatment with a mood stabilizer before and during pregnancy may be the safest option. If the patient decides to attempt conception, accepting the small absolute increase in teratogenic risk with first-trimester exposure to lithium or lamotrigine with or without antipsychotic, for example, may be justified because such patients are at highest risk for clinical deterioration if pharmacological treatment is withdrawn. Many patients who are treated with sodium valproate or other newer anticonvulsants, such as gabapentin, for which there are particularly sparse reproductive safety data, may never have received a lithium trial before pregnancy. For such patients, a lithium trial before pregnancy may be a particularly reasonable option.

Even if all psychotropics have been safely discontinued, pregnancy in a woman with BPD should be considered as a high-risk pregnancy, because the risk of major psychiatric illness during pregnancy is increased in the absence of treatment with a mood-stabilizing medication and it is even higher in the postpartum period. Extreme vigilance is required for early detection of an impending relapse of illness, and rapid intervention can significantly reduce morbidity and improve overall prognosis. Therefore, close monitoring with assessment of mood, sleep, and other symptoms are urged throughout pregnancy and the immediate postpartum period.

POSTPARTUM MOOD AND ANXIETY DISORDERS: DIAGNOSIS AND TREATMENT

The postpartum period has typically been considered a time of risk for the development of affective illness.[107] Although several studies have suggested that rates of depression during the postpartum period are equal to those in nonpuerperal controls, other research has identified subgroups of women at particular risk for postpartum worsening of mood.[108–111] At highest risk are women with a history of postpartum psychosis; up to 70% of women who have had 1 episode of puerperal psychosis experience another episode following a subsequent pregnancy.[107,111] Similarly, women with a history of postpartum depression are at significant risk, with rates of postpartum recurrence as high as 50%.[112] Women with BPD also seem to be particularly vulnerable during the postpartum period, with rates of postpartum relapse ranging from 30% to 50%.[19,110,113] The extent to which a history of MDD influences the risk for postpartum illness is less clear. However, in all women (with or without a history of MDD) the emergence of depressive symptoms during pregnancy significantly increases the likelihood of postpartum depression.[108]

During the postpartum period, about 85% of women experience some mood disturbance. For most women the symptoms are mild; however, 10% to 15% of women experience clinically significant symptoms. Postpartum depressive disorders typically are divided into 3 categories: (1) postpartum blues, (2) nonpsychotic major depression, and (3) puerperal psychosis. Because there may be some overlap across these 3 diagnostic subtypes, it is not clear if they actually represent 3 distinct disorders. It may be more useful to conceptualize these subtypes as existing along a continuum, on which postpartum blues is the mildest and postpartum psychosis the most severe form of puerperal psychiatric illness.

Postpartum blues does not indicate psychopathology; it is common and occurs in approximately 50% to 85% of women following delivery.[114,115] Symptoms of reactivity of mood, tearfulness, and irritability are, by definition, time limited and typically remit by the 10th postpartum day. As postpartum blues is associated with no significant impairment of function and is time limited, no specific treatment is indicated. Symptoms that persist beyond 2 weeks require further evaluation and may suggest an evolving depressive disorder. In women with a history of recurrent mood disorder, the blues may herald the onset of postpartum MDD.[108,116]

Several studies describe a prevalence of postpartum MDD of between 10% and 15%.[114,117] The signs and symptoms of postpartum depression usually appear in the first 2 to 3 months following delivery and are indistinguishable from the characteristics of MDD that occur at other times in a woman's life. The presenting symptoms of postpartum depression include depressed mood, irritability, and loss of interest in usual activities. Insomnia, fatigue, and loss of appetite are frequently described. Postpartum depressive symptoms also commingle with anxiety and obsessional symptoms, and women may present with generalized anxiety, panic disorder, or hypochondriasis.[118,119] Although it may sometimes be difficult to diagnose depression in the acute puerperium given the normal occurrence of symptoms suggestive of depression (eg, sleep and appetite disturbance, low libido), it is an error to dismiss neurovegetative symptoms (such as severe decreased energy, profound anhedonia, and guilty ruminations), as normal features of the puerperium. In its most severe form, postpartum depression may result in profound dysfunction. Risk factors for postpartum depression include antenatal depression, antenatal anxiety, and a history of depression.

A wealth of literature on this topic indicates that postpartum depression, especially when left untreated, may have a significant effect on the child's well-being and development.[120,121] In addition, the syndrome demands aggressive treatment to avoid the sequelae of an untreated mood disorder, such as chronic depression and recurrent disease. Treatment should be guided by the type and severity of the symptoms and by the degree of functional impairment. However, before initiating psychiatric treatment, medical causes for mood disturbances (eg, thyroid dysfunction and anemia) must be excluded. Initial evaluation should include a thorough history, physical examination, and routine laboratory tests.

Although postpartum depression is common, few studies have systematically assessed the efficacy of nonpharmacological and pharmacological therapies in the treatment of this disorder. Nonpharmacological therapies are useful in the treatment of postpartum depression, and several preliminary studies have yielded encouraging results. Appleby and colleagues[122] have shown in a randomized study that short-term CBT was as effective as treatment with fluoxetine in women with postpartum depression. IPT has also been shown to be effective for the treatment of women with mild to moderate postpartum depression.[123]

These nonpharmacological interventions may be particularly attractive to those patients who are reluctant to use psychotropics (eg, women who are breastfeeding) or for patients with milder forms of depressive illness. Further investigation is required to determine the efficacy of these treatments in women who suffer from more severe forms of postpartum mood disturbances. Women with more severe postpartum depression may choose to receive pharmacological treatment, either in addition to or instead of nonpharmacological therapies.

To date, only a few studies have systematically assessed the pharmacological treatment of postpartum depression. Conventional antidepressants (eg, fluoxetine, sertraline, and venlafaxine) have shown efficacy in the treatment of postpartum depression.[73,122,124–127] In all of these studies, standard antidepressant doses were effective and well tolerated. The choice of an antidepressant should be guided by the patient's prior response to antidepressants and the side-effect profile of a given medication. SSRIs are ideal first-line agents because some are anxiolytic, nonsedating, and well tolerated; bupropion is also another good option, particularly for anergic patients. TCAs are used frequently and, because they tend to be more sedating, may be more appropriate for women who have prominent sleep disturbances. Given the prevalence of anxiety in women with postpartum depression, adjunctive use of a benzodiazepine (eg, clonazepam or lorazepam) may be helpful.

Some investigators have also explored the role of hormonal manipulation in women who suffer from postpartum depression. The postpartum period is associated with rapid shifts in the reproductive hormonal environment, most notably a dramatic decrease in estrogen and progesterone levels, and postpartum mood disturbance has not infrequently been attributed to a deficiency (or change in the levels) in these gonadal steroids. However, clear evidence supporting this hypothesis regarding the cause of postpartum mood disorder is sparse. Although early reports suggested that progesterone may be helpful,[128] no systematically derived data exist to support its use in this setting. Two studies have described the benefit of exogenous estrogen therapy, either alone or in conjunction with an antidepressant in women with postpartum depression.[129–131] Although these studies suggest a role for estrogen in the treatment of women with postpartum depression, these treatments remain understudied. Estrogen delivered during the acute postpartum period is not without risk and has been associated with changes in breast-milk production and more significant thromboembolic events. Antidepressants are safe, well tolerated, and highly effective; they remain the first choice for women with moderate to severe postpartum depression in particular.

In cases of severe postpartum depression, inpatient hospitalization may be required, particularly for patients who are at risk for suicide. In Great Britain, innovative treatment programs involving joint hospitalization of the mother and the baby have been successful; however, mother-infant units are less common in the United States. Women with severe postpartum illness should be considered candidates for ECT. The option should be considered early in treatment because it is safe and highly effective. In choosing any treatment strategy, it is important to consider the effect of prolonged hospitalization or incomplete response to treatment by the mother on infant development and attachment.

Although symptoms of postpartum panic attacks and obsessive compulsive disorder (OCD) symptoms are frequently included in the description of postpartum mood disturbance, several studies support the likelihood that postpartum anxiety disorders are discrete diagnostic entities.[119,132] Several investigators have described postpartum worsening of panic disorder in women with pregravid histories of this anxiety disorder but with an absence of comorbid depressive illness. Postpartum OCD has also been described in the absence of comorbid postpartum MDD. Symptoms often include intrusive obsessional thoughts to harm the newborn in the absence of psychosis. Treatment with antiobsessional agents, such as fluoxetine or clomipramine, has been effective.[133]

Postpartum psychosis is a psychiatric emergency. The clinical picture is most frequently consistent with mania or a mixed state consistent with an episode of BPD[24] and may include symptoms of restlessness, agitation, sleep disturbance, paranoia, delusions, disorganized thinking, impulsivity, and behaviors that place mother and infant at risk. The typical onset is within the first 2 weeks after delivery, and symptoms may appear as early as the first 72 hours post partum. Although investigators have debated whether postpartum psychosis is a discrete diagnostic entity or a manifestation of BPD, treatment should follow the same algorithm to treat acute manic psychosis, including hospitalization and potential use of mood stabilizers, antipsychotics, benzodiazepines, and ECT.

Although it is difficult to reliably predict which women will experience a postpartum mood disturbance, it is possible to identify certain subgroups of women (ie, women with a history of mood disorder) who are more vulnerable to postpartum affective illness. Several investigators have explored the potential efficacy of prophylactic interventions in these women at risk.[134–137]

Several studies report that women with a history of BPD or puerperal psychosis benefit from prophylactic treatment with lithium, instituted either before delivery (at 36 weeks' gestation) or no later than the first 48 hours following delivery.[134–137] Prophylactic lithium seems to significantly reduce relapse rates and diminish the severity and duration of puerperal illness.

For women with a history of postpartum depression, Wisner and Wheeler[138] have described a beneficial effect of a prophylactic antidepressant (either a TCA or an SSRI) administered after delivery. However, a subsequent randomized, placebo-controlled study from the same group did not report a positive effect in women treated prophylactically with nortriptyline.[139] These investigators have suggested that nortriptyline may be less effective than SSRIs for the treatment of postpartum depression. The efficacy of prophylactic treatment with SSRIs in this population is under investigation.

SUMMARY

Postpartum depressive illness may be conceptualized along a continuum, in which some women are at lower risk for puerperal illness and others are at higher risk. Although a less aggressive, wait-and-see approach is appropriate for women with no history of postpartum psychiatric illness, women with BPD or a history of postpartum psychiatric illness deserve not only close monitoring but also specific prophylactic measures.

REFERENCES

1. Zajicek E. Psychiatric problems during pregnancy. In: Wolkind S, Zajicek E, editors. Pregnancy: a psychological and social study. London: Academic; 1981. p. 57–73.
2. Evans J, Heron J, Francomb H, et al. Cohort study of depressed mood during pregnancy and after childbirth. Br Med J 2001;323:257–60.
3. Cohen LS, Sichel DA, Dimmock JA, et al. Impact of pregnancy on panic disorder: a case series. J Clin Psychiatry 1994;55:284–8.
4. Cohen LS, Sichel DA, Faraone SV, et al. Course of panic disorder during pregnancy and the puerperium: a preliminary study. Biol Psychiatry 1996;39:950–4.
5. Cohen LS, Altshuler LL, Harlow BL, et al. Relapse of major depression during pregnancy in women who maintain or discontinue antidepressant treatment. JAMA 2006;295:499–507.
6. O'Hara MW. Social support, life events, and depression during pregnancy and the puerperium. Arch Gen Psychiatry 1986;43:569–73.
7. Frank E, Kupfer DJ, Jacob M, et al. Pregnancy related affective episodes among women with recurrent depression. Am J Psychiatry 1987;144:288–93.
8. Kessler RC, McGonagle KA, Swartz M, et al. Sex and depression in the national comorbidity survey I: lifetime prevalence, chronicity and recurrence. J Affect Disord 1993;29:85–96.
9. Eaton WW, Kessler RC, Wittchen HU, et al. Panic and panic disorder in the United States. Am J Psychiatry 1994;151:413–20.
10. Orr S, Miller C. Maternal depressive symptoms and the risk of poor pregnancy outcome. Review of the literature and preliminary findings. Epidemiol Rev 1995; 17:165–71.

11. Steer RA, Scholl TO, Hediger ML, et al. Self-reported depression and negative pregnancy outcomes. J Clin Epidemiol 1992;45:1093–9.
12. Wisner KL, Sit DK, Hanusa BH, et al. Major depression and antidepressant treatment: impact on pregnancy and neonatal outcomes. Am J Psychiatry 2009; 166(5):557–66.
13. Kupfer D, Frank E, Perel J, et al. Five-year outcome for maintenance therapies in recurrent depression. Arch Gen Psychiatry 1992;49(10):769–73.
14. Suppes T, Baldessarini RJ, Faedda GL, et al. Risk of recurrence following discontinuation of lithium treatment in bipolar disorder. Arch Gen Psychiatry 1991;48:1082–8.
15. Dencker SJ, Malm U, Lepp M. Schizophrenic relapse after drug withdrawal is predictable. Acta Psychiatr Scand 1986;73:181–5.
16. Roy-Byrne PP, Dager SR, Cowley DS, et al. Relapse and rebound following discontinuation of benzodiazepine treatment of panic attacks: alprazolam versus diazepam. Am J Psychiatry 1989;146:860–5.
17. Neziroglu F, Anemone R, Yaryura-Tobias JA. Onset of obsessive-compulsive disorder in pregnancy. Am J Psychiatry 1992;149:947–50.
18. Wisner KL, Zarin DA, Holmboe ES, et al. Risk-benefit decision making for treatment of depression during pregnancy. Am J Psychiatry 2000;157: 1933–40.
19. Viguera AC, Nonacs R, Cohen LS, et al. Risk of recurrence of bipolar disorder in pregnant and nonpregnant women after discontinuing lithium maintenance. Am J Psychiatry 2000;157:179–84.
20. Viguera AC, Whitfield T, Baldessarini RJ, et al. Risk of recurrence in women with bipolar disorder during pregnancy: prospective study of mood stabilizer discontinuation. Am J Psychiatry 2007;164:1817–24 [quiz: 923].
21. Flynn HA, O'Mahen HA, Massey L, et al. The impact of a brief obstetrics clinic-based intervention on treatment use for perinatal depression. J Womens Health (Larchmt) 2006;15:1195–204.
22. Marcus SM, Flynn HA. Depression, antidepressant medication, and functioning outcomes among pregnant women. Int J Gynaecol Obstet 2008; 100:248–51.
23. Frautschi S, Cerulli A, Maine D. Suicide during pregnancy and its neglect as a component of maternal mortality. Int J Gynaecol Obstet 1994;47:275–84.
24. Appleby L. Suicide during pregnancy and in the first postnatal year. BMJ 1991; 302:137–40.
25. Marzuk M, Tardiff K, Leon AC, et al. Lower risk of suicide during pregnancy. Am J Psychiatry 1997;154:122–3.
26. Altshuler L, Cohen LS, Moline M, et al. Treatment of depression in women: a summary of the expert consensus guidelines. J Psychiatr Pract 2001;7(3): 185–208.
27. Cohen L, Altshuler L, Heller V, et al. Psychotropic drug use in pregnancy. In: Bassuk GA, editor. The practitioner's guide to psychoactive drugs. New York: Plenum Publishing Corporation; 1998. p. 417–40.
28. Cohen LS, Rosenbaum J. Psychotropic drug use during pregnancy: weighing the risks. J Clin Psychiatry 1998;59:18–28.
29. Cott A, Wisner K. Psychiatric disorders during pregnancy. Int Rev Psychiatry 2003;15:217–30.
30. Einarson TR, Einarson A. Newer antidepressants in pregnancy and rates of major malformations: a meta-analysis of prospective comparative studies. Pharmacoepidemiol Drug Saf 2005;14:823–7.

31. Hallberg P, Sjoblom V. The use of selective serotonin reuptake inhibitors during pregnancy and breast-feeding: a review and clinical aspects. J Clin Psychopharmacol 2005;25:59–73.
32. Altshuler LL, Cohen L, Szuba MP, et al. Pharmacologic management of psychiatric illness during pregnancy: dilemmas and guidelines. Am J Psychiatry 1996; 153:592–606.
33. Cohen L, Altshuler L. Pharmacologic management of psychiatric illness during pregnancy and the postpartum period. In: Dunner D, Rosenbaum J, editors. The psychiatric clinics of North America annual of drug therapy. Philadelphia: WB Saunders Company; 1997. p. 21–60.
34. Wisner KL, Gelenberg AJ, Leonard H, et al. Pharmacologic treatment of depression during pregnancy. JAMA 1999;282:1264–9.
35. Pastuszak A, Schick-Boschetto B, Zuber C, et al. Pregnancy outcome following first-trimester exposure to fluoxetine (Prozac). JAMA 1993;269:2246–8.
36. Altshuler LL, Hendrick VC. Pregnancy and psychotropic medication: changes in blood levels. J Clin Psychopharmacol 1996;16:78–80.
37. Chambers C, Johnson K, Dick L, et al. Birth outcomes in pregnant women taking fluoxetine. N Engl J Med 1996;335:1010–5.
38. Nulman I, Rovet J, Stewart D, et al. Neurodevelopment of children exposed in utero to antidepressant drugs. N Engl J Med 1997;336:258–62.
39. Kulin N, Pastuszak A, Sage S, et al. Pregnancy outcome following maternal use of the new selective serotonin reuptake inhibitors: a prospective controlled multicenter study. JAMA 1998;279:609–10.
40. Einarson A, Fatoye B, Sarkar M, et al. Pregnancy outcome following gestational exposure to venlafaxine: a multicenter prospective controlled study. Am J Psychiatry 2001;158:1728–30.
41. Alwan S, Reefhuis J, Rasmussen SA, et al. Use of selective serotonin-reuptake inhibitors in pregnancy and the risk of birth defects. N Engl J Med 2007;356: 2684–92.
42. Louik C, Lin AE, Werler MM, et al. First-trimester use of selective serotonin reuptake inhibitors and the risk of birth defects. N Engl J Med 2007;356: 2675–83.
43. Pregnancy and Lactation Labeling. Available at: http://www.fda.gov/CDER/regulatory/pregnancy_labeling/default.htm. Accessed February 3, 2010.
44. Yonkers KA, Wisner KL, Stewart DE, et al. The management of depression during pregnancy: a report from the American Psychiatric Association and the American College of Obstetricians and Gynecologists. Gen Hosp Psychiatry 2009;31:403–13.
45. Freeman M, Davis M, Sinha P, et al. Omega-3 fatty acids and supportive psychotherapy for perinatal depression: a randomized placebo-controlled study. J Affect Disord 2008;110(1–2):142–8.
46. Beck AT, Rush AJ, Shaw BF, et al. Cognitive therapy of depression. New York: Guilford; 1979.
47. Klerman GL, Weissman MM, Rounsaville BJ, et al. Interpersonal psychotherapy of depression. New York: Basic Books Inc Publishers; 1984.
48. Spinelli M. Interpersonal psychotherapy for depressed antepartum women: a pilot study. Am J Psychiatry 1997;154:1028–30.
49. Cohen LS, Altshuler LL, Stowe ZN, et al. Reintroduction of antidepressant therapy across pregnancy in women who previously discontinued treatment. A preliminary retrospective study. Psychother Psychosom 2004;73: 255–8.

50. Brandes M, Soares CN, Cohen LS. Postpartum onset obsessive-compulsive disorder: diagnosis and management. Arch Womens Ment Health 2004;7: 99–110.
51. Heikkinen T, Ekblad U, Palo P, et al. Pharmacokinetics of fluoxetine and norfluoxetine in pregnancy and lactation. Clin Pharmacol Ther 2003;73:330–7.
52. Hostetter A, Stowe ZN, Strader JR Jr, et al. Dose of selective serotonin uptake inhibitors across pregnancy: clinical implications. Depress Anxiety 2000;11:51–7.
53. Freeman MP, Nolan PE Jr, Davis MF, et al. Pharmacokinetics of sertraline across pregnancy and postpartum. J Clin Psychopharmacol 2008;28:646–53.
54. Sit DK, Perel JM, Helsel JC, et al. Changes in antidepressant metabolism and dosing across pregnancy and early postpartum. J Clin Psychiatry 2008;69: 652–8.
55. Ericson A, Källén B, Wilhom B. Delivery outcome after the use of antidepressants in early pregnancy. Eur J Clin Pharmacol 1999;55:503–8.
56. New safety information regarding paroxetine: findings suggest increased risk over other antidepressants, of congenital malformations, following first trimester exposure to paroxetine. 2005. Available at: http://www.gsk.ca/en/health_info/PAXIL_PregnancyDHCPL_E-V4.pdf. Accessed June 15, 2006.
57. New safety information regarding paroxetine: second large study shows an increased risk of cardiac defects, over other antidepressants, following first trimester exposure to paroxetine, 2005. Available at: http://www.womensmentalhealth.org/resources/PDFs/GSK_Canada_Paxil_Letter.pdf. Accessed June 15, 2006.
58. Gentile S. Pregnancy exposure to serotonin reuptake inhibitors and the risk of spontaneous abortions. CNS Spectr 2008;13:960–6.
59. Einarson A, Pistelli A, DeSantis M, et al. Evaluation of the risk of congenital cardiovascular defects associated with use of paroxetine during pregnancy. Am J Psychiatry 2008;165:749–52.
60. Updated preliminary report on bupropion and other antidepressants, including paroxetine, in pregnancy and the occurrence of cardiovascular and major congenital malformation 2005. Available at: http://www.gsk.com/media/paroxetine/ingenix_study.pdf. Accessed February 3, 2010.
61. Chun-Fai-Chan B, Koren G, Fayez I, et al. Pregnancy outcome of women exposed to bupropion during pregnancy: a prospective comparative study. Am J Obstet Gynecol 2005;192:932–6.
62. Cole JA, Modell JG, Haight BR, et al. Bupropion in pregnancy and the prevalence of congenital malformations. Pharmacoepidemiol Drug Saf 2007;16: 474–84.
63. Verbeeck W, Tuinier S, Bekkering GE. Antidepressants in the treatment of adult attention-deficit hyperactivity disorder: a systematic review. Adv Ther 2009;26: 170–84.
64. Humphreys C, Garcia-Bournissen F, Ito S, et al. Exposure to attention deficit hyperactivity disorder medications during pregnancy. Can Fam Physician 2007;53:1153–5.
65. Henshaw S. Unintended pregnancy in the United States. Fam Plann Perspect 1998;30:24–9.
66. Djulus J, Koren G, Einarson TR, et al. Exposure to mirtazapine during pregnancy: a prospective, comparative study of birth outcomes. J Clin Psychiatry 2006;67:1280–4.
67. Krauer B. Pharmacotherapy during pregnancy: emphasis on pharmacokinetics. In: Eskes TK, Finster M, editors. Drug therapy during pregnancy. London: Butterworths; 1985. p. 9–31.

68. Jeffries WS, Bochner F. The effect of pregnancy on drug pharmacokinetics. Med J Aust 1988;149:675–7.
69. Wisner K, Perel J, Wheeler S. Tricyclic dose requirements across pregnancy. Am J Psychiatry 1993;150:1541–2.
70. Zeskind P, Stephens L. Maternal selective serotonin reuptake inhibitor use during pregnancy and newborn neurobehavior. Pediatrics 2004;113:368–75.
71. Simon GE, Cunningham ML, Davis RL. Outcomes of prenatal antidepressant exposure. Am J Psychiatry 2002;159:2055–61.
72. Nulman I, Rovet J, Stewart DE, et al. Child development following exposure to tricyclic antidepressants or fluoxetine throughout fetal life: a prospective, controlled study. Am J Psychiatry 2002;159:1889–95.
73. Suri R, Altshuler L, Hendrick V, et al. The impact of depression and fluoxetine treatment on obstetrical outcome. Arch Womens Ment Health 2004;7: 193–200.
74. Levinson-Castiel R, Merlob P, Linder N, et al. Neonatal abstinence syndrome after in utero exposure to selective serotonin reuptake inhibitors in term infants. Arch Pediatr Adolesc Med 2006;160:173–6.
75. Chambers CD, Hernandez-Diaz S, Van Marter LJ, et al. Selective serotonin-re-uptake inhibitors and risk of persistent pulmonary hypertension of the newborn. N Engl J Med 2006;354:579–87.
76. Källén B, Otterblad OP. Maternal use of selective serotonin reuptake inhibitors in early pregnancy and infant congenital malformations. Birth Defects Res A Clin Mol Teratol 2007;79:301–8.
77. Andrade SE, McPhillips H, Loren D, et al. Antidepressant medication use and risk of persistent pulmonary hypertension of the newborn. Pharmacoepidemiol Drug Saf 2009;18:246–52.
78. Hernandez-Diaz S, Van Marter LJ, Werler MM, et al. Risk factors for persistent pulmonary hypertension of the newborn. Pediatrics 2007;120:e272–82.
79. Moses-Kolko EL, Bogen D, Perel J, et al. Neonatal signs after late in utero exposure to serotonin reuptake inhibitors: literature review and implications for clinical applications. JAMA 2005;293:2372–83.
80. Misri S, Reebye P, Kendrick K, et al. Internalizing behaviors in 4-year-old children exposed in utero to psychotropic medications. Am J Psychiatry 2006; 163:1026–32.
81. Goldstein H, Weinberg J, Sankstone M. Shock therapy in psychosis complicating pregnancy, a case report. Am J Psychiatry 1941;98:201–2.
82. Impasato DJ, Gabriel AR, Lardara M. Electric and insulin shock therapy during pregnancy. Dis Nerv Syst 1964;25:542–6.
83. Remick RA, Maurice WL. ECT in pregnancy [letter]. Am J Psychiatry 1978;135: 761–2.
84. Miller LJ. Use of electroconvulsive therapy during pregnancy. Hosp Community Psychiatry 1994;45:444–50.
85. Wise MG, Ward SC, Townsend-Parchman W, et al. Case report of ECT during high-risk pregnancy. Am J Psychiatry 1984;141:99–101.
86. Repke JT, Berger NG. Electroconvulsive therapy in pregnancy. Obstet Gynecol 1984;63:39S–40S.
87. Sherer DM, D'Amico LD, Warshal DP, et al. Recurrent mild abruption placentae occurring immediately after repeated electroconvulsive therapy in pregnancy. Am J Obstet Gynecol 1991;165:652–3.
88. Ferrill MJ, Kehoe WA, Jacisin JJ. ECT during pregnancy: physiologic and pharmacologic considerations. Convuls Ther 1992;8:186–200.

89. Anderson EL, Reti IM. ECT in pregnancy: a review of the literature from 1941 to 2007. Psychosom Med 2009;71:235–42.
90. Viguera AC, Cohen LS, Baldessarini RJ, et al. Managing bipolar disorder during pregnancy: weighing the risks and benefits. Can J Psychiatry 2002;47:426–36.
91. Faedda GL, Tondo L, Baldessarini RJ, et al. Outcome after rapid vs gradual discontinuation of lithium treatment in bipolar disorders. Arch Gen Psychiatry 1993;50:448–55.
92. Tohen M, Waternaux CM, Tsuang MT. Outcome in mania. A 4-year prospective follow-up of 75 patients utilizing survival analysis. Arch Gen Psychiatry 1990;47: 1106–11.
93. Suppes T, Baldessarini R, Faedda G, et al. Discontinuation of maintenance treatment in bipolar disorder: Risks and implications. Harv Rev Psychiatry 1993;1:131–44.
94. Newport DJ, Stowe ZN, Viguera AC, et al. Lamotrigine in bipolar disorder: efficacy during pregnancy. Bipolar Disord 2008;10:432–6.
95. Cohen LS, Heller VL, Rosenbaum JF. Treatment guidelines for psychotropic drug use in pregnancy. Psychosomatics 1989;30:25–33.
96. Weinstein MR, Goldfield MD. Cardiovascular malformations with lithium use during pregnancy. Am J Psychiatry 1975;132:529–31.
97. Schou M, Goldfield MD, Weinstein MR, et al. Lithium and pregnancy, I: Report from the register of lithium babies. Br Med J 1973;2:135–6.
98. Cohen LS, Friedman JM, Jefferson JW, et al. A reevaluation of risk of in utero exposure to lithium. JAMA 1994;271:146–50.
99. Tennis P. Preliminary results on pregnancy outcome in women using lamotrigine. Epilepsia 2002;43:1161–7.
100. Messenheimer J, Wiel J. Thirteen year interim results from an international observational study of pregnancy outcomes following exposure to lamotrigine. In: 58th annual meeting of the American Academy of Neurology. San Diego (CA), April 1–8, 2006.
101. Cunnington M, Tennis P. Lamotrigine and the risk of malformations in pregnancy. Neurology 2005;64:955–60.
102. Meador KJ, Baker GA, Finnell RH, et al. In utero antiepileptic drug exposure: fetal death and malformations. Neurology 2006;67:407–12.
103. Holmes LB, Wyszynski DF, Baldwin EJ, et al. Increased risk for non-syndromic cleft palate among infants exposed to lamotrigine during pregnancy. In: 46th annual meeting of the Teratology Society. Tucson (AZ), June 24–29, 2006.
104. Wyszynski D, Nambisan M, Surve T, et al. Increased rate of major malformations in offspring exposed to valproate during pregnancy. Neurology 2005;64: 291–5.
105. Lammer EJ, Sever LE, Oakley GP. Teratogen update: valproic acid. Teratology 1987;35:465–73.
106. Omtzigt JG, Los FJ, Grobbee DE, et al. The risk of spina bifida aperta after first-trimester exposure to valproate in a prenatal cohort. Neurology 1992;42:119–25.
107. Kendell RE, Chalmers JC, Platz C. Epidemiology of puerperal psychoses. Br J Psychiatry 1987;150:662–73.
108. O'Hara MW. Postpartum depression: causes and consequences. New York: Springer-Verlag; 1995.
109. Bratfos O, Haug JO. Puerperal mental disorders in manic depressive females. Acta Psychiatr Scand 1966;42:285–94.
110. Reich T, Winokur G. Postpartum psychosis in patients with manic depressive disease. J Nerv Ment Dis 1970;151:60–8.

111. Davidson J, Robertson E. A follow-up study of postpartum illness. Acta Psychiatr Scand 1985;71:451–7.
112. Kupfer DJ, Frank E. Relapse in recurrent unipolar depression. Am J Psychiatry 1987;144:86–8.
113. Dean C, Williams RJ, Brockington IF. Is puerperal psychosis the same as bipolar manic-depressive disorder? A family study. Psychol Med 1989;19:637–47.
114. O'Hara MW, Zekoski EM, Philipps LH, et al. Controlled prospective study of postpartum mood disorders: comparison of childbearing and nonchildbearing women. J Abnorm Psychol 1990;99:3–15.
115. Handley SL, Dunn TL, Waldron G, et al. Tryptophan, cortisol and puerperal mood. Br J Psychiatry 1980;136:498–508.
116. Parekh RI. Prospective study of postpartum blues. In: Annual meeting of the American Psychiatric Association. New York, May 6, 1996.
117. Gotlib IH, Whiffen VE, Mount JH, et al. Prevalence rates and demographic characteristics associated with depression in pregnancy and the postpartum period. J Consult Clin Psychol 1989;57:269–74.
118. Hendrick V, Altshuler L, Strouse T, et al. Postpartum and nonpostpartum depression: differences in presentation and response to pharmacologic treatment. Depress Anxiety 2000;11:66–72.
119. Buttolph ML, Holland A. Obsessive compulsive disorders in pregnancy and childbirth. In: Jenike M, Baer L, Minichiello WE, editors. Obsessive compulsive disorders, theory and management. 2nd edition. Chicago: Yearbook Medical Publishers; 1990. p. 89–97.
120. Murray L. Postpartum depression and child development. Psychol Med 1997; 27:253–60.
121. Hayworth J, Little BC, Carter SB, et al. A predictive study of post-partum depression: some predisposing characteristics. Br J Med Psychol 1980;53: 161–7.
122. Appleby L, Warner R, Whitton A, et al. A controlled study of fluoxetine and cognitive-behavioural counselling in the treatment of postnatal depression. BMJ 1997; 314:932–6.
123. O'Hara MW, Stuart S, Gorman LL, et al. Efficacy of interpersonal psychotherapy for postpartum depression. Arch Gen Psychiatry 2000;57:1039–45.
124. Suri R, Burt VK, Altshuler LL, et al. Fluvoxamine for postpartum depression. Am J Psychiatry 2001;158:1739–40.
125. Stowe ZN, Casarella J, Landrey J, et al. Sertraline in the treatment of women with postpartum major depression. Depression 1995;3:49–55.
126. Cohen LS, Viguera AC, Bouffard SM, et al. Venlafaxine in the treatment of postpartum depression. J Clin Psychiatry 2001;62:592–6.
127. Nonacs RM, Soares CN, Viguera AC, et al. Bupropion SR for the treatment of postpartum depression: a pilot study. Int J Neuropsychopharmacol 2005;8: 445–9.
128. Dalton K. Progesterone prophylaxis used successfully in postnatal depression. Practitioner 1985;229:507–8.
129. Gregoire AJ, Kumar R, Everitt B, et al. Transdermal oestrogen for treatment of severe postnatal depression. Lancet 1996;347:930–3.
130. Gregoire A. Estrogen supplementation in postpartum depression. In: Biennial Conference of the Marcé Society. Cambridge (UK), September 25–28, 1994.
131. Ahokas A, Kaukoranta J, Wahlbeck K, et al. Estrogen deficiency in severe postpartum depression: successful treatment with sublingual physiologic 17beta-estradiol: a preliminary study. J Clin Psychiatry 2001;62:332–6.

132. Cohen LS, Sichel DA, Dimmock JA, et al. Postpartum course in women with preexisting panic disorder. J Clin Psychiatry 1994;55:289–92.
133. Sichel DA, Cohen LS, Rosenbaum JF, et al. Postpartum onset of obsessive-compulsive disorder. Psychosomatics 1993;34:277–9.
134. Austin MP. Puerperal affective psychosis: is there a case for lithium prophylaxis? Br J Psychiatry 1992;161:692–4.
135. Stewart DE, Klompenhouwer JL, Kendall RE, et al. Prophylactic lithium in puerperal psychosis: the experience of three centers. Br J Psychiatry 1991;158: 393–7.
136. Sichel DA, Cohen LS, Rosenbaum JF. High dose estrogen prophylaxis in 11 women at risk for recurrent postpartum psychosis and severe non-psychotic depression. In: Annual meeting of the Marcé Society. Einthoven, the Netherlands; November 5, 1993.
137. Cohen LS, Sichel DA, Robertson LM, et al. Postpartum prophylaxis for women with bipolar disorder. Am J Psychiatry 1995;152:1641–5.
138. Wisner KL, Wheeler SB. Prevention of recurrent postpartum major depression. Hosp Community Psychiatry 1994;45:1191–6.
139. Wisner P. Prevention of recurrent postpartum depression: a randomized clinical trial. J Clin Psychiatry 2001;62:82–6.

Challenges and Opportunities to Manage Depression During the Menopausal Transition and Beyond

Claudio N. Soares, MD, PhD, FRCPC[a,b,c],*, Benicio N. Frey, MD, PhD[a,c]

KEYWORDS

- Menopause • Depression • Anxiety • Vasomotor symptoms
- Perimenopause • Estrogen

Women are at higher risk than men of developing depression and such risk is particularly high during the reproductive years.[1] Although the risk for developing a major depressive disorder (MDD) among women during their lifetime is 1.7 times higher than that observed in men, no significant differences have been observed in the childhood years[2] or among the elderly, when women are predominantly postmenopausal.[3] Similarly, anxiety disorders have been reported to be more prevalent in women compared with men.[4] Given that gender differences in mood and anxiety disorders seem to emerge after puberty and decline during the postmenopausal years, it has

Disclosures for Dr Soares: No direct financial conflicts with regard to this manuscript. Dr Soares has received grant/research support from Eli Lilly, AstraZeneca, Physicians Services Incorporated (PSI) Foundation, Allergen National Centre of Excellence, Hamilton Community Foundation, Lundbeck, Wyeth, Pfizer, Canadian Institute of Health Research (CIHR). He has worked as research consultant for Wyeth, Lundbeck, Pfizer, and Bayer Healthcare Pharmaceuticals. He is a member of Speakers' Bureau of AstraZeneca, Wyeth, Bayer Healthcare Pharmaceuticals and an Advisory Board member of AstraZeneca, Wyeth, Pfizer, and Bayer Healthcare Pharmaceuticals.
Disclosures for Dr Frey: No direct financial conflicts with regard to this manuscript. Dr Frey has received research support from the Canadian Institutes of Health Research, Stanley Research Center, and Wyeth Pharmaceuticals, as well as speaker/advisory honoraria from Wyeth Pharmaceuticals and AstraZeneca.
[a] Department of Psychiatry and Behavioural Neurosciences, McMaster University, ON, Canada
[b] Department of Obstetrics and Gynecology, McMaster University, ON, Canada
[c] Mood Disorders Division, Women's Health Concerns Clinic, St Joseph's Healthcare, 301 James Street South, Suite F614, FB 638, Hamilton, ON L8P 3B6, Canada
* Corresponding author. Mood Disorders Division, Women's Health Concerns Clinic, St Joseph's Healthcare, 301 James Street South, Suite F614, FB 638, Hamilton, ON L8P 3B6, Canada.
E-mail address: csoares@mcmaster.ca

been postulated that the fluctuation of gonadal hormones might exert a modulatory effect on women's vulnerability to these disturbances. A closer look at women's mood during the reproductive years reveals that about 20% to 40% of women report moderate to severe premenstrual symptoms (PMS) and that 10% to 12% of post-partum women meet criteria for postpartum depression (PPD); these 2 windows of risk corroborate the notion that some women are particularly sensitive to developing mood symptoms when facing normal changes in the hormonal milieu.

Estrogen receptors are widely distributed throughout the brain[5,6] and the effects of estrogen have been observed in the hypothalamus, prefrontal cortex, hippocampus and brain stem, and cerebral regions known to be closely associated with mood and cognitive regulation.[6] Much of the interaction between estrogen and mood is believed to be associated with the effects of estrogen on monoaminergic neurotransmitters, especially serotonin and norepinephrine.[7] Estrogen regulates serotonin neuronal firing, increases serotonin and norepinephrine synthesis, and modulates the availability and gene expression of serotonin and norepinephrine receptors.[5,8]

More recently, the modulatory effect of estrogen on serotonin and noradrenaline neurotransmission has been linked to the development of depressive symptoms. Studies in vivo and in vitro have provided good evidence that there is a close recip-rocal relationship between estrogen and serotonin transmission. For instance, studies revealed selective estrogen-induced changes in serotonin transmission, binding, and metabolism in cerebral regions such as the amygdala. Studies on estrogen add-back in ovariectomized animals show that the administration of estrogen affects serotonin neurons and its afferent and target neurons. Moreover, it has been shown that estro-gens selectively increased serotonin receptor density in brain regions containing estrogen receptors, such as the hypothalamus, the preoptic area, and the amygdala. The noradrenergic system is also under the influence of estrogen. It has been observed that estrogen increases noradrenaline availability and synthesis while reducing its turnover. It has recently been shown that, compared with young repro-ductive women, postmenopausal women not on hormone therapy have a blunted serotonin response measured by either the serotonin agonist metachlorophenylpiper-azine or abnormal prolactin responses to the specific serotonin-releasing and reup-take inhibiting agent, d-fenfluramine. Estrogen therapy had a positive effect on serotonin tone because both acute and long-term estrogen therapy were associated with increased serotonin responsivity. The results from animal models revealed that estrogen enhances neurogenesis, synaptic plasticity, dendritic spine density, and connectivity in hippocampal formation, suggesting that estrogen may have neuropro-tective effects and may modulate neuronal plasticity. In addition, the ability of estrogen to act as a neutrophic factor may be associated with the activation of a brain-derived neurotrophic factor (BDNF) signaling system. BDNF levels seem to be higher with higher estrogen levels during the menstrual cycle and while using hormone therapy following menopause. These results corroborate the neurotrophin hypothesis of depression, which is based on the effect of recurrent stress and a putative antidepres-sant effect associated with the BDNF cascade; however, this hypothesis has never been investigated in the context of menopausal transition.

The presence of vasomotor symptoms (VMS, namely hot flashes and night sweats), believed to be related to the dysregulation of the thermoregulatory center, seem to be associated with fluctuations in estrogen levels and increased noradrenergic tone in the hypothalamus.[9] Curiously, selective serotonin reuptake inhibitors (SSRIs) and selec-tive serotonin and norepinephrine reuptake inhibitors (SNRIs) are efficacious for the management of depression and VMS. These data suggest that the brain in women is constantly challenged to adapt to hormonal variations, which could render some women vulnerable to developing mood and anxiety symptoms during times of chaotic or unpredictable hormone fluctuations such as the menopausal transition.

The transition to menopause is typically characterized by a complex set of emotional and physical symptoms associated with the progressive decline of ovarian function.[10] Population studies have demonstrated that vasomotor symptoms, sleep disturbances, and vaginal dryness are particularly prevalent in peri- and postmenopausal compared with premenopausal women.[11] Several community-based prospective studies have clearly shown that menopause transition is a period of heightened risk for recurrent and new-onset depression (as discussed in detail later), which is in line with current hypothesis suggesting that the transition to menopause represents a window of vulnerability for depression.[12,13] Moreover, accumulated evidence shows that hormonal and nonhormonal interventions are useful for the management of affective disorders in perimenopausal women.[14,15] In this article, some of the most relevant studies that have investigated the emergence of depressive and anxiety states during the menopausal transition are highlighted and available evidence-based strategies in the treatment of anxiety and depression in this population are presented.

COMMUNITY-BASED EPIDEMIOLOGIC STUDIES

Data from community-based cross-sectional studies that assessed psychological distress or depression in women during menopausal transition revealed mixed results.[16–18] Bromberger and colleagues (2001)[17] found higher scores of psychological distress in early perimenopausal women compared with pre- and postmenopausal women in a large multiethnic study of women aged 40 to 55 years across the United States (N = 10,374). In another study of 1434 women between 45 and 55 years of age depressive symptoms were found to be significantly higher in postmenopausal compared with premenopausal women.[16] Slaven and Lee,[19] on the other hand, reported no association between depression and menopausal transition in a community sample of 304 women from Australia who were assessed with the Women's Health Questionnaire and the Profile of Mood States scales. Juang and colleagues[18] examined a sample of 1273 women between the ages of 40 and 54 years using the Hospital Anxiety and Depression Scale and demonstrated that anxiety and depression were significantly associated with the presence of hot flashes in peri- and postmenopausal women. Several other studies reported anxiety (traits and state) as being significantly correlated with the severity of sleep disturbance in women during the menopause transition.[20–22] No such association was found in premenopausal women,[20] suggesting that perhaps the effect of anxiety on sleep disturbance may be caused by the higher incidence of hot flashes and night sweats in this period.

Joffe and colleagues[23] have recently shown that the interactions between sleep, vasomotor symptoms, and depression can be more complex than initially believed. By using objective and subjective sleep parameters in perimenopausal and postmenopausal women with and without depression, they demonstrated that depressed women spent less time in bed and had shorter total sleep time, longer sleep-onset latency, and a tendency toward lower sleep efficiency compared with women who were not depressed; however, measurements of sleep interruption (wake time after sleep onset, number of awakenings, duration of awakenings) did not differ between depressed and nondepressed participants. When vasomotor symptoms were taken into consideration, depressed women with VMS reported poorer perceived sleep quality than nondepressed women with VMS. The association between depression and worse sleep was seen despite a similar frequency of nocturnal VMS in the 2 groups. No increased frequency of nocturnal VMS, more awakenings, or more time spent awake after sleep onset were observed among depressed women; therefore, the domino hypothesis that explains the development of depression in menopausal women as a result of the sleep disruption caused by VMS was not supported.

Other factors that have been associated with anxiety and depressive symptoms during the menopause transition are: history of stressful live events, history of PMS and/or mood disorders, poor social support, lower education, age, and living in a rural region.[16,18,24,25] Some but not all cross-sectional studies suggest that the menopausal transition may be associated with a higher risk for developing depression and anxiety. However, cross-sectional studies are not suitable for the investigation of temporal changes in mood and anxiety during the menopausal transition and early postmenopausal years.

Unlike the cross-sectional studies, most prospective studies[26–30] confirmed the transition to menopause as a period of heightened risk for development of depressive symptoms and/or depression, perhaps with the exception of Kaufert and colleagues.[31] The Penn Ovarian Aging Study followed 436 women from the community across the menopausal transition for an average of 4 years[28]; in this study, the severity of depressive symptoms, as measured by the Center for Epidemiologic Studies Depression Scale (CES-D) was higher during the transition to menopause and decreased after menopause; this increased risk remained significant after controlling for past history of depression, age, PMS, poor sleep, hot flashes, race, and employment status.[28] The investigators proposed that depressive and menopause-related symptoms may be mechanistically related, given that a history of severe PMS and the presence of hot flashes and sleep disturbance were independent predictors of depressive symptoms and diagnosed MDD. The Massachusetts Women's Health Study was a community-based study that investigated 2356 middle-age women for 5 years using the CES-D scale for the assessment of depressive symptoms in the transition to menopause.[26] Perimenopausal women exhibited an increased risk for depression and such risk was even higher among those with menopause-related vasomotor symptoms. Two other independent community-based studies evaluated large samples of middle-age women: the Study of Women's Health Across the Nation (SWAN; N = 3302)[27] and the Seattle Midlife Women's Health Study (N = 508).[30] Both studies also revealed a heightened risk for depression during the perimenopausal period, with the presence of hot flashes being an independent risk factor.

To assess whether the transition to menopause increases the risk for new-onset depression, 2 long-term prospective studies followed women with no history of depression across the menopause transition.[32,33] In the Harvard Study of Moods and Cycles, 460 never-depressed women were followed up for 6 to 8 years and those who entered the perimenopause were nearly twice as likely (odds ratio [OR]=1.8 [1.0–3.2]) to develop significant depressive symptoms compared with those who remained premenopausal. In this study, the presence of vasomotor symptoms and history of significant life events were independent predictors of higher risk for depression.[32] In the Penn Ovarian Aging Study, 231 women with no history of depression were followed for 8 years; perimenopausal women were 4 times more likely to have high CES-D scores and twice as likely to meet criteria for MDD than premenopausal women.[33] In addition, greater variation of estradiol and follicle-stimulating hormone levels (calculated from the standard deviation of hormonal levels) was associated with higher depressive scores and diagnosis of MDD; this particular finding is indicative that fluctuations of hormonal levels, rather than their absolute levels, may play a significant role as a trigger for depressive symptoms in biologically vulnerable women. This result is consistent with previous studies reporting that hormone fluctuations, rather than absolute hormonal levels, are more likely to be associated with the onset of depressive symptoms during certain female reproductive life events.[30,34] Several other factors have also been associated with depression during menopausal transition, including age, ethnicity (higher risk in African American, lower risk in Asian population), education, family history of depression, postpartum blues or depression, body mass index, use of hormone therapy or antidepressants, cigarette smoking, and stressful life events[26–30] reinforcing the complex, multifaceted aspect of depression.

Rocca and colleagues[35] examined a cohort of women who underwent oophorectomy before the onset of menopause (average follow-up was 25 years) and an aged-matched sample from the same community who had not undergone the same surgical procedure. In this study, those who underwent surgery (bilateral oophorectomy, N = 666) had a significant increased risk for developing depressive symptoms (hazard ration [HR] = 1.54, 95% confidence interval [CI] = 1.04–2.26) and anxiety symptoms (HR = 2.29, 5% CI = 1.33–3.95) compared with the referent group (N = 673). These results remained significant after adjusting for age, education, and type of surgery; moreover, the risks were even greater among those who underwent surgery at younger age.[35] The investigators speculated that these findings could be associated with the early loss of putative neuroprotective effects of estrogen levels throughout the reproductive life, and with the deficiency of testosterone and progesterone after surgery, resulting in an adverse effect on the hypothalamus-pituitary-gonadal axis; putative genetic variants could also increase the risk for these outcomes (ovarian disorders and psychiatric disturbances) independently.

Longitudinal studies looking specifically at the risk for anxiety in perimenopausal women indicated that natural (ie, nonsurgical) transition to menopause is associated with increased risk for anxiety, after controlling for the presence or severity of depression. Freeman and colleagues (2005)[36] followed up 436 midlife women for 6 years and found that hot flashes were strongly associated with anxiety, especially in women who were in the early menopausal transition. There was a dose-response effect between the severity of anxiety and the presence of hot flashes, with women with high anxiety scores being 4 times more likely to report hot flashes compared with women with no anxiety; those with moderate anxiety scores had a 3-fold increased risk for hot flashes. Anxiety remained strongly associated with hot flashes after controlling for depression, age, race, menopause stage, body mass index, smoking, and estradiol levels. More recently, the same group investigated the relationship between menopausal stage and anxiety, depression, mood swings, headache, and concentration difficulties in the same cohort after 9 years of follow-up.[37] Anxiety achieved its peak during early menopausal transition and returned to premenopausal levels in the postmenopausal years. In addition, women with a history of premenstrual syndrome were twice as likely to report anxiety compared with those with no history of premenstrual syndrome. In the SWAN study, the association between vasomotor symptoms and several health and lifestyle factors was examined in 3198 midlife women during a 6-year follow-up.[38] This study suggested a mutual relationship between anxiety and vasomotor symptoms; at baseline, women reporting more vasomotor symptoms were more likely to be anxious than women with fewer vasomotor symptoms (53.6% vs 19.1%; $P<.0001$). Conversely, more baseline anxiety was an independent factor for more vasomotor symptoms at the end of the 6-year follow-up (OR = 3.10; CI = 2.33–4.12).[38] Long-term, community-based longitudinal studies provide strong evidence that the menopausal transition is a period of higher risk for depression and anxiety. Although multiple risk factors seem to independently modulate such risk, the presence of vasomotor symptoms and hormonal fluctuation seem to be closely associated with emotional disturbance. Thus, it is likely that treatment strategies to ameliorate menopause-related symptoms can not only improve women's quality of life but may also decrease the likelihood of emotional disturbance in this population at risk.

TREATMENT STRATEGIES

Treatment strategies specifically targeting the management of depression and anxiety during menopausal transition are scarce. The few randomized placebo-controlled trials (RCTs) conducted to date have primarily focused on the efficacy of hormone therapies in depressed women. Although several open trials have suggested that SSRIs and SNRIs can be effective in the treatment of depression in perimenopausal women, large RCTs are lacking. In addition, most treatment studies assessed anxiety symptoms as secondary outcomes or included populations with low anxiety levels. Nevertheless, as further discussed, available evidence suggests that hormonal and nonhormonal agents are useful tools for the management of depression and anxiety in perimenopausal women.

DEPRESSION

The few RCTs that investigated the antidepressant effects of estrogen found that estradiol can be efficacious for the treatment of depressive disorders. Transdermal 17β-estradiol, 50 to 100 μg, has been used in clinical trials (6–12-week trials) for the treatment of major depression, minor depression, or dysthymia in perimenopausal women, with remission rates of 68% to 80% compared with 20% to 22% with placebo.[14,15] Transdermal estradiol 100 μg for 8 weeks was not effective in the treatment of depression in postmenopausal women,[39] suggesting that the menopausal transition might not only be a critical window of risk for depression but also a window of opportunity for the use of hormonal strategies in the management of depression.[12]

The initial findings from the Women's Health Initiative (WHI) had a significant negative effect on physicians' and patients' perception of the long-term safety and benefits of hormone replacement therapies (HRT)[40]; as a result, many health professional and their patients became more cautious or reluctant to initiate HRT or to stay on HRT for longer periods of time; others started seeking nonhormonal strategies to improve menopause-related physical and psychological discomforts.[41,42] In Ontario, Canada, for example, right after the interruption of the WHI study, a sharp decrease in prescriptions of HRT occurred in parallel with a marked increase in prescriptions of antidepressants to women 40 years of age or older[43]; such change in prescription patterns was suggestive of the development of depressive and/or anxiety states in some women following abrupt HRT interruption and/or a switch in patients and doctors' preference toward nonhormonal strategies to manage menopause-related symptoms.

Several open trials have provided evidence that SSRIs and SNRIs are efficacious for the management of depression[44,45] and vasomotor symptoms[46–48] in perimenopausal and/or postmenopausal women. Remission rates of depressive symptoms were considerably high after monotherapy with citalopram and escitalopram (86.6% and 75%, respectively).[45,49] In addition to the alleviation of depression, there was a significant improvement in menopause-related symptoms (eg, hot flashes, night sweats, and somatic complaints). Mirtazapine and citalopram were tested as adjunctive treatments to estrogen therapy in depressed peri- and postmenopausal women, with remission rates of 87.5% with mirtazapine and 91.6% with citalopram.[45,50]

More recently, a pooled analysis of 8 RCT studies showed higher remission rates with the SNRI venlafaxine (48%) compared with SSRIs (28%) among depressed women more than 50 years of age who were not receiving estrogen therapies; the difference between the 2 treatment groups, however, was significantly reduced among depressed women receiving estrogen-based therapies.[51] These results led many to speculate that reproductive-aging women might benefit from the priming/synergistic effects of estrogens while on SSRIs. Conversely, during times of unstable estrogen levels (ie, perimenopause) or in the absence of menopause-related estrogen therapies during postmenopausal years, some women would not sustain the same response to SSRIs and could have a more robust response to antidepressants that act preferably on noradrenergic neurotransmission. Although intriguing, this hypothesis still warrants further investigation and should not discourage physicians or patients from using SSRIs to manage MDD during the postmenopausal years. In a recent study investigating the use of the SNRI duloxetine in the treatment of depression in postmenopausal women, remission rates of 78.6% were obtained after 8 weeks of treatment.[44] Duloxetine also showed a positive effect in the amelioration of menopause-related symptoms.

Botanical agents have been investigated as nonhormonal alternatives for the treatment of menopause-associated symptoms, with limited evidence that these agents may in fact reduce the frequency and severity of vasomotor symptoms. Two small RCTs suggested that black cohosh (*Actaea racemosa*) is more effective than placebo in the treatment of mild to moderate vasomotor symptoms.[52,53] In a recent meta-analysis of 43 RCTs, soy isoflavone extracts showed a small positive effect over placebo after 12 weeks of treatment.[54] Newton and colleagues[55] tested the efficacy of 3 herbal regimens, hormone therapy, and placebo for the relief of vasomotor symptoms in a 1-year randomized double-blind trial (N = 353). Treatment groups included black cohosh alone (160 mg/d), multibotanical preparation including black cohosh (200 mg) and 9 other ingredients, multibotanical plus dietary soy counseling, conjugated equine estrogen, 0.625 mg (with or without medroxyprogesterone acetate), and placebo. At 12 months, symptom intensity was significantly worse with the use of multibotanical plus soy intervention than with placebo. Moreover, the difference in vasomotor symptoms between placebo and any of the herbal treatments at any time point in the study was minimal at less than 1 symptom per day. The only intervention that appeared to be efficacious compared with placebo was estrogen therapy.

To date, no studies have investigated the efficacy of botanical agents in the treatment of peri- and postmenopausal women with a major depressive episode. Nonetheless, 1 RCT that investigated 301 women with climacteric complaints showed a 41.8% improvement in Hamilton Depression Rating Scale (HAM-D) scores from baseline (18.9 ± 2.2) to 16 weeks (11.0 ± 3.8) with a combination of black cohosh and St. John's wort (*Hypericum perforatum*).[56] These results are consistent with those from a 12-week open trial with St John's wort in 111 women (aged between 43 and 65 years) with climacteric symptoms, in which participants showed significant improvement of psychological and somatic symptoms.[57]

The available evidence indicates that transdermal estrogen, SSRIs, and SNRIs are effective in the treatment of depression during the menopausal transition; antidepressants, however, remain the first choice for the management of depression in any given age/reproductive staging group. More systematic data on botanical agents and other nonhormonal treatment strategies for depression in peri- and postmenopausal women are lacking. Women with a lifetime history of depression who are unable or unwilling to use hormone therapies may benefit from the mild effects of nonhormonal, nonpharmacological strategies for menopause-related symptoms. The presence of vasomotor symptoms and other menopause-related complaints seems to be associated with a higher risk for new onset or reemergence of depression during the menopausal transition.[27,30]

MANAGING ANXIETY DURING MIDLIFE

To date, no studies have systematically investigated the effects of hormonal therapies for the treatment of anxiety in perimenopausal or postmenopausal women. Some studies have assessed the effect of hormone therapies on symptoms of anxiety through secondary outcome measures. In a study of 70 women with climacteric symptoms, those who opted to receive HRT (N = 35) reported lower anxiety, sleep and somatic complaints compared with women who chose not to receive HRT (N = 35).[58] Three RCTs that assessed the secondary effects of HRT on anxiety symptoms in peri- and postmenopausal women reported little or no effects.[59–61] A large trial that randomized 419 postmenopausal women to 4 different HRT regimens found only modest effects of hormone treatments on anxiety scores after a long (up to 9 years) follow-up period.[62] However, these negative findings may be explained in part by a floor effect, because most study participants revealed relatively low anxiety scores at study entry.

Two studies investigated the effects of tibolone, a selective estrogen receptor modulator (SERM), on symptoms of anxiety and depression. One study compared 19 postmenopausal women using tibolone for 6 months with 25 women on no medication and found that tibolone had a positive effect in decreasing anxiety scores.[63] However, Hamilton Anxiety Rating Scale (HAM-A) scores decreased from 7.8 ± 7.7 at baseline to 5.5 ± 4.3 at 6 months, which may not have been clinically significant. In an RCT of 75 women who underwent surgical menopause for benign conditions, participants were randomized to receive tibolone, transdermal estradiol, or placebo and followed for 6 months. Improvement in anxiety and depression scores was observed with both active treatments compared with placebo; no differences between tibolone and transdermal estradiol were documented.[64] The relatively low baseline anxiety scores (HAM-A scores approximately 9–10) limit the generalization of these results. Studies including women with well-defined reproductive staging and high anxiety scores at study entry are necessary to better investigate the potential benefits of hormone therapies for the treatment of anxiety in midlife women.

Scarce data are available on the effects of antidepressants for the management of anxiety disorders in peri- and postmenopausal women; most data are derived from studies of healthy or depressed subpopulations. Nonetheless, existing evidence suggests that antidepressants may have a positive effect in alleviating anxiety symptoms among midlife postmenopausal women. Two open trials observed a modest anxiolytic effect with trazodone and paroxetine for the management of menopausal symptoms in otherwise healthy peri- and postmenopausal women.[65,66] Three open trials evaluated the effects of citalopram, venlafaxine, and duloxetine in peri- and postmenopausal women with major depression and reported reduction in anxiety scores as secondary outcome measures.[44,45,67] In all these studies, beneficial effects on depressive and anxiety scores were observed after 8 weeks of therapy. These antidepressants also had a positive effect in alleviating menopause-related symptoms, such as hot flashes and night sweats. Consistently, a study of perimenopausal women with depression reported a significant improvement in depression, anxiety, and menopause scores after 3 months of treatment with fluvoxamine (N = 53) or paroxetine (N = 52).[68] Although results with antidepressants are encouraging, future studies examining the efficacy of antidepressants in women with primary anxiety disorders in the context of menopause transition are warranted.

Several studies have investigated the use of botanical agents in the management of anxiety symptoms in peri- and postmenopausal women. In 1 RCT, 149 individuals (67% women) with a primary diagnosis of somatoform disorder were allocated to St. John's wort or placebo and the HAM-A total score was used as the primary outcome measure.[69] A significant decrease in total HAM-A scores was observed after 42 days of treatment with St. John's wort. Two small RCTs evaluated the effects of kava extract on anxiety symptoms in peri-[70] and postmenopausal women[71]; the efficacy of kava extract plus calcium supplementation in reducing anxiety symptoms was superior than calcium supplementation only (control group).[70] The combination of kava extract + hormone therapy was more efficacious than hormone alone to alleviate anxiety symptoms in 40 postmenopausal women and this effect was maintained after 6 months of treatment.[71] Although preliminary, these findings suggest that kava extract may be a useful option in the management of anxiety during menopausal transition and the postmenopausal years. However, clinicians should be aware of the potential hepato-toxicity of kava extract as well as its various drug-drug interactions.[72] A small open trial tested the efficacy of Korean red ginseng on anxiety scores in 12 postmenopausal women with menopausal symptoms and found a small effect of this compound for the reduction of anxiety symptoms after 1 month of treatment.[73] Negative effects of *Ginko biloba* and *Panax ginseng* (Gincosan) on anxiety, mood, and menopausal symptoms were reported in an RCT involving 70 postmenopausal women.[74] More recently, 64 peri- and postmenopausal women were randomly allocated to either black cohosh or transdermal estradiol, and both treatments were equally effective in decreasing anxiety, depressive, and vasomotor symptoms.[75] Negative effects of isoflavones and valerian extract were reported by 2 RCTs.[76,77] In summary, studies investigating the effects of botanical agents in the management of anxiety in peri- and postmenopausal women are limited, given that anxiety scores were part of secondary outcome measures in most studies. Therefore, RCTs assessing peri- and postmenopausal women with well-defined anxiety disorders as primary diagnosis are necessary.

SUMMARY

Increasing evidence supports the notion that the menopausal transition may constitute a window of vulnerability for the development of mood and anxiety disorders; little is known, however, about the underlying mechanisms that contribute to the occurrence of this phenomenon. Moreover, more tailored treatment strategies to address the spectrum of physical and psychological complaints at this stage in life are lacking. In the post-WHI era, it is imperative that health professionals become aware of the putative effect of menopause (natural or surgical) on psychological well-being, particularly among those who are unable or unwilling to use hormone therapies. More research on nonhormonal options (ie, SERMs, herbal supplements, and psychotropic agents) should be strongly encouraged to expand the portfolio of treatment strategies available for this population.

TREATMENT RECOMMENDATIONS

It is crucial that physicians and health professionals incorporate questions regarding reproductive status and past reproductive-related psychiatric events into their medical and psychiatric history. Antidepressants remain the treatment of choice for the management of most depressive and anxiety disorders during the perimenopausal and postmenopausal years. Nonetheless, the use of hormonal strategies, particularly estrogen-based therapies, has shown to not only improve depressive symptoms but also to promote alleviation of menopause-related complaints (eg, vasomotor symptoms, sexual dysfunction, sleep disruption) and better overall functioning and quality of life. Thus, the use of menopause-related hormone therapies, either as an augmenting strategy or as a monotherapy (the latter for those who failed to have a considerable response/tolerability with conventional treatments), should be carefully considered.

Women are at a higher risk than men for developing depression and anxiety and such increased risk might be particularly associated with reproductive cycle events. Evidence suggests that the menopause transition constitutes a window of vulnerability for some women for new-onset and/or recurrent depression. Existing data supporting such risk and the putative underlying mechanisms contributing to this window of vulnerability are examined in this article. Moreover, hormonal and nonhormonal treatment strategies are critically reviewed, although more tailored treatment options for this population are still needed.

REFERENCES

1. Kessler RC, McGonagle KA, Swartz M, et al. Sex and depression in the National Comorbidity Survey. I: lifetime prevalence, chronicity and recurrence. J Affect Disord 1993;29(2–3):85–96.
2. Birmaher B, Ryan ND, Williamson DE, et al. Childhood and adolescent depression: a review of the past 10 years. Part I. J Am Acad Child Adolesc Psychiatry 1996;35(11):1427–39.
3. Bebbington P, Dunn G, Jenkins R, et al. The influence of age and sex on the prevalence of depressive conditions: report from the National Survey of Psychiatric Morbidity. Int Rev Psychiatry 2003;15(1–2):74–83.
4. Kessler RC, McGonagle KA, Zhao S, et al. Lifetime and 12-month prevalence of DSM-III-R psychiatric disorders in the United States. Results from the National Comorbidity Survey. Arch Gen Psychiatry 1994;51(1):8–19.
5. McEwen BS. Invited review. Estrogens effects on the brain: multiple sites and molecular mechanisms. J Appl Phys 2001;91(6):2785–801.
6. Morrison JH, Brinton RD, Schmidt PJ, et al. Estrogen, menopause, and the aging brain: how basic neuroscience can inform hormone therapy in women. J Neurosci 2006;26(41):10332–48.
7. McEwen BS, Alves SE. Estrogen actions in the central nervous system. Endocr Rev 1999;20(3):279–307.
8. Deecher D, Andree TH, Sloan D, et al. From menarche to menopause: exploring the underlying biology of depression in women experiencing hormonal changes. Psychoneuroendocrinology 2008;33(1):3–17.
9. Freedman RR. Pathophysiology and treatment of menopausal hot flashes. Semin Reprod Med 2005;23(2):117–25.
10. Santoro N. The menopausal transition. Am J Med 2005;118(Suppl 12B):8–13.
11. Nelson HD. Menopause. Lancet 2008;371(9614):760–70.
12. Soares CN. Depression during the menopausal transition: window of vulnerability or continuum of risk? Menopause 2008;15(2):207–9.
13. Soares CN, Zitek B. Reproductive hormone sensitivity and risk for depression across the female life cycle: a continuum of vulnerability? J Psychiatry Neurosci 2008;33(4):331–43.
14. Soares CN, Almeida OP, Joffe H, et al. Efficacy of estradiol for the treatment of depressive disorders in perimenopausal women: a double-blind, randomized, placebo-controlled trial. Arch Gen Psychiatry 2001;58(6):529–34.
15. Schmidt PJ, Nieman L, Danaceau MA, et al. Estrogen replacement in perimenopause-related depression: a preliminary report. Am J Obstet Gynecol 2000; 183(2):414–20.

16. Amore M, Di Donato P, Berti A, et al. Sexual and psychological symptoms in the climacteric years. Maturitas 2007;56(3):303–11.
17. Bromberger JT, Meyer PM, Kravitz HM, et al. Psychologic distress and natural menopause: a multiethnic community study. Am J Public Health 2001;91(9):1435–42.
18. Juang KD, Wang SJ, Lu SR, et al. Hot flashes are associated with psychological symptoms of anxiety and depression in peri- and post- but not premenopausal women. Maturitas 2005;52(2):119–26.
19. Slaven L, Lee C. Mood and symptom reporting among middle-aged women: the relationship between menopausal status, hormone replacement therapy, and exercise participation. Health Psychol 1997;16(3):203–8.
20. Baker A, Simpson S, Dawson D. Sleep disruption and mood changes associated with menopause. J Psychosom Res 1997;43(4):359–69.
21. Kloss JD, Tweedy K, Gilrain K. Psychological factors associated with sleep disturbance among perimenopausal women. Behav Sleep Med 2004;2(4):177–90.
22. Thurston RC, Blumenthal JA, Babyak MA, et al. Association between hot flashes, sleep complaints, and psychological functioning among healthy menopausal women. Int J Behav Med 2006;13(2):163–72.
23. Joffe H, Soares CN, Thurston RC, et al. Depression is associated with worse objectively and subjectively measured sleep, but not more frequent awakenings, in women with vasomotor symptoms. Menopause 2009;16(4):671–9.
24. Binfa L, Castelo-Branco C, Blumel JE, et al. Influence of psycho-social factors on climacteric symptoms. Maturitas 2004;48(4):425–31.
25. Malacara JM, Canto de Cetina T, Bassol S, et al. Symptoms at pre- and postmenopause in rural and urban women from three States of Mexico. Maturitas 2002; 43(1):11–9.
26. Avis NE, Brambilla D, McKinlay SM, et al. A longitudinal analysis of the association between menopause and depression. Results from the Massachusetts Women's Health Study. Ann Epidemiol 1994;4(3):214–20.
27. Bromberger JT, Matthews KA, Schott LL, et al. Depressive symptoms during the menopausal transition: the Study of Women's Health Across the Nation (SWAN). J Affect Disord 2007;103(1–3):267–72.
28. Freeman EW, Sammel MD, Liu L, et al. Hormones and menopausal status as predictors of depression in women in transition to menopause. Arch Gen Psychiatry 2004;61(1):62–70.
29. Maartens LW, Knottnerus JA, Pop VJ. Menopausal transition and increased depressive symptomatology: a community based prospective study. Maturitas 2002;42(3):195–200.
30. Woods NF, Smith-DiJulio K, Percival DB, et al. Depressed mood during the menopausal transition and early postmenopause: observations from the Seattle Midlife Women's Health Study. Menopause 2008;15(2):223–32.
31. Kaufert PA, Gilbert P, Tate R. The Manitoba Project: a re-examination of the link between menopause and depression. Maturitas 1992;14(2):143–55.
32. Cohen LS, Soares CN, Vitonis AF, et al. Risk for new onset of depression during the menopausal transition: the Harvard Study of Moods and Cycles. Arch Gen Psychiatry 2006;63(4):385–90.
33. Freeman EW, Sammel MD, Lin H, et al. Associations of hormones and menopausal status with depressed mood in women with no history of depression. Arch Gen Psychiatry 2006;63(4):375–82.
34. Bloch M, Schmidt PJ, Danaceau M, et al. Effects of gonadal steroids in women with a history of postpartum depression. Am J Psychiatry 2000; 157(6):924–30.

35. Rocca WA, Grossardt BR, Geda YE, et al. Long-term risk of depressive and anxiety symptoms after early bilateral oophorectomy. Menopause 2008;15(6): 1050–9.

36. Freeman EW, Sammel MD, Lin H, et al. The role of anxiety and hormonal changes in menopausal hot flashes. Menopause 2005;12(3):258–66.

37. Freeman EW, Sammel MD, Lin H, et al. Symptoms in the menopausal transition: hormone and behavioral correlates. Obstet Gynecol 2008;111(1):127–36.

38. Gold EB, Colvin A, Avis N, et al. Longitudinal analysis of the association between vasomotor symptoms and race/ethnicity across the menopausal transition: study of women's health across the nation. Am J Public Health 2006; 96(7):1226–35.

39. Morrison MF, Kallan MJ, Ten Have T, et al. Lack of efficacy of estradiol for depression in postmenopausal women: a randomized, controlled trial. Biol Psychiatry 2004;55(4):406–12.

40. Rossouw JE, Anderson GL, Prentice RL, et al. Risks and benefits of estrogen plus progestin in healthy postmenopausal women: principal results from the Women's Health Initiative randomized controlled trial. JAMA 2002;288(3):321–33.

41. Hackley B, Rousseau ME. CEU: managing menopausal symptoms after the women's health initiative. J Midwifery Womens Health 2004;49(2):87–95.

42. Kessel B, Kronenberg F. The role of complementary and alternative medicine in management of menopausal symptoms. Endocrinol Metab Clin North Am 2004; 33(4):717–39.

43. McIntyre RS, Konarski JZ, Grigoriadis S, et al. Hormone replacement therapy and antidepressant prescription patterns: a reciprocal relationship. CMAJ 2005; 172(1):57–9.

44. Joffe H, Soares CN, Petrillo LF, et al. Treatment of depression and menopause-related symptoms with the serotonin-norepinephrine reuptake inhibitor duloxetine. J Clin Psychiatry 2007;68(6):943–50.

45. Soares CN, Poitras JR, Prouty J, et al. Efficacy of citalopram as a monotherapy or as an adjunctive treatment to estrogen therapy for perimenopausal and postmenopausal women with depression and vasomotor symptoms. J Clin Psychiatry 2003;64(4):473–9.

46. Evans ML, Pritts E, Vittinghoff E, et al. Management of postmenopausal hot flushes with venlafaxine hydrochloride: a randomized, controlled trial. Obstet Gynecol 2005;105(1):161–6.

47. Speroff L, Gass M, Constantine G, et al. Efficacy and tolerability of desvenlafaxine succinate treatment for menopausal vasomotor symptoms: a randomized controlled trial. Obstet Gynecol 2008;111(1):77–87.

48. Stearns V, Beebe KL, Iyengar M, et al. Paroxetine controlled release in the treatment of menopausal hot flashes: a randomized controlled trial. JAMA 2003; 289(21):2827–34.

49. Soares CN, Arsenio H, Joffe H, et al. Escitalopram versus ethinyl estradiol and norethindrone acetate for symptomatic peri- and postmenopausal women: impact on depression, vasomotor symptoms, sleep, and quality of life. Menopause 2006;13(5):780–6.

50. Joffe H, Groninger H, Soares CN, et al. An open trial of mirtazapine in menopausal women with depression unresponsive to estrogen replacement therapy. J Womens Health Gend Based Med 2001;10(10):999–1004.

51. Thase ME, Entsuah R, Cantillon M, et al. Relative antidepressant efficacy of venlafaxine and SSRIs: sex-age interactions. J Womens Health (Larchmt) 2005;14(7): 609–16.

52. Osmers R, Friede M, Liske E, et al. Efficacy and safety of isopropanolic black cohosh extract for climacteric symptoms. Obstet Gynecol 2005;105(5 Pt 1): 1074–83.
53. Wuttke W, Jarry H, Christoffel V, et al. Chaste tree (Vitex agnus-castus)–pharmacology and clinical indications. Phytomedicine 2003;10(4):348–57.
54. Nelson HD, Vesco KK, Haney E, et al. Nonhormonal therapies for menopausal hot flashes: systematic review and meta-analysis. JAMA 2006;295(17):2057–71.
55. Newton KM, Reed SD, LaCroix AZ, et al. Treatment of vasomotor symptoms of menopause with black cohosh, multibotanicals, soy, hormone therapy, or placebo: a randomized trial. Ann Intern Med 2006;145(12):869–79.
56. Uebelhack R, Blohmer JU, Graubaum HJ, et al. Black cohosh and St. John's wort for climacteric complaints: a randomized trial. Obstet Gynecol 2006;107(2 Pt 1): 247–55.
57. Grube B, Walper A, Wheatley D. St. John's Wort extract: efficacy for menopausal symptoms of psychological origin. Adv Ther 1999;16(4):177–86.
58. Boyle GJ, Murrihy R. A preliminary study of hormone replacement therapy and psychological mood states in perimenopausal women. Psychol Rep 2001; 88(1):160–70.
59. Gambacciani M, Ciaponi M, Cappagli B, et al. Effects of low-dose, continuous combined estradiol and noretisterone acetate on menopausal quality of life in early postmenopausal women. Maturitas 2003;44(2):157–63.
60. Haines CJ, Yim SF, Chung TK, et al. A prospective, randomized, placebo-controlled study of the dose effect of oral oestradiol on menopausal symptoms, psychological well being, and quality of life in postmenopausal Chinese women. Maturitas 2003;44(3):207–14.
61. Khoo SK, Coglan M, Battistutta D, et al. Hormonal treatment and psychological function during the menopausal transition: an evaluation of the effects of conjugated estrogens/cyclic medroxyprogesterone acetate. Climacteric 1998;1(1): 55–62.
62. Heikkinen J, Vaheri R, Timonen UA. 10-year follow-up of postmenopausal women on long-term continuous combined hormone replacement therapy: update of safety and quality-of-life findings. J Br Menopause Soc 2006; 12(3):115–25.
63. Gulseren L, Kalafat D, Mandaci H, et al. Effects of tibolone on the quality of life, anxiety-depression levels and cognitive functions in natural menopause: an observational follow-up study. Aust N Z J Obstet Gynaecol 2005;45(1):71–3.
64. Baksu A, Ayas B, Citak S, et al. Efficacy of tibolone and transdermal estrogen therapy on psychological symptoms in women following surgical menopause. Int J Gynaecol Obstet 2005;91(1):58–62.
65. Pansini F, Albertazzi P, Bonaccorsi G, et al. Trazodone: a non-hormonal alternative for neurovegetative climacteric symptoms. Clin Exp Obstet Gynecol 1995; 22(4):341–4.
66. Stearns V, Isaacs C, Rowland J, et al. A pilot trial assessing the efficacy of paroxetine hydrochloride (Paxil) in controlling hot flashes in breast cancer survivors. Ann Oncol 2000;11(1):17–22.
67. Ladd CO, Newport DJ, Ragan KA, et al. Venlafaxine in the treatment of depressive and vasomotor symptoms in women with perimenopausal depression. Depress Anxiety 2005;22(2):94–7.
68. Ushiroyama T, Ikeda A, Ueki M. Evaluation of double-blind comparison of fluvoxamine and paroxetine in the treatment of depressed outpatients in menopause transition. J Med 2004;35(1–6):151–62.

69. Volz HP, Murck H, Kasper S, et al. St John's wort extract (LI 160) in somatoform disorders: results of a placebo-controlled trial. Psychopharmacology (Berl) 2002; 164(3):294–300.
70. Cagnacci A, Arangino S, Renzi A, et al. Kava-Kava administration reduces anxiety in perimenopausal women. Maturitas 2003;44(2):103–9.
71. De Leo V, la Marca A, Morgante G, et al. Evaluation of combining kava extract with hormone replacement therapy in the treatment of postmenopausal anxiety. Maturitas 2001;39(2):185–8.
72. Geller SE, Studee L. Botanical and dietary supplements for mood and anxiety in menopausal women. Menopause 2007;14(3 Pt 1):541–9.
73. Tode T, Kikuchi Y, Hirata J, et al. Effect of Korean red ginseng on psychological functions in patients with severe climacteric syndromes. Int J Gynaecol Obstet 1999;67(3):169–74.
74. Hartley DE, Elsabagh S, File SE. Gincosan (a combination of Ginkgo biloba and Panax ginseng): the effects on mood and cognition of 6 and 12 weeks' treatment in post-menopausal women. Nutr Neurosci 2004;7(5–6):325–33.
75. Nappi RE, Malavasi B, Brundu B, et al. Efficacy of Cimicifuga racemosa on climacteric complaints: a randomized study versus low-dose transdermal estra-diol. Gynecol Endocrinol 2005;20(1):30–5.
76. Andreatini R, Sartori VA, Seabra ML, et al. Effect of valepotriates (valerian extract) in generalized anxiety disorder: a randomized placebo-controlled pilot study. Phytother Res 2002;16(7):650–4.
77. Casini ML, Marelli G, Papaleo E, et al. Psychological assessment of the effects of treatment with phytoestrogens on postmenopausal women: a randomized, double-blind, crossover, placebo-controlled study. Fertil Steril 2006;85(4): 972–8.

Depressive Symptoms Related to Infertility and Infertility Treatments

Kirsten M. Wilkins, MD[a],*, Julia K. Warnock, MD, PhD[a],
Elka Serrano, MD[b]

KEYWORDS

- Depression • Infertility • Mood disorders
- Assisted reproductive technology • In vitro fertilization

By definition, infertility is unprotected heterosexual intercourse for a duration of 1 year without conception.[1] Although rates of infertility in the United States have remained stable at about 10% to 14%, this number will likely increase as the average age of first-time mothers also increases. In 1975, less than 20% of women attempted their first pregnancy between the ages of 35 and 39 years. In 1995, this number increased to 44%.[1] To date, 9.3 million American women are using or have sought some form of infertility treatment.[2] With rapid advancement in assisted reproductive technology (ART), more couples have access to effective forms of infertility treatment. However, the financial cost of these treatments can be astonishingly high. Some couples pay up to $12,400 for 1 cycle of in vitro fertilization (IVF), and insurance companies rarely cover the cost of such services. In addition to the financial burden of infertility and the associated treatment, there is also an associated emotional cost. The evaluation and treatment of infertility is considered by many women to be the most upsetting experience of their lives.[3] Although the prognosis for an infertile couple is arguably less bleak than in years past as a result of recent technological advances, it is still not uncommon for women with infertility to experience a wide range of emotions including grief, anger, anxiety, and denial. Infertility has also been shown to affect self-esteem, sexual function, and marital relationships.[4] A literature search reveals many articles that provide data on the prevalence of depression among couples with infertility. However, the data are equivocal and likely confounded by the presence of preexisting psychiatric disorders and treatment-related variables. This article reviews the common causes

Disclosures: Dr Wilkins has no financial relationships to disclose. Dr Warnock has no financial relationships to disclose. Dr Serrano has no financial relationships to disclose.
[a] Department of Psychiatry, The University of Oklahoma College of Medicine-Tulsa, 4502 East 41st Street, Tulsa, OK 74135, USA
[b] Family and Children's Services, 2325 South Harvard Avenue Suite 400, Tulsa, OK 74114, USA
* Corresponding author.
E-mail address: Kirsten-Wilkins@ouhsc.edu

of infertility. The second part of the article presents the literature on depressive symptoms in women as they relate to infertility. Depressive symptoms in infertile women before infertility treatment are reviewed, and this is followed by a discussion of depressive symptoms in women undergoing infertility treatments. Recommendations are made from a psychiatric perspective of how to manage depressive symptoms in the context of infertility in women.

COMMON CAUSES OF INFERTILITY

As with the advances in treatment-related technology, significant progress has been made in elucidating the causes of infertility. As recently as the 1950s, approximately 50% of infertility cases were of unknown cause or were attributed to psychosomatic causes.[2] Currently, investigators are able to identify a cause for infertility in 90% of cases. Of these identifiable causes, 50% are related to female reproductive factors and 35% are related to male reproductive factors, with the remainder caused by both partners. Most sources recommend a medical work-up for infertility after 1 year of unsuccessful attempts at conception. An evaluation should be pursued even earlier if the couple or 1 of the individuals has a previous history of infertility. The work-up for infertility usually includes a history and physical evaluation, documentation of ovulation, semen analysis, and a hysterosalpingogram. The more common causes of infertility are described in the following sections.

Causes Related to Anovulation

Polycystic ovarian syndrome (PCOS) affects more than 6% of women of reproductive age and is the most common cause of female infertility.[5] The primary characteristics of this syndrome are hyperandrogenism, ovulatory dysfunction, insulin resistance, and metabolic syndrome.[6] Although the specific pathophysiology of PCOS has yet to be determined, some potential factors contributing to its development include emotional, nutritional, and physical stress. Women with PCOS have an increased frequency of pulsatile gonadotropin-releasing hormone (GnRH), which leads to increases in luteinizing hormone (LH) synthesis and impaired follicle maturation. Tan and colleagues[5] found that although individuals with this condition have higher rates of depression and lower levels of life satisfaction than control subjects, distress related specifically to involuntary childlessness was not high. The treatment of PCOS involves conservative measures such as weight loss; more aggressive therapy involves the use of medications such as metformin, clomiphene, or oral contraceptives. Recent studies have also examined the efficacy of recombinant follicle-stimulating hormone (FSH) for ovulation induction in patients with PCOS.[7]

Hypothalamic amenorrhea is related to 5% of cases of anovulation and is similar to PCOS in that it is caused by severe emotional stress and nutritional stress. In contrast to PCOS, women with hypothalamic amenorrhea have a low frequency of pulsatile GnRH secretion, which impairs the stimulation of follicles. Hypothalamic amenorrhea has been linked to major depressive disorder (MDD), and there is evidence to suggest that a direct correlation exists between elevated stress hormones and reproductive dysfunction. Smeenk and colleagues[8] studied levels of adrenaline, noradrenaline, and cortisol metabolites in infertile women undergoing in vitro fertilization. They reported that women with lower levels of depression as indicated on rating instruments had lower levels of urinary adrenaline and that rates of successful IVF were greater in this group compared with women with higher levels of urinary adrenaline. This study further supports the connection between the hypothalamic-pituitary-adrenal-axis and fertility.

Hyperprolactinemia is another cause of infertility and accounts for 5% of the cases of female anovulation.[9] Whether related to tumor secretion or medication-related effects of dopamine antagonists, elevated prolactin suppresses ovulation and can be treated with dopamine agonists. A less frequent cause of anovulation in women is premature ovarian failure, which may occur as a result of the development of anti-ovarian antibodies or as a result of cancer treatments such as chemotherapy or radiation.[9]

Anatomical Abnormalities

Anatomical anomalies range from hereditary uterine dysmorphology to fallopian tube damage related to a history of pelvic inflammatory disease. Fibroids are a more common cause of infertility in women in the third and fourth decades of life. Most of these conditions can be successfully treated with surgical procedures and/or IVF. Endometriosis is another common cause of infertility. This condition is discovered in 21% to 48% of women undergoing laparoscopy for infertility.[1] Endometriosis can be treated medically or surgically.

Male Factors Associated with Infertility

Some of the more common causes of infertility in men include impaired shape and movement of sperm, low sperm count, and low testosterone levels inhibiting sexual functioning. Male fertility can also be affected abnormal anatomy such as varicocele, undescended testes, or a blockage of the epididymis. Treatment of these various conditions may include interventions ranging from lifestyle modification to surgery. Some of the lifestyle modifications recommended include smoking cessation, abstaining from alcohol and drug use, engaging in regular sexual activity with a partner, vitamin supplementation, and stress management. From the treatment perspective, IVF with intracytoplasmic sperm injection (ICSI) has provided a highly effective means of treating most male infertility problems. Men with infertility have been reported to have high levels of depression but seldom identify themselves as depressed or seek treatment for depression.[10]

DEPRESSIVE MOOD SYMPTOMS IN INFERTILE WOMEN BEFORE INFERTILITY TREATMENT

Women with a history of depression are more than twice as likely as nondepressed women to experience infertility.[11] Numerous studies have suggested a strong correlation between depression and infertility. As early as 1950, Selye[12] observed ovarian atrophy in a study of rats exposed to stress. Although a single causal link between depression and infertility has yet to be identified, there are several studies that correlate stress hormones and their effect on sex hormones and ultimately fertility. One study by Arcuri and colleagues[13] identified an association between the activity of 11β-hydroxysteroid dehydrogenase, the ovarian enzyme that catalyzes cortisol, and fertility. Schenker and colleagues[14] proposed that stress hormones interfere with gamete transport through the fallopian tubes by interacting directly with receptors in the fallopian tubes, diminishing blood flow to these structures.

Considering this evidence, a relationship is suggested between depressive mood symptoms, associated stress factors, and the onset of infertility. However, the likelihood of infertility causing clinically significant depressive mood symptoms is less clear and is confounded by numerous variables. Some of these variables include, but are not limited to, a history of preexisting mood disorder, the stage of treatment, and the coping skills and attitudes of the individual. Most research to this point has yielded equivocal results on whether there is a generalized increased rate of new-onset depression in women diagnosed with infertility. A study by Domar and colleagues[15] found that infertile women were twice as likely to experience depressive symptoms as the control group. They reported higher depression scores in women with an identified causative factor for their infertility, compared with those with unexplained or undiagnosed infertility. Higher depression scores were also noted among women with a 2- to 3-year history of infertility, compared with women with infertility lasting less than 1 year or more than 6 years.

Guerra and colleagues[16] studied the prevalence of psychiatric morbidity in patients attending a fertility clinic who were referred to a psychosomatic medicine specialist. They reported that 69% of women in this group had a psychiatric disorder, with adjustment disorders and anxiety being most common. Demyttenaere and colleagues[17] found that at the onset of IVF, 19.4% of infertile women had moderate to severe depressive symptoms and 54% were mildly depressed. Downey and colleagues[18] reported that among infertile women, there was no difference in psychiatric symptoms or in the percentage of patients with current or past MDD. However, most women did endorse mood changes (74.6%) and change in sense of self-worth (49.2%).

Meller and colleagues[19] gave the Structured Clinical Interview for the DSM-III-R (SCID)[20] and the Beck Depression Inventory (BDI)[21] to 19 women with unexplained infertility and 20 community controls. There were significantly more women with current or past history of depression in the infertile group compared with the control group; most of these women experienced their first episode of depression before they received the diagnosis of infertility. Chen and colleagues[22] gave women presenting for infertility treatment the Mini-International Neuropsychiatric Interview.[23] They reported that 40.2% of women had a psychiatric illness, including generalized anxiety disorder (23.2%), MDD (17%), and dysthymia (9.8%). Other investigators have reported the rate of depression among infertile women to be comparable with rates of depression in individuals with chronic medical illness.[24]

A small study by Brasile and colleagues[25] reported that only a minority of infertile women presenting for infertility treatment had depressive symptoms as measured by the BDI, and which were of mild severity only. However, these investigators acknowledged that only 5% of new patients voluntarily participated in the study and that women with moderate to severe depression may have declined to participate. Paulson and colleagues[26] concluded that, based on psychometric tests, infertile women had no higher prevalence of significant emotional maladjustment compared with women without infertility. Similarly, Hearn and colleagues[27] reported that, based on measures of personality, coping skills, emotional status, family environment, and quality of life, couples undergoing IVF reported good quality of life without depression and anxiety.

Although the prevalence of clinically relevant mood disorders in infertile women before infertility treatment remains debatable, the diagnosis of infertility undoubtedly poses a considerable stressor. Psychosocial factors associated with infertility can play a significant role in the development of mood symptoms following such a diagnosis. Although women may not develop clinical depression, multiple studies indicate that a significant number of women experience a grief reaction to the loss of the hope of parenthood. Some women compare the severity of this grief with that of the loss of a loved one or divorce.[15] Men may experience this grief as well, but women describe greater global distress related to social issues, sexual concerns, and need for parenthood.[28] However, as the technology in the treatment of infertility has improved in the past decade, resulting in significant increases in pregnancy rates, perhaps patients' stress levels have diminished as they contemplate their diagnosis and embark on their treatment.

DEPRESSIVE MOOD SYMPTOMS AND INFERTILITY TREATMENTS

There are now more than 40 ways to conceive a child without having intercourse.[2] Technology has allowed many couples to realize their dream of having a child, when just a few years ago, it would have been impossible. Despite the advantages that these treatments provide to infertile couples, they also come at a cost. Many of these treatments have direct and common psychiatric side effects that may manifest as depression, anxiety, irritability, and even psychosis. Some affect individuals more indirectly by the nature of their invasiveness and associated physical discomfort. Of course, there is also the disappointment experienced when treatment fails. Some of the more common forms of infertility treatments and their associated psychiatric side effects are presented in the following sections.

Oral Contraceptives

Contrary to logic, oral contraceptive medications can aide in treating infertility. These medications are commonly used in conjunction with IVF to down-regulate the hypothalamus and prevent premature ovulation.[2] Oral contraceptives that contain predominantly higher concentrations of progesterone have been associated with side effects such as increased rates of depression (5%–50%).[29] Warnock and Blake[30] reviewed psychiatric aspects of hormonal contraception, noting that some of the earlier associations between oral contraceptive pills (OCPs) and depression have been challenged given the multiple limitations of clinical trials involving these medications. They did note that a minority of women may suffer mood disturbance from OCPs (possibly triggered by fluctuations in hormone levels) and that, for women with a mood diathesis, monophasic pills are suggested.

GnRH Agonists

GnRH agonists are prescribed in conjunction with IVF and are also used to prevent a premature LH surge. GnRH agonists such as leuprolide acetate have a strong association with increased rates of depressive symptoms. Warnock and colleagues[31,32] found that 80% of women taking leuprolide experienced significant depressive symptoms using a cutoff score of 20 on the 21-item Hamilton Depression Rating Scale.[33] In addition, sertraline was found to be significantly helpful in the treatment of depressive mood symptoms during the course of GnRH agonist therapy.[31] Steingold and colleagues[34] found that 75% of patients using GnRH agonist medication suffered depressive symptoms. In another study by Eyal and colleagues,[35] it was reported that ovarian suppression with a GnRH agonist was associated with elevated scores on the Hamilton Rating Scales for depression and anxiety. They also identified a down-regulatory effect of GnRH agonists on the platelet serotonin transporter, which may provide a biochemical explanation for the clinical effects of this class of medications.

An interesting study by de Clerk and colleagues[36] compared the effects of treating women with a standard GnRH agonist long-protocol ovarian stimulation and double-embryo transfer versus a milder ovarian stimulation including GnRH antagonist cotreatment and single-embryo transfer. The standard protocol included 2 weeks of GnRH agonist administration beginning in the midluteal phase of the preceding cycle, followed by ovarian stimulation with recombinant FSH, oocyte retrieval, IVF, and eventual transfer of a maximum of 2 embryos. The milder protocol included no GnRH agonist administration and began with ovarian stimulation with recombinant FSH on day 5 of the current cycle, followed by use of a GnRH antagonist to commence ovarian stimulation once a follicle greater than or equal to 14 mm was observed. This was followed by oocyte retrieval, IVF, and eventual transfer of just 1 embryo. It was found that the milder form of treatment caused the patient less stress and fewer short-term symptoms of depression, even if the treatment failed to achieve conception.

Clomiphene Citrate

Clomiphene is the most commonly used medication to treat infertility because of its cost effectiveness and safety profile.[37] This medication is commonly used to treat infertility associated with PCOS. Clomiphene is a competitive estrogen receptor antagonist that interferes with estrogen negative feedback and ultimately drives follicular development. Psychiatric symptoms associated with clomiphene include anxiety, sleep disturbances, irritability, mood lability, and symptoms similar to premenstrual syndrome.[38]

Dopamine Agonists

Dopamine agonists, such as bromocriptine and cabergoline, can be used to treat infertility associated with hyperprolactinemia. Because these medications act directly on the dopamine receptors, they may have psychiatric side effects. Individuals taking dopamine agonists may experience psychiatric symptoms such as depression, somnolence or insomnia, delirium, and even psychosis.[39]

ART

ART is a broad term encompassing numerous forms of in vitro fertilization (IVF). Psychiatric symptoms in patients undergoing these procedures have been studied extensively. The results of these studies are typically divided into phases of treatment: before IVF, during IVF, and after IVF. Beutel and colleagues[40] reported that women undergoing IVF or ICSI were significantly more depressed than age-matched female controls. A study by Volgsten and colleagues[41] involving 862 male and female subjects undergoing IVF revealed that although mood disorders in infertile women are common, undiagnosed, and untreated, the prevalence rates are similar to those in gynecological outpatients.

Lok and colleagues[42] administered the BDI to women before and after ART. They reported that 8% of women had BDI scores greater than 20, indicating moderate-severe depression before treatment and after failed treatment. They noted that depression severity was associated with longer duration of infertility. Another study found that BDI scores increased after unsuccessful infertility treatment and decreased after successful infertility treatment.[43]

Some studies have examined the emotional response of individuals who have failed to conceive with IVF. A cross-sectional analysis by Berg and Wilson[44] investigated the psychological functioning of couples undergoing fertility treatment after 1, 2 and 3 years. This study did not identify the specific form of fertility treatment, but interesting trends in emotional responses were noted. Emotional strain was evident during the first year of treatment, but then remitted during the second year. The emotional strain then returned and markedly increased in year 3. This study also noted that marital adjustment and sexual satisfaction were stable during years 1 and 2 but then deteriorated in the third year.

A systematic review by Verhaak and colleagues[45] in 2007 examined the literature for trends in women's responses to IVF before, during, and after treatment. Based on the findings, these investigators concluded that most women adjust well to multiple cycles of IVF. Before treatment, women did not exhibit significantly increased levels of state-dependent anxiety or depression, which may be explained by the chronic nature of the stress of infertility and by the hope engendered by actively engaging in a solution to their problem. This review also identified that when IVF resulted in pregnancy, negative emotions abated, which emphasizes that the treatment-induced stress is strongly associated with threats of failure. In an earlier article, Verhaak and colleagues[46] identified several risk factors for the development of depression and anxiety following failed fertility treatment; these risk factors included neuroticism, feelings of helplessness, and marital dissatisfaction. Based on these articles, attention to the psychosocial implications of infertility and childlessness can be as important as the biological factors affecting depression/anxiety in infertile couples.

The effect of depression and stress on the outcome of IVF has been examined in several studies. However, the literature is inconclusive. Lintsen and colleagues[47] highlighted the contradictory data on this issue in their recent article on the effect of anxiety and depression on cancellation (defined by the authors as having started ovarian stimulation without reaching oocyte retrieval) and pregnancy rates of a first IVF or ICSI. They reported that neither baseline nor procedural anxiety nor depression affected cancellation or pregnancy rates. The authors acknowledged that women with higher levels of distress may have declined to participate in the study.

TREATMENT OF DEPRESSIVE SYMPTOMS ASSOCIATED WITH INFERTILITY
Assessment and Treatment of Depressive Symptoms Before Infertility Treatment

A 2007 review of the literature on mood disorders and fertility reported that most studies found increased rates of depressive symptoms in infertile women presenting for treatment and that many studies, although not all, found that depressive symptoms may decrease the success rate of infertility treatment.[48] In a review on psychiatric aspects of infertility, Burns[2] reported that women with a history of depression were twice as likely to experience a recurrence of depression during treatment of infertility. In light of these findings, it is reasonable to suggest that at the outset of an infertility evaluation, before treatment begins, the patient's past medical and psychiatric history should be reviewed, with attention paid to any past or present symptoms of a mood disorder. Some patients may be reluctant to spontaneously disclose psychiatric histories for fear of being refused infertility treatment. Patients should be asked directly about mood and anxiety symptoms so that any current identifiable psychiatric disorders can be assessed. Any current identifiable psychiatric syndromes, such as mood and anxiety disorders, should be further evaluated and treated. Patients should be encouraged to adopt a healthy lifestyle, including avoidance of alcohol, illicit drugs, or tobacco.

Researchers have found that certain personality types, coping styles, and cognitive beliefs may affect adjustment to the diagnosis of infertility. Concerning personality characteristics, lower levels of neuroticism and higher levels of extroversion and optimism seem to predict a more positive emotional adjustment.[49] Avoidant coping styles seem to be correlated with a more negative emotional response, whereas active coping seems to aid in acceptance. Cognitions of helplessness are associated with a greater amount of distress in individuals with infertility, whereas greater perceived control over a stressor is associated with better adjustment.[50] In an article on the topic of stress and fertility, Campagne[51] suggests that treatment of infertility should include very early measurement of stress. Assessment instruments that may be useful include the Holmes and Rahe Stress Scale[52] or the FertiQol.[53] The FertiQol is the first internationally validated instrument that surveys infertile patients to assess their quality of life. It measures major domains and dimensions of life and has been translated into 10 languages. For those individuals with high levels of stress, stress reduction techniques (cognitive-behavioral therapy, relaxation techniques, fertility sabbatical, and so forth) before beginning infertility treatment are suggested.

Treatment of Depressive Symptoms During Infertility Treatment

Patients, in particular those with a history of depression, should be monitored for any depressive symptoms that may occur following the diagnosis of infertility, as a result of the direct effects of the treatments themselves, or as a result of the ensuing stress and marital conflict. If depressive symptoms are clinically significant and cause distress, psychiatric referral may be indicated to help determine if a patient's symptoms represent an adjustment disorder with depressed mood, substance-induced mood disorder, or a major depressive episode. Numerous treatment options are available for individuals experiencing grief, depression, and/or anxiety related to infertility and its treatment.

When deciding on treatment, it is important to take into consideration that the individual may be pregnant or soon become pregnant. Therapies that pose no potential risk to the fetus should be used first in this population of patients. Psychotherapy is an excellent, first-line treatment with a high rate of efficacy in the treatment of mild to moderate depression with no risk to the fetus. Some studies have suggested that psychological interventions for depression and psychological distress not only reduce depressive symptoms and distress but also increase the likelihood of successful conception.[54,55] Cognitive-behavioral therapy (CBT) and interpersonal therapy are short-term treatments that have been studied in patients with infertility.[2] Pook and colleagues[56] recommend short-term goals for therapy such as reducing the feelings of helplessness, changing sexual behavior, modifying negative cognitions about infertility, acquiring knowledge about infertility, and improving marital communication skills. Infertility support groups (such as RESOLVE) and informational Web sites (such as http://www.sart.org and http://www.asrm.org) are available to couples undergoing treatment.

A few studies have looked at specific psychopharmacologic treatments of depressive symptoms associated with infertility and infertility treatments. Certainly any medication must be carefully considered in this patient population given the possibility of pregnancy. The selective serotonin reuptake inhibitors are theoretically attractive for use in this population given their tolerability, minimal drug-drug interactions, and apparent lack of teratogenicity. Warnock and colleagues[32] examined the efficacy of sertraline versus placebo for depressive symptoms associated with ovarian suppression during GnRH agonist therapy. A statistically significant difference was noted between the 2 groups, with the sertraline-treated group manifesting fewer depressive symptoms (as measured by the Hamilton Rating Scale for Depression) than the control group. Noorbala and colleagues[57] compared the effect of a combined psychological intervention given to depressed infertile couples before beginning infertility treatment versus during infertility treatment. They found that a 6-month intervention of CBT, supportive therapy, and 20 to 60 mg of fluoxetine before infertility treatment significantly reduced depressive symptoms as measured by the BDI, to a greater degree than those given psychiatric intervention during the infertility treatment. Faramarzi and colleagues[58] compared treatment with 10 sessions of CBT, fluoxetine 20 mg daily for 90 days, and placebo in women suffering from mild to moderate depression and infertility. Resolution of depression occurred in 79% of the CBT group, 50% of the fluoxetine group, and 10% of the placebo group. The investigators concluded that CBT was a reliable alternative to pharmacotherapy and superior to fluoxetine in the treatment of depression and anxiety in infertile women. What has yet to be examined is whether treatment of depression with medication before infertility treatments increases the chance of later conception.

Additional treatment considerations for depressed infertile women may include nonpsychotropic somatic treatments such as omega-3 fatty acids, given the available literature suggesting their effect on mood stabilization.[59] Similarly,

S-adenosylmethionine (SAM-e) has shown promise in reducing mood symptoms in patients with major depression.[60] Light therapy is another avenue to consider for the depressed infertile woman, given its reported benefit in patients with nonseasonal depression and its minimal risks (notably, hypomania).[61] Women with moderate to severe depression, with or without psychotic features, will require psychiatric monitoring, hopefully in concert with the reproductive endocrinologist. It would be premature at this time to recommend any standard psychiatric treatments for depression in women undergoing infertility interventions. Psychiatric assessments and recommendations must be individualized. However, there is enough evidence to suggest that depression is frequent enough in this population that additional research in these areas is needed.

Treatment of Depressive Symptoms Following Failure to Achieve Pregnancy

Failure to achieve a pregnancy following IVF leaves other options such as donor eggs, adopting an embryo, child-free living or adopting a child, among others. In situations where the female has medical issues that cannot be mediated, as in the case of extreme hypertension or uterine anomalies, gestational surrogacy is another option allowed in some states. In cases of oocyte donations, typically the donor and the patient undergo evaluation by a mental health professional. Unsuccessful treatment with IVF often results in a range of emotions including sadness, anger, and grief in many couples. Thus, they may be open to counseling and education on these remaining family planning options. Supportive counseling at this point may facilitate some couples to decide to accept childlessness and pursue other life goals. Although not necessary for all couples, individual therapy, marital therapy, and/or support groups may assist in the healing process and allow some couples to better use appropriate resources, should they continue to pursue alterative family planning options. Psychiatric referral may be indicated for an individual who manifests evidence of an MDD.

SUMMARY

Infertility is a problem that 1 in 10 women will face at some point in their lives. Although it is a common condition and technological advances in treatment have certainly improved the prognosis, individuals suffering from infertility can feel isolated, defective, and helpless. Although the nature of the relationship between depression and infertility has yet to be elucidated, few would argue that they affect each other. A causal link between infertility and clinically significant depression is likely to have direct and indirect aspects. Additional research in this area is indicated to further clarify this multifaceted relationship. Technological advances have allowed more and more couples to conceive successfully. However, infertility treatments themselves can bring about symptoms of depression, anxiety, and irritability. For this reason, it is imperative that we understand the potential risk of such treatments and the alternative treatments available so that patients and their providers may collaborate to choose the best treatment. The literature suggests that psychotherapy and psychopharmacologic treatments may be effective in the treatment of depression in infertile women. Future research should not only further explore effective treatment options for depression in infertile women but also examine the effect of treatment of depression on the outcome of infertility treatment.

ACKNOWLEDGMENTS

The authors would like to acknowledge the assistance of Faye Biggs in the preparation of the manuscript.

REFERENCES

1. Scott JR, Gibbs RS, Karlan BY, et al. Danforth's obstetrics and gynecology. 9th edition. Philadelphia: Lippincott, Williams, and Wilkins; 2003.
2. Burns LH. Psychiatric aspects of infertility and infertility treatments. Psychiatr Clin North Am 2007;30(4):689–716.
3. Freeman EW, Boxer AS, Rickels K, et al. Psychological evaluation and support in a program of in vitro fertilization and embryo transfer. Fertil Steril 1985;43(1):49–53.
4. Stanton AL, Dunker-Schetter L. Psychological reactions to infertility. In: Stanton AL, Dunker-Schetter L, editors. Infertility: perspectives from stress and coping research. New York: Plenum Press; 1991. p. 29–57.
5. Tan S, Hahn S, Benson OE, et al. Psychological implications of infertility in women with polycystic ovary syndrome. Humanit Rep 2008;23(9):2064–71.
6. Azziz R. PCOS: a diagnostic challenge. Reprod Biomed Online 2004;8:644–8.
7. Bayram N, van Wely M, Van der Veen F. Recombinant FSH versus urinary gonadotrophins or recombinant FSH for ovulation induction in subfertility associated with polycystic ovary syndrome. Cochrane Database Syst Rev 2001;(2):CD002121.
8. Smeenk JMJ, Verhaak CM, Vingerhoets CGJ, et al. Stress and outcome success in IVF: the role of self-reports and endocrine variables. Humanit Rep 2005;20(4): 991–6.
9. Managing anovulatory infertility. Drug Ther Bull 2004;42(4):28–32.
10. Natchigall RD, Quiroga SS, Tschann JM, et al. Stigma, disclosure, and family functioning among parents with children conceived through donor insemination. Fertil Steril 1997;68:1–7.
11. Lapane KL, Zierler S, Lasater TM, et al. Is a history of depressive symptoms associated with an increased risk of infertility in women? Psychosom Med 1995;57(6): 509–13.
12. Selye H. Stress. A treatise based on the concepts of the general-adaptation-syndrome and the disease of adaptation. Montreal (QC): Acta Inc; 1950.
13. Arcuri F, Moner C, Lockwood CJ, et al. Expression of 11b-hydroxysteroid dehydrogenase during decidualization of human endometrial stromal cells. Endocrinology 1996;137:595–600.
14. Schenker JG, Meirow D, Schenker E. Stress and human reproduction. Eur J Obstet Gynecol Reprod Biol 1992;45:1–8.
15. Domar AD, Broome A, Zuttermeister PC, et al. The prevalence and predictability of depression in infertile women. Fertil Steril 1992;58:1158–63.
16. Guerra D, Llobera A, Veiga A, et al. A prospective study of stress among women undergoing in vitro fertilization or gamete intrafallopian transfer. Fertil Steril 2001; 76:75–97.
17. Demyttenaere K, Bonte L, Gheldorf M, et al. Coping style and depression level influence outome in in vitro fertilization. Fertil Steril 1998;69:1026–33.
18. Downey J, Yingling S, McKinney M, et al. Mood disorders, psychiatric symptoms, and distress in women presenting for an infertility evaluation. Fertil Steril 1989; 52(3):425–32.
19. Meller W, Burns LH, Crow S, et al. Major depression in unexplained fertility. J Psychosom Obstet Gynaecol 2002;23:27–30.
20. Spitzer RL, Williams JB, Gibbon M, et al. Structured clinical interview for DSM-III-R (SCID-P). Biometrics Research Department. New York: New York State Psychiatric Institute; 1988. 722 West 168th Street, NY 10032.
21. Beck A, Steir R. Beck depression inventory manual. San Antonio (TX): The Psychological Corporation; 1987.

22. Chen TH, Chang SP, Tsai CF, et al. Prevalence of depressive and anxiety disorders in an assisted reproductive technique clinic. Humanit Rep 2004;19(10): 2313–8.
23. Sheehan DV, Lacrudiber Y, Sheehan KH, et al. The Mini-International Neuropsychiatric Interview (MINI): the development and validation of a structured diagnostic psychiatric interview for the DSM-IV and ICD-10. J Clin Psychiatry 1998; 59(Suppl 20):22–33.
24. Domar AD, Zuttermeister PC, Friedman R. The psychological impact of infertility: a comparison with patients with other medical conditions. J Psychosom Obstet Gynaecol 1993;14:45–52.
25. Brasile D, Katsoff B, Check JH. Moderate or severe depression is uncommon in women seeking infertility therapy according to the Beck Depression Inventory. Clin Exp Obstet Gynecol 2006;33(1):16–8.
26. Paulson JD, Haarman BS, Salerno RL, et al. An investigation of the relationship between emotional maladjustment and fertility. Fertil Steril 1988;49(2):258–62.
27. Hearn MT, Yuzpe AA, Brown SE, et al. Psychological characteristics of in vitro fertilization participants. Am J Obstet Gynecol 1987;156(2):269–74.
28. Newton CR, Sherrard W, Glavac I. The fertility problem inventory: measuring perceived infertility-related stress. Fertil Steril 1999;72(1):54–62.
29. Jensvold MF. Nonpregnant reproductive age women. Part II: exogenous sex steroid hormones and psychopharmacology. In: Jensvold MF, Halbreich U, Hamilton JA, editors. Psychopharmacology and women: sex, gender and hormones. Washington, DC: American Psychiatric Press; 1996. p. 171–90.
30. Warnock JK, Blake CF. Psychiatric aspects of hormonal contraception. Dir Psychiatry 2002;22:233–41.
31. Warnock JK, Bundren JC, Morris DW. Sertraline in the treatment of depression associated with gonadotropin-releasing hormone agonist therapy. Biol Psychiatry 1998;43:464–5.
32. Warnock JK, Bundren JC, Morris DW. Depressive mood symptoms associated with ovarian suppression. Fertil Steril 2000;74(5):984–6.
33. Hamilton M. A rating scale for depression. J Neurol Neurosurg Psychiatr 1960;23: 56–62.
34. Steingold KA, Cedars M, Lu JK, et al. Treatment of endometriosis with a long-acting gonadotropin-releasing hormone agonist. Obstet Gynecol 1987;69(3 pt 1):403–11.
35. Eyal S, Weizman A, Toren P, et al. Chronic GnRH agonist administration down-regulates platelet serotonin transporter in women undergoing assisted reproductive treatment. Psychopharmacology 1996;125:141–5.
36. De Clerk C, Macklon NS, Heijnen EM, et al. The psychological impact of IVF failure after two or more cycles of IVF with a mild versus standard treatment strategy. Humanit Rep 2007;22(9):2554–8.
37. Fauser BCJM, Macklon NS. Medical approaches to ovarian stimulation for infertility. In: Strauss JF, Barbieri RL, editors. Yen and Jaffe's reproductive endocrinology. 5th edition. Philadelphia, PA: Elsevier Saunders; 2004. p. 965–1012.
38. Blenner J. Clomiphene-induced mood swings. J Obstet Gynecol Neonatal Nurs 1991;20:321–7.
39. Bromocriptine Mesylate DrugPoint Summary. Micromedex Healthcare Series [intranet database]. Version 5.1. Greenwood Village, Colo: Thomson Reuters (Healthcare) Inc. Accessed September 13, 2009.
40. Beutel M, Kupfer J, Kirchmeyer P, et al. Treatment-related stresses and depression in couples undergoing assisted reproductive treatment by IVF or ICSI. Andrologia 1999;31(1):27–35.

41. Volgsten H, Svanberg A, Ekselius O, et al. Prevalence of psychiatric disorders in infertile women and men undergoing in vitro fertilization treatment. Humanit Rep 2008;23(9):2056–63.
42. Lok IH, Lee DT, Cheung LP, et al. Psychiatric morbidity amongst infertile Chinese women undergoing treatment with assisted reproductive technology and the impact of treatment failure. Gynecol Obstet Invest 2002;53(4):195–9.
43. Khamedi A, Alleyssin A, Aghahosseini M, et al. Pretreatment Beck Depression Inventory score is an important predictor for post-treatment score in infertile patients. BMC Psychiatry 2005;5(1):25.
44. Berg B, Wilson J. Psychological functioning across stages of treatment for infertility. J Behav Med 1991;14(1):11–26.
45. Verhaak CM, Smeenk JMJ, Evers AWM, et al. Women's emotional adjustment to IVF: a systematic review of 25 years of research. Hum Reprod Update 2007; 13(1):27–36.
46. Verhaak C, Smeenk J, Evers A, et al. Predicting emotional response to unsuccessful fertility treatment: a prospective study. J Behav Med 2005;28(2): 181–90.
47. Lintsen AME, Verhaak CM, Eijkemans MJC, et al. Anxiety and depression have no influence on the cancellation and pregnancy rates of a first IVF or ICSI treatment. Humanit Rep 2009;24(5):1092–8.
48. Williams KE, Marsh WK, Rasgon NL. Mood disorders and fertility in women: a critical review of the literature and implications for future research. Hum Reprod Update 2007;13(6):607–16.
49. Carver CS, Pozo CP, Harris SD, et al. How coping mediates the effect of optimism on distress: a study of women with early stage breast cancer. J Pers Soc Psychol 1993;65:375–90.
50. Miller-Campbell S, Dunkel-Schetter C, Peplau LA. Perceived control and adjustment to infertility among women undergoing in vitro fertilization. In: Stanton AL, Dunkel-Schetter C, editors. Infertility: perspectives from stress and coping research. New York: Plenum; 1991. p. 133–56.
51. Campagne DM. Should fertilization treatment start with reducing stress? Humanit Rep 2006;21(7):1651–8.
52. Holmes TH, Rahe RH. The social readjustment rating scale. J Psychosom Res 1967;11(2):213–8.
53. European Society of Human Reproduction and Embryology. American Society of Reproductive Medicine (ASRM), and Merck-Serono International. Fertiqol Website. Available at: http://www.fertiqol.org. Accessed September 27, 2009.
54. Domar AD, Seibel MM, Benson H. The mind/body program for infertility: a new behavioral treatment approach for women with infertility. Fertil Steril 1990;53(2): 246–9.
55. Domar AD, Clapp D, Slawsby EA, et al. Impact of group psychological interventions on pregnancy rates in infertile women. Fertil Steril 2000;73(4):805–11.
56. Pook M, Kraus W, Rohrle B. Coping with infertility: distress and changes in sperm quality. Humanit Rep 1999;14:1487–92.
57. Noorbala AA, Ramazanzadeh F, Malekafzali H, et al. Effects of a psychological intervention on depression in infertile couples. Int J Gynaecol Obstet 2008;101: 248–52.
58. Faramarzi M, Alipor A, Esmaelzadeh S, et al. Treatment of depression and anxiety in infertile women: cognitive behavioral therapy versus fluoxetine. J Affect Disord 2008;108(1–2):159–64.

59. Ross BM, Seguin J, Sieswerda LE. Omega-3 fatty acids as treatments for mental illness: which disorder and which fatty acid? Lipids Health Dis 2007;6:21.
60. Williams AL, Girard C, Jui D, et al. S-Adenosylmethionine (SAMe) as treatment for depression: a systematic review. Clin Invest Med 2005;28(3):132–9.
61. Tuunainen A, Kripke DF, Endo T. Light therapy for non-seasonal depression. Cochrane Database Syst Rev 2004;(2):CD004050.

Female Sexual Dysfunction

Anita H. Clayton, MD[a],*, David V. Hamilton, MD, MA[b]

KEYWORDS

- Female sexual dysfunction • Sexual disorders
- Hypoactive sexual desire disorder
- Female sexual arousal disorder

The past 20 years has seen an explosion of research into female sexuality. Although rigorous epidemiologic study of female sexuality essentially began with publication of *Sexual Behavior of the Human Female*[1] in 1953, the specific study of postmenopausal sexuality did not begin in earnest until the 1990s. With the research, practitioners have come to understand that healthy, even satisfying, sexual function may extend throughout the life cycle.

SEXUAL RESPONSE CYCLE

Three models of the female sexual response cycle have been postulated: Masters and Johnson described stimulation leading to excitement, plateau, orgasm, and resolution, Kaplan articulated sexual desire, arousal, and orgasm as a pattern, and Basson suggested some women may participate in sexual activity for reasons other than desire, for example, motivated by a wish for emotional intimacy. In a study by Sand and Fisher, equal numbers of women endorsed each model, suggesting that the female sexual response is heterogenous,[2] with sexual dysfunction as measured by the Female Sexual Function Index (FSFI) more likely to occur in those identifying with the Basson model.

FEMALE SEXUAL PHYSIOLOGY

Regulation of the hormonal cycle involves complex interplay along the HPG axis: the hypothalamus, the anterior pituitary gland, and the ovaries. The hypothalamus releases gonadotropin-releasing hormone (GnRH), which induces the release of

An advance version of this article was published in *Obstetric and Gynecology Clinics of North America* 2009;36(4):861–76.

[a] Department of Psychiatry and Neurobehavioral Sciences, University of Virginia, PO Box 801210, Charlottesville, VA 22908-1210, USA

[b] Department of Psychiatry and Neurobehavioral Sciences, Institute for Law, Psychiatry, and Public Policy, University of Virginia, Charlottesville, VA, USA

* Corresponding author.

E-mail address: ahc8v@virginia.edu

luteinizing hormone (LH) and follicle-stimulating hormone (FSH) from the anterior pituitary gland. LH stimulates ovarian theca cells to produce testosterone, some of which is converted to estrogen by the granulosa cells before release into circulation. FSH acts on granulosa cells in the ovary, producing estrogens and inhibin. As a regulating feedback mechanism, estrogen inhibits release of LH in the anterior pituitary, while inhibin decreases release of FSH (also at the anterior pituitary), keeping the system in balance.

Several factors complicate the detection of sexual dysfunction due to androgen insufficiency. Only bioavailable testosterone traverses the blood-brain barrier to exert an influence on the brain structures involved in sexual function (eg, hypothalamus, pituitary, amygdala). The majority of circulating testosterone is bound to the protein, sex hormone-binding globulin (SHBG). This chemical complex, too large to cross the blood-brain barrier, does not influence the central nervous system directly. Little is known about androgen effects in women relative to men. Assays used in determining the amount of both free and bound testosterone have relative ranges defined by androgen levels measured in men.[3]

Several neurotransmitters influence sexual function, evidenced by the number of centrally active medications that produce sexual side effects. Dopamine seems to mediate sexual desire and the subjective sense of arousal, as well as the drive to continue sexual activity once it begins.[4] In both the brain and the genitalia,[5] norepinephrine is the principal neurotransmitter regulating sexual arousal, which depends on central nervous system arousal via norepinephrine increases in excitation in the ventromedial hypothalamus.[6] Increased serotonergic transmission modulates dopamine and norepinephrine, diminishing the excitatory effects of both.[7] Serotonin seems to affect sexual arousal in peripheral tissues, by way of effects on vascular tone and blood flow. Serotonin may mediate uterine contractions during orgasm, may also interfere with arousal via negative effects on sensation and inhibition of the synthesis of nitric oxide (NO).[8] Finally, serotonin inhibits orgasm in some people by stimulation of 5-HT2 receptors, evidenced by selective serotonin reuptake inhibitor (SSRI)-induced anorgasmia and other problems with orgasm.[9]

Once sexual stimulation begins, the vasocongestion of clitoral tissue during arousal is positively mediated by NO[10] and vasoactive intestinal peptide (VIP).[11] Sufficient levels of free testosterone[12] are also required for NO to initiate vasocongestion with sexual stimulation. Acetylcholinergic nerve fibers innervate vascular smooth muscle in the vagina, allowing for vaginal engorgement during arousal, and subsequent lubrication.[13]

Multiple neurotransmitters must act in concert for adequate sexual functioning to occur. Drugs affecting sex steroids, such as estrogen and prolactin, or neurotransmitter function (eg, norepinephrine, serotonin, NO) also run the risk of impairing the ability to orgasm.[14,15] The most common medical conditions affecting these neurotransmitters include neurologic disorders, endocrine dysfunction, cardiovascular disease, and pelvic conditions. Depression, anxiety disorders, and eating disorders are also associated with sexual dysfunction. Medications that contribute to sexual dysfunction include histamine receptor (H2) blockers, narcotics, NSAIDs, oral contraceptives, thiazide diuretics, non-selective beta antagonists, and psychotropics such as antidepressants, antipsychotics, and benzodiazepines.[16] Studies have found that the SSRI antidepressants (ie, citalopram, escitalopram, fluvoxamine, fluoxetine, paroxetine, and sertraline), along with the serotonin-norepinephrine reuptake inhibiting (SNRI) antidepressant venlafaxine, confer the greatest risk of sexual dysfunction. Antidepressants that do not exploit serotonin reuptake as their primary therapeutic action, including bupropion, mirtazapine, and transdermal selegiline, do not significantly inhibit sexual function.[17,18] A special case appears to be the SNRI duloxetine, which has been demonstrated to have effects on sexual function intermediate to SSRIs and placebo (**Figs. 1** and **2**).[19]

DYSFUNCTIONS AND DISORDER

To properly detect and diagnose the presence of sexual disorders, it is critical to discern the distinction between *dysfunction* and *disorder*. Dysfunction describes the presence of medically relevant symptoms or signs of sexual function that is in some way not consistent with the medical understanding of healthy sexual functioning. However, the diagnosis of female sexual dysfunction (FSD) requires not only the presence of clinically significant sexual dysfunction but also that this dysfunction causes *distress* in the woman experiencing it. In brief, a diagnosis of FSD is not indicated if a putative symptom or sign of sexual dysfunction is not associated with distress. This necessity for distress in making the diagnosis of a sexual disorder is part of the *Diagnostic and Statistical Manual of Mental Disorders* (Fourth Edition, Text Revised) (DSM-IV-TR) diagnostic criteria for each FSD, typically delineated as criterion B.[20]

EPIDEMIOLOGY

Unfortunately, discussions regarding sexual functioning have not been a routine part of health care. Nusbaum and colleagues[21] found that only 14% to 17% of women reported that their doctor had brought up the subject of sexual function, and that most women had never spoken with their doctor about sex. If the topic had been raised, the patient was nearly twice as likely as the physician to have initiated the discussion, regardless of age group. The majority of women in each age category believed that their physician would not be receptive to discussing their sexual concerns, either because they felt their doctor simply lacked interest or they would be too embarrassed.

Few studies in the United States have specifically addressed the incidence and prevalence of sexual dysfunction among women. In one of the few studies to address

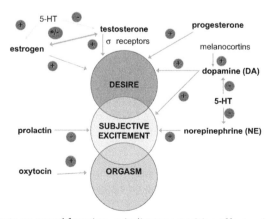

Fig. 1. Central effects on sexual function. + indicates a positive effect; − indicates a negative effect. (*Modified from* Clayton AH. Sexual function and dysfunction in women. Psychiatr Clin North Am 2003;26:673–82; with *Data from* Cohen AJ. Antidepressant-induced sexual dysfunction associated with low serum free testosterone. Mental Health Today 2000. http://www.mental-health-today.com/rx/testos.htm; with permission.)

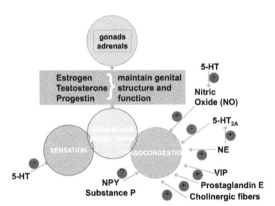

Fig. 2. Peripheral effects on sexual function. + indicates a positive effect; − indicates a negative effect. (*Modified from* Clayton AH. Sexual function and dysfunction in women. Psychiatr Clin North Am 2003;26:673–82; with permission.)

the issue, Bancroft and colleagues[22] found that among Caucasian and African American women between 20 and 65 years old who were asked about their degree of
distress associated with sexual problems, 24% of women reported distress about
their sexual relationship, their own sexuality, or both. Although this study provided
valuable preliminary results, it did not address whether menopausal status was associated with changes in sexual function.

A recent meta-analysis of international epidemiologic studies of the prevalence of
FSD suggested that sexual dysfunctions are highly prevalent across cultures, with
the incidence of sexual dysfunctions increasing directly with age for both men and
women.[23] Whereas the frequency of symptoms increases with age, personal distress
about those symptoms seems to diminish as women age.[24] Finally, the role of culture
was not as important as the medical problems suffered by respondents in determining
likelihood of participation in sexual activity.[23]

A large, recent epidemiologic survey, the Prevalence and Correlates of Female
Sexual Disorders and Determinants of Treatment Seeking (PRESIDE), queried a representative sample of 50,002 United States women (n = 31,581 with 63% response rate)
using the Changes in Sexual Functioning Questionnaire (CSFQ) to determine sexual
dysfunctions, and the Female Sexual Distress Scale (FSDS) to evaluate level of
distress.[25] Complaints of desire, arousal, and orgasm were reported in 38.7%,
26.1%, and 20.5%, respectively, with 44.2% of women describing any sexual
problem. When marked distress was assessed as a cofactor, consistent with DSM-
IV-TR criterion B, the prevalence rates decreased to 10%, 5.4%, and 4.7%, respectively, with 12% reporting any distressing sexual problem.

NEUROIMAGING

Recent advances in neuroimaging have demonstrated regions of the brain involved in
sexual activity. Functional magnetic resonance imaging (fMRI) of 20 women with no
history of sexual dysfunction (NHSD) was compared with 16 women with hypoactive
sexual desire disorder (HSDD). Subjective arousal to erotic stimuli was significantly
greater in the NHSD women, with different areas of the brain activated in women
with NHSD versus HSDD. Cognitive/central sexual response or brain activation
patterns were not significantly associated with peripheral sexual response in either
group.[26]

In another study, positron emission tomography (PET) suggested that activation of the left lateral orbital frontal cortex is related to the level of behavioral inhibition during sex, with deactivation of the temporal lobe directly reflecting the level of arousal. The prefrontal cortex and the left temporal lobe showed decreased regional blood flow during orgasm in women. Glucose metabolism in the deep cerebellar nuclei was associated with orgasm-specific muscle contractions, with ventral midbrain and right caudate dopamine-containing areas also involved.[27] Other PET scans, coupled with magnetic resonance imaging (MRI), have shown increased activation at orgasm, compared with pre-orgasm sexual arousal in the paraventricular nucleus of the hypothalamus, the periaqueductal gray area of the midbrain, the hippocampus, and the cerebellum.[28] Subsequent hormonal spikes in prolactin and oxytocin have been associated with an overall sense of well-being, and perhaps facilitate bonding with a sexual partner.

GENETICS

Recent data support both a genetic and an environmental contribution to sexual function. Twin studies of 4037 women from the United Kingdom and 3080 Australian women supported a significant genetic influence on orgasmic capacity.[29,30] One-third of the women reported never or infrequently achieving orgasm during intercourse and 21% during masturbation. Genetic influences accounted for 34% and 32% among UK and Australian women, respectively of the variance in achieving orgasm with intercourse, with an estimated heritability of 45% and 51%, respectively for orgasm during masturbation. These results suggest that the wide variation in orgasmic function in women has a strong genetic basis, and cannot be attributed solely to sociocultural influences. However, high variability in traits suggests limited selection for functionality. For example, clitoral length is highly variable, whereas vaginal length is not. Given the association between the size of clitoral structures and ability to achieve orgasm, the marked variability in clitoral size is not suggestive of evolutionary selection bias for clitoral structure, and by inference, on female orgasm.[31]

Vulnerability to sexual dysfunction with antidepressant medications is also subject to genetic influences, related to 5-HT2A receptor polymorphisms.[32] Women with the ll genotype for the SLC6A4 promoter region (5HTTLPR) were nearly 8 times more likely to have SSRI-associated sexual dysfunction if they were taking oral contraceptives.[33] In addition, dopamine (D4) receptor polymorphisms influence all phases of the sexual response cycle.[34]

HYPOACTIVE SEXUAL DESIRE DISORDER

The 2 key criteria for the diagnosis of HSDD are (1) the experiencing of difficulty in the desire phase of the sexual response cycle and (2) that this difficulty causes marked distress. Data from the PRESIDE study suggest rates of distressing low sexual desire (ie, HSDD) in the general population of 10%.[25] The most common co-occurring conditions were psychiatric (depression and anxiety), followed by thyroid problems and urinary incontinence. Comorbid arousal problems increased dramatically in postmenopausal women, with surgically induced menopause rates 54% higher and 34% higher in natural menopause women than in premenopausal women. In the Women's International Study of Health and Sexuality (WISHeS), Leiblum and colleagues[35] reported on HSDD from data collected from 952 partnered United States women (46% response rate), employing 2 valid and reliable psychometric instruments to determine women with or without HSDD: the Profile of Female Sexual Function (PFSF) to assess sexual desire in women, and the Personal Distress Scale (PDS) to assess distress experienced by women due to low sexual desire. The WISHeS data demonstrated that HSDD ranged in prevalence from 14% in premenopausal women to 26% in surgically postmenopausal women aged 20 to 49 years. No significant differences were found in the prevalence of HSDD between surgically postmenopausal women, aged 50 to 70 years, and naturally postmenopausal women in the same age cohort. In addition, HSDD was associated with significantly lower sexual and partner satisfaction, as well as significant decrements in general health status, including aspects of mental and physical health.

A 5-question diagnostic screening tool for HSDD, the Decreased Sexual Desire Screener (DSDS), has been recently validated and found to be easy to use by clinicians who are not experts in sexual health, with an accuracy rate of greater than 85% compared with an expert clinician interview.[36,37]

FEMALE SEXUAL AROUSAL DISORDER

The central diagnostic feature of female sexual arousal disorder (FSAD) as defined by DSM-IV-TR criteria is the inability to achieve, or maintain during sexual activity, an adequate genital lubrication-swelling response.[38] As discussed earlier, arousal in women has 2 parts: a central/cognitive sense of excitement and genital lubrication-swelling. This physiologic arousal response in women consists of vasocongestion of the pelvic vasculature, vaginal lubrication, and expansion and swelling of the external genitalia and breast tissues. If dysfunction of both desire and arousal are present, a diagnosis of both HSDD and FSAD should be made.

Quirk and colleagues[39] have recently shown that the Sexual Function Questionnaire (SFQ) is able to discriminate various sexual dysfunctions, including FSAD. The FSFI has also demonstrated discriminant validity for FSD.[40] The rate of FSAD in the general population found in the PRESIDE study was 5.4%.[25]

FEMALE ORGASMIC DISORDER

The critical factor in the making the diagnosis is criterion A: there must be delay or absence of orgasm *following a normal excitement phase*. Although a lack of sexual excitement may, in turn, lead to the inability to achieve orgasm, this would not correctly be diagnosed female orgasmic disorder (FOD). Another important part of criterion A is the clinician's judgment that the woman's orgasmic capacity is "less than should be reasonable for her age, sexual experience..."[38] Data indicate that, unlike men, women typically find it easier to orgasm as they age, which seems to be related to increased sexual experience.[41] Finally, a woman must have adequate stimulation to achieve orgasm. The diagnosis of FOD would not be indicated in a woman whose sexual partner suffers from premature ejaculation, thus depriving her of sufficient stimulation to reach orgasm. As discussed earlier, for orgasmic dysfunction to be diagnosed as FOD it must cause *distress* to fulfill DSM-IV-TR criterion B.

SEXUAL PAIN DISORDERS: DYSPAREUNIA AND VAGINISMUS

Dyspareunia is the occurrence of recurrent or persistent genital pain during intercourse, and, like all FSDs, it must cause distress to be diagnosed.[38] Dyspareunia cannot be due exclusively to the presence of FSAD (ie, an inadequate lubrication-swelling response to subjective arousal) or vaginismus. Dyspareunia is relatively uncommon in premenopausal women (approximately 5%). While the prevalence of dyspareunia is known to increase among postmenopausal women, estimations of the rate vary widely between 12% and 45%.[42]

Vaginismus has been defined by recurrent or persistent involuntary spasm of the musculature of the outer third of vagina. These spasms interfere with, or even prevent, sexual intercourse. This sexual dysfunction must cause distress, must not be due to another Axis I disorder (eg, somatization disorder), and not caused exclusively by the direct physiologic effects of a medical condition.[38] The SFQ, in addition to being able to discriminate between HSDD, FSAD, and FOD, is also able to detect the presence of sexual pain disorders and discriminate between them.

THE INFLUENCE OF CULTURE

The Study of Women's health Across the Nation (SWAN) used phone and clinic-based interviews to establish the rates of sexual dysfunction in 3167 white, African American, Hispanic, Chinese, and Japanese women, aged 42 to 52 years, who were not using hormones.[43] Researchers found that premenopausal women reported less pain with intercourse than perimenopausal women ($P = .01$), but these 2 groups did not differ in frequency of intercourse, desire, arousal, or physical or emotional satisfaction. Relationships factors, the perceived importance of sex, attitudes toward aging, and vaginal dryness were the variables having the greatest association across all outcomes. Controlling for sociodemographic factors such as income, amount of education, and geography, significant ethnic differences were identified. African American women reported higher frequency of sexual intercourse than white women. Hispanic women reported lower physical pleasure and arousal. Both Chinese and Japanese women reported more pain, less desire, and less arousal that white women, although only the difference in arousal was statistically significant.

SEXUALITY THROUGHOUT THE DEVELOPMENTAL CONTINUUM: PERIMENOPAUSAL AND POSTMENOPAUSAL SEXUALITY

The end of the childbearing years often means the end of discussions about reproductive health between patient and provider. Although much has been made of how contraception has impacted women of childbearing age, few physicians have received adequate training in how to monitor a woman's sexual health through the menopausal transition and beyond, much less how to treat the sexual problems that can arise during this time. Apart from the menopause itself, women at mid-life are also subject to the typical diseases of both men and women in this demographic, and sexual functioning may be affected by the pathophysiology of these disease processes, as well as their treatment.

The Transition Defined

Reproductive stages are classified by changes in menstrual patterns and FSH levels.[44] The onset of the menopausal transition begins with fluctuations in GnRH, which alters the release of FSH and LH. Over the course of a woman's life, as ovulation proceeds, there is a steady decline in the number of follicles present in the ovaries. In general, sometime after age 40 years, the number of follicles is low enough to cause changes in menstruation. When increased release of FSH and LH can no longer compensate for the diminishing number of ovarian follicles, several hormonal changes emerge: androgen synthesis decreases in the theca cells (though the adrenals continue to produce a relatively small amount of androgens), estrogen levels decrease, and progesterone synthesis in the corpus luteum is reduced.[45] The final menstrual period (FMP) in the naturally menopausal woman signals ovarian failure.

One year after FMP, a woman is considered to be postmenopausal. The hypothalamus and anterior pituitary gland continue to function throughout a woman's life. In early menopause FSH and LH levels increase to as much as 20 times their premenopausal levels as LH and FSH attempt to stimulate the production of hormones in the follicle-depleted ovaries.[46] FSH and LH levels decline steadily after age 55, and continue to decline until age 70 years.

Decreased estrogen leads to atrophy in genital tissues. The uterus decreases in size, and the vulva and vagina lose thickness and vascularity. Secretions from the cervix and Bartholin glands decrease, contributing to vaginal dryness. Changes in vaginal flora lead to decreased acid production and increased pH. Vaginal atrophy and dryness may lead to pruritus, dyspareunia, and increased rates of infection. Estrogen is essential in maintaining the integrity of pelvic connective tissue, and its withdrawal during menopause can result in decreased strength in pelvic ligaments, increasing the risk of urinary stress incontinence and prolapse of both the uterus and bladder.[47]

The relationship between vaginal atrophy due to diminishing estrogen levels during menopause and the increased occurrence of dyspareunia is also unclear. Postmenopausal dyspareunia is usually thought to result from atrophy of the vaginal wall tissue, leading to difficulty in lubrication. However, a 1997 Danish study found that while decreasing estrogen levels during menopause were significantly associated with vaginal atrophy, there was not an association with vaginal dryness or dyspareunia.[48]

Breast tissues are also sensitive to the withdrawal of estrogen. Many postmenopausal women experience decreased tactile sensitivity in their breasts. Decreased estrogen leads to diminished fat content in the breasts, as well as decreased nipple sensitivity and erection during sexual arousal. These changes mean that greater stimulation is required to achieve sexual excitement.[49]

Decreased levels of bioavailable testosterone may lead to symptoms of androgen insufficiency, characterized by a diminished sense of well-being or dysphoric mood, persistent and unexplained fatigue, and sexual function changes such as decreased libido, diminished sexual receptivity, and reduced pleasure.[50] Overall, these changes in brain and genital function and anatomy may contribute to an increase in the prevalence of sexual disorders among postmenopausal women.

A prevailing myth about the menopausal transition is that the end of a woman's fertility signals the end of her sex life. Although many women experience problems with sexual function, recent advances in the understanding of FSD allow effective interventions for many of these problems. Recent studies have suggested that the prevalence of sexual complaints increases during the menopausal transition, and that hormonal changes that occur during the menopausal transition have a negative impact on sexual function.[51] From early to late in the menopausal transition, the percentage of women with scores on the McCoy Female Sexuality Questionnaire indicating sexual dysfunction was found to increase from 42% to 88%. More severe sexual dysfunction was correlated with decreasing estrogen, but not with level of free testosterone. By the postmenopausal period, significant decline was found in several areas of sexual response, including: sexual excitement and interest, frequency of sexual intercourse, and overall satisfaction with sexual function. Significant increases were reported in vaginal dryness and dyspareunia. Low satisfaction with partner sexual function was also significantly correlated with poor sexual function. Women with low scores on the Sexuality Questionnaire were more likely to report distress about their sexuality.[52]

However, the results of recent trials investigating the role of testosterone in postmenopausal sexual function have not yet yielded concise clinical recommendations.

A recent Australian study of 1021 women aged 18 to 75 years seen in a community-based setting examined the role of multiple androgens in female sexual function. A low PFSF domain score for sexual responsiveness for women aged 45 years or older was associated with higher odds of having a serum dehydroepiandrosterone sulfate (DHEAS) level below the 10th percentile for this age group (odds ratio 3.90, $P = .004$). However, the majority of women with low DHEAS levels did not have low sexual function. No single androgen level, including free testosterone, was found to be predictive of sexual function.

To better examine the role of relationship factors in women's sexual functioning at mid-life, a recent Australian study interviewed 438 women ages 45 to 55 years who were still menstruating at the time of their baseline interview.[53] Eight years of longitudinal data were available for 336 of these women, none of whom underwent surgical or medication-induced menopause. Sexual response was found to be predicted by prior level of sexual function, change in partner status, feelings for partner, and estrogen level. Significant predictors of dyspareunia included premenopausal history of dyspareunia and, contrary to the 1997 Danish study cited earlier, estrogen levels. Frequency of sexual activity was predicted by prior level of sexual function and response, change in partner status, and feelings for partner. In all, prior sexual function and relationship factors were found to be more important than hormonal determinants of sexual function in perimenopausal women.

INTERVENTIONS
Psychological Treatment

For both the contemporary clinician and women suffering from FSD, the most important first step is education about anatomy, physiology, and expectations. Disparities in sexual desire between partners can be addressed in couple's therapy, and should not necessarily be interpreted as a problem with low desire. Duration of sexual activity is an important factor in determining if a woman has received adequate stimulation. For women that have never, or rarely, been able to experience orgasm, either alone or with a partner, directed masturbation (DM) is a technique that has been shown to be highly effective,[54] with success rates of greater than 65%.[55] Other women are able to orgasm while masturbating, but find the pressure of a sexual encounter with their partner too anxiety provoking. Masters and Johnson addressed this problem with *sensate focus* (SF), which dictated programmatic, progressive levels of touching, starting with nonsexual touching, progressing to more sexual touching, and eventual intercourse or other direct genital stimulation. Various other techniques have attempted to reduce the anxiety surrounding sexual encounters, falling under the moniker of systematic desensitization (SD), which entails exposure to sexually explicit material.

Some women experience pervasive anxiety, or other mood symptoms, that are also manifest during sexual activity. Cognitive-behavioral therapy (CBT) uses thought records to capture the cognitions that accompany these emotions. McCabe found that the use of CBT in conjunction with SF, SD, and DM reduced anorgasmia in a sample of sexually dysfunctional women from 66% to 11%.[56]

Lubricants

Lubricants can clearly help with vaginal dryness and resulting dyspareunia, and subsequently improve orgasmic function without any long-term safety concerns. In addition, lubricants can be used in combination with other treatments for sexual dysfunction associated with the menopausal transition. The primary objection to this intervention is displeasure with the mechanical interruption to sexual activity required for vaginal application.

Pharmacotherapy

Various agents have been tested to address FSD, and some have shown a degree of preliminary success. The vasoactive agent, sildenafil, demonstrated efficacy in the treatment of FOD, though larger subsequent studies failed to demonstrate separation from placebo.[57] In a recent study, 50 to 100 mg/d of sildenafil was found to be superior to placebo in effects on arousal and orgasmic dysfunction in premenopausal women with SSRI-induced arousal or orgasmic problems. Better results were seen in women with higher levels of thyroxine and testosterone, which enhances NO function. Despite more than 80% of the women complaining of decreased desire at study baseline, low desire was unaffected by sildenafil treatment.[58]

The non-SSRI bupropion has been studied in women with FSD, and has been found superior to placebo in improving sexual desire and decreasing distress in nondepressed premenopausal women with HSSD.[59,60] Results with bupropion in FOD were less robust.[61] Studies of women with SSRI-induced sexual dysfunction have demonstrated statistical improvements in desire, and clinical improvements in arousal and orgasm with bupropion SR 300 to 400 mg/d.[62] Some of the difficulties in demonstrating superiority of new treatments to placebo may be related to difficulties in defining the study population, lack of validation of outcome measures, and problems obtaining long-term safety data. Unfortunately, Food and Drug Administration (FDA)-approved treatments for FSD remain an unaccomplished goal of medical science.

Hormones

The increase in vasomotor symptoms and FSD during menopause is due, in part, to decreasing levels of available sex steroids. Providing an exogenous source for these hormones is the most straightforward approach to ameliorating these symptoms, with a goal of returning a woman's body to an endocrine milieu closer to its premenopausal state. A meta-analysis of 192 randomized controlled trials showed that estrogen therapy, alone or in a combination form, remains the most reliable, effective therapy for relieving the vasomotor symptoms of menopause, as well as, the associated sexual dysfunction.[63]

However, controversy stemming from the publication of the Women's Health Initiative (WHI) findings has led to concerns that a small percentage of women who use hormone replacement therapy (HRT) may suffer an increased rate of cardiovascular disease, cerebrovascular disease, blood clots, and breast and ovarian cancers.[64–66] Since the publication of the WHI, many clinicians and patients have determined that the increased risk of these serious side effects is small for the individual patient, and in some cases the severity of postmenopausal symptoms may warrant the use of exogenous hormones as a treatment, at least through the perimenopause.[67]

Although several trials have reported that estrogen replacement therapy (ERT) leads to increased desire for sex in postmenopausal women,[68] there have been few randomized placebo-controlled trials in this cohort.[69] A Danish study showed that long-term HRT positively and significantly affected hot flushes, sleep difficulties, sexual problems of decreased libido and dyspareunia, and blood pressure.[70] Libido and problems with mood swings improved in the HRT group more than in the placebo group.

For women experiencing vaginal atrophy and who do not wish to take systemic estrogen, topical estrogen creams may be a solution. Limited randomized controlled trials have shown that low-dose local vaginal estrogen delivery as treatment for vaginal atrophy is effective and well tolerated.[71] All approved vaginal estrogen products in the United States seem equally effective at the doses recommended in their labeling.

Transdermal delivery is another effective route of estrogen administration. Pharmacodynamic differences between oral and transdermal routes of estrogen administration suggest that transdermal estrogen exerts minimal effects on the concentrations of total and bioavailable testosterone, thyroxine, and cortisol, compared with oral estrogen.[72] In particular, free testosterone levels were higher by 16.4% with transdermal estrogen.

Although putative natural progestin-containing creams are efficacious in the treatment of menopausal symptoms when combined with estrogen, patients should be cautioned that these creams may increase sex hormones to levels seen with oral preparations. Although it is unlikely that topical estrogen preparations will affect serum estrogen levels to the same degree as oral HRT, perhaps due to differences in first-pass metabolism with these 2 routes of administration, care should still be taken to avoid using these products in women who should not be exposed to any exogenous sources of estrogen (eg, women with a history of estrogen-receptor positive breast cancer).

A testosterone patch was studied in the early 2000s for the treatment of HSDD in surgically menopausal women. A randomized placebo-controlled study found statistically significant increases in sexual desire and frequency of satisfying sexual encounters among the group of women received the 300 μg/d dose.[73] The 150 μg/d dose showed no significant improvement in either of these outcomes, whereas the 450 μg/d showed no improvement in these outcomes greater than those achieved at the 300 μg/d dose. Another study assessed the efficacy and safety of the 300 μg/d testosterone patch during 24 weeks of administration in surgically menopausal women with HSDD on concomitant estrogen therapy.[74] In this cohort, the 300 μg/d patch was found to significantly increase satisfying sexual activity and sexual desire, and decrease personal distress. Although the incidence of adverse events was similar in both groups ($P > .05$), the incidence of androgenic adverse events (eg, acne, hirsutism) was higher in the testosterone group, though most were mild. While being approved for use in postmenopausal women in the European Union, the testosterone patch failed to gain FDA approval in 2004 due to concerns over long-term safety.

Tibolone

Tibolone is a synthetic steroid sex hormone with estrogenic, androgenic, and progestogenic effects, available in the European Union. In a recent study, 48 postmenopausal women were randomized to tibolone versus estrogen-progesterone HRT for a 3-month treatment period.[75] Based on subjective qualitative scores on the Greene Climacteric Scale (GCS) and McCoy Female Sexuality Questionnaire, tibolone treatment was found to be at least as effective as HRT in improving quality of life. Tibolone was superior to HRT in perceived improvement of sexual performance, including general sexual satisfaction, sexual interest, sexual fantasies, sexual arousal, and orgasm, with decreased frequency of vaginal dryness and dyspareunia. Another study compared tibolone to transdermal estradiol (E2)/norethisterone (NETA) (50 μg/120 μg) in naturally postmenopausal women with FSD.[76] Self-reported FSFI scores, and FSDS scores indicated that both treatments resulted in improved overall sexual function, evidenced by increased frequency of sexual events, and reduction in sexuality-related personal distress. A significantly larger increase in FSFI total scores was seen in the tibolone group compared with the E2/NETA group, with nonsignificant group differences in FSDS scores, although decreases in distress were found in both groups.

SUMMARY

Problems with desire, arousal, and orgasmic function are common in women, but associated distress reduces the rates of sexual disorders to less than 10% of the general population. Comorbid sexual disorders and medical/psychiatric conditions may complicate diagnosis and treatment, particularly in peri- and postmenopausal women. Currently available interventions include psychotherapy, targeted sexual therapies, and pharmacologic treatments. Further research into diagnosis and potential treatments for sexual disorders in women are anticipated to enhance sexual function and satisfaction throughout women's lives.

REFERENCES

1. Kinsey A. Sexual behavior in the human female. Philadelphia: Saunders; 1953.
2. Sand M, Fisher WA. Women's endorsement of models of female sexual response: the nurses' sexuality study. J Sex Med 2007;4:708–19.
3. Braunstein GD. Androgen insufficiency in women: summary of critical issues. Fertil Steril 2002;77(Suppl 4):S94–9.
4. Hull EM, Eaton RC, Moses J, et al. Copulation increases dopamine activity in the medial preoptic area of male rats. Life Sci 1993;52:935–40.
5. Segraves RT. Effects of psychotropic drugs on human erection and ejaculation. Arch Gen Psychiatry 1989;46:275–84.
6. Lee AW, Pfaff DW. Hormone effects on specific and global brain functions. J Physiol Sci 2008;58(4):213–20.
7. Done CJ, Sharp T. Evidence that 5-HT2 receptor activation decreases noradrenaline release in rat hippocampus in vivo. Br J Pharmacol 1992;107:240–5.
8. Frolich PF, Meston CM. Evidence that serotonin affects female sexual functioning via peripheral mechanisms. Physiol Behav 2000;71:383–93.
9. Watson NV, Gorzalka BB. Concurrent wet dog shaking and inhibition of male rat copulation after ventromedial brainstem injection of the 5-HT2 agonist DOI. Neurosci Lett 1992;141:25–9.
10. D'Amati G, di Gioia CRT, Bologna M, et al. Type 5 phosphodiesterase expression in the human vagina. Urology 2002;60:191–5.
11. Palle C, Bredkajer HE, Ottesen B, et al. Vasoactive intestinal polypeptide in human vaginal blood flow: comparison between transvaginal and intravenous administration. Clin Exp Pharmacol Physiol 1990;17:61–8.
12. Marin R, Escrig A, Abreu P, et al. Androgen-dependent nitric oxide release in rat penis correlates with levels of constitutive nitric oxide synthetase isoenzymes. Biol Reprod 2002;61:1012–6.
13. Giuliano F, Allard J, Compagnie S, et al. Vaginal physiological changes in a model of sexual arousal in anesthetized rats. Am J Physiol Regul Integr Comp Physiol 2001;281(1):R140–9.
14. Kruger TH, Hartmann U, Schedlowski M. Prolactinergic and dopaminergic mechanisms underlying sexual arousal and orgasm in humans. World J Urol 2005; 23(2):130–8.
15. Stahl SM. The psychopharmacology of sex, part 2, effects of drugs and disease on the 3 phases of human sexual response. J Clin Psychiatry 2001; 62(3):147–8.
16. Clayton A, Ramamurthy S. The impact of physical illness on sexual dysfunction. In: Balon R, editor. Sexual Dysfunction: the brain body connection. Adv Psychosom Med Basel: Karger; 2008. p. 70–88.

17. Montejo AL, Llorca G, Izquierdo JA, et al. Incidence of sexual dysfunction associated with antidepressant agents: a prospective multicenter study of 1022 outpatients. J Clin Psychiatry 2001;62(Suppl 3):10–21.
18. Clayton AH, Pradko JF, Croft HA, et al. Prevalence of sexual dysfunction among newer antidepressants. J Clin Psychiatry 2002;63:357–66.
19. Clayton A, Kornstein S, Prakash A, et al. Changes in sexual functioning associated with duloxetine, escitalopram and placebo in the treatment of patients with major depressive disorder. J Sex Med 2007;4:917–29.
20. American Psychiatric Association. Diagnostic and statistical manual of mental disorders. Text revision. 4th edition. Washington, DC: American Psychiatric Association; 2000.
21. Nusbaum MRH, Helton MR, Ray N. The changing nature of women's sexual health concerns through the midlife years. Maturitas 2004;49:283–91.
22. Bancroft J, Loftus J, Long JS. Distress about sex: a national survey of women in heterosexual relationships. Arch Sex Behav 2003;32:193–208.
23. Derogatis LR, Burnett AL. The epidemiology of sexual dysfunctions. J Sex Med 2008;5(2):289–300.
24. Hayes RD, Dennerstein L, Bennett CM, et al. Relationship between hypoactive sexual desire disorder and aging. Fertil Steril 2007;87(1):107–12.
25. Shifren JL, Monz BU, Russo PA, et al. Sexual problems and distress in United States women. Obstet Gynecol 2008;112(5):970–8.
26. Arnow BA, Millheiser L, Garrett A, et al. Women with hypoactive sexual desire disorder compared to normal females: a functional magnetic resonance imaging study. Neuroscience 2009;158:484–502.
27. Georgiadis JR, Kortekaas R, Kuipers R, et al. Regional cerebral blood flow changes associated with clitorally induced orgasm in healthy women. Eur J Neurosci 2006;24:3305–16.
28. Komisaruk BR, Whipple B, Crawford A, et al. Brain activity (fMRI and PET) during orgasm in women, in response to vaginocervical self-stimulation. Abstr Soc Neurosci 2002;841:17.
29. Dunn KM, Cherkas LF, Spector TD. Genetic influences on variation in female orgasmic function: a twin study. Biol Lett 2005;1(3):260–3.
30. Dawood K, Kirk KM, Bailey JM, et al. Genetic and environmental influences on the frequency of orgasm in women. Twin Res Hum Genet 2006;9(4):603–8.
31. Wallen K, Lloyd EA. Clitoral variability compared with penile variability supports nonadaptation of female orgasm. Evol Dev 2008;10(1):1–2.
32. Bishop JR, Moline J, Ellingrod VL, et al. Serotonin 2A-1438 G-A and G-protein beta3 subunit C825T polymorphisms in patients with depression and SSRI-associated sexual side effects. Neuropsychopharmacology 2006;31:2281–8.
33. Bishop JR, Ellingrod VL, Akroush M, et al. The association of serotonin transporter genotypes and selective serotonin reuptake inhibitor (SSRI)-associated sexual side effects: possible relationship to oral contraceptives. Hum Psychopharmacol 2009;24:207–15.
34. Ben Zion IZ, Tessler R, Cohen L, et al. Polymorphisms in the dopamine D4 receptor gene (DRD4) contribute to individual differences in human sexual behavior: desire arousal, and sexual function. Mol Psychiatry 2006;11(8):782–6.
35. Leiblum SR, Koochaki PE, Rodenberg CA, et al. Sexual desire disorder in postmenopausal women: US results from the Women's International Study of Health and Sexuality (WISHeS). Menopause 2006;13(1):46–56.
36. Clayton AH, Goldfischer ER, Goldstein I, et al. Validation of the decreased sexual desire screener (DSDS): a brief diagnostic instrument for generalized

acquired female hypoactive sexual desire disorder (HSDD). J Sex Med 2009;6: 730–8.

37. Goldfischer ER, Clayton AH, Goldstein I, et al. Decreased sexual desire screener (DSDS) for diagnosis of hypoactive sexual desire disorder in women. Obstet Gynecol 2008;111:109.

38. American Psychiatric Association. Diagnostic and statistical manual of mental disorders. 4th edition, text revision. Washington, DC: American Psychiatric Association; 2000. p. 543, 549, 556, 558.

39. Quirk F, Haughie S, Symonds T. The use of the sexual function questionnaire as a screening tool for women with sexual dysfunction. J Sex Med 2005;2:469–77.

40. Sand M, Rosen R, Meston C, et al. The female sexual function index (FSFI): a potential "gold standard" measure for assessing sexual function in women, Poster 24, 3rd International Consultation on Sexual Medicine. Paris, July 10–13, 2009.

41. Levin RJ. Sexual desire and the deconstruction and reconstruction of the human female response model of Masters and Johnson. In: Everaerd W, Laan E, Both S, editors. Sexual appetite, desire and motivation: energetics of the sexual system. Amsterdam (The Netherlands): Royal Netherlands Academy of Arts and Sciences; 2001. p. 63–93.

42. Gregersen N, Jensen PT, Giraldi AGE. Sexual dysfunction in the peri- and postmenopause. Status of incidence, pharmacological treatment and possible risks. A secondary publication. Dan Med Bull 2006;53(3):349–53.

43. Avis NE, Zhao X, Johannes CB, et al. Correlates of sexual function among multiethnic middle-aged women: results from the Study of Women's Health Across the Nation (SWAN). Menopause 2005;12(4):385–98.

44. Arroyo A, Yeh J. Understanding the menopause transition and managing its clinical challenges. Sex Reprod Menopause 2006;3:12–7.

45. Weismiller D. The perimenopause and menopause experience: an overview. Clin Geriatr Med 2003;20:565–70.

46. Hall J. Neuroendocrine physiology of the early and late menopause. Endocrinol Metab Clin North Am 2004;33:637–59.

47. Wilson MM. Menopause. Clin Geriatr Med 2003;19(3):483–506.

48. Laan E, van Lunsen RH. Hormones and sexuality in postmenopausal women: a psychophysiological study. J Psychosom Obstet Gynaecol 1997;18(2):126–33.

49. Phillips NA. Female sexual dysfunction: evaluation and treatment. Am Fam Physician 2000;62(1):127–36, 141–2.

50. Bachmann G, Bancroft J, Braunstein G, et al. Female androgen insufficiency: the Princeton consensus statement on definition, classification, and assessment. Fertil Steril 2002;77(4):660–5.

51. Bachmann GA, Leiblum SR. The impact of hormones on menopausal sexuality: a literature review. Menopause 2004;11:120–30.

52. Dennerstein L, Alexander JL, Kotz K. The menopause and sexual functioning: a review of the population-based studies. Annu Rev Sex Res 2003;14:64–82.

53. Dennerstein L, Lehert P, Burger H. The relative effects of hormones and relationship factors on sexual function of women through the natural menopausal transition. Fertil Steril 2005;84(1):174–80.

54. Heiman JR. Orgasmic disorders in women. In: Leiblum SR, Rosen RC, editors. Principles and practice of sex therapy. 3rd edition. New York: Guildford Press; 2000. p. 84–123.

55. McMullen S, Rosen RC. Self-administered masturbation training in the treatment of primary orgasmic dysfunction. J Consult Clin Psychol 1979;47:912–8.

56. McCabe MP. Evaluation of a cognitive behavioral therapy program for people with sexual dysfunction. J Sex Marital Ther 2001;27:259–71.
57. Shields KM, Hrometz SL. Use of sildenafil for female sexual dysfunction. Ann Pharmacother 2006;40(5):931–4.
58. Nurnberg HG, Hensley PL, Heiman JR, et al. Sildenafil treatment of women with antidepressant-associated sexual dysfunction: a randomized controlled trial. JAMA 2008;300(4):395–404.
59. Segraves RT, Croft H, Kavoussi R, et al. Bupropion sustained release (SR) for the treatment of hypoactive sexual desire disorder (HSDD) in nondepressed women. J Sex Marital Ther 2001;27(3):303–16.
60. Modell JG, May RS, Katholi CR. Effect of bupropion-SR on orgasmic dysfunction in nondepressed subjects: a pilot study. J Sex Marital Ther 2000;26(3): 231–40.
61. Seagraves RT, Clayton AH, Croft H, et al. A multicenter, double-blind, placebo-controlled study of bupropion XL in females with orgasm disorder. Abstracts of the 19th Annual U.S. Psychiatric & Mental Health Congress, November, 2006.
62. Clayton AH, Warnock JK, Kornstein SG, et al. A placebo-controlled trial of bupropion SR as an antidote for selective serotonin reuptake inhibitor-induced sexual dysfunction. J Clin Psychiatry 2004;65:62–7.
63. Nelson H, Haney H, Miller J, et al. Management of menopause-related symptoms: summary. (Evidence Rep Technology Assessment No. 120, AHQR Publ. No. 05-E016-1), Rockville (MD): agency for Healthcare Research and Quality. As cited by Petersen M. In: Tepper MS, Owens AF, editors. Menopause and sexuality in sexual health. Westport (CT): Praeger Press; 2007.
64. Rossouw JE, Prentice RL, Manson JE, et al. Postmenopausal hormone therapy and risk of cardiovascular disease by age and years since menopause. JAMA 2007;297(13):1465–77.
65. Wassertheil-Smoller S, Hendrix SL, Limacher M, et al. Effect of estrogen plus progestin on stroke in postmenopausal women: the Women's Health Initiative: a randomized trial. JAMA 2003;289(20):2673–84.
66. Rossouw JE, Anderson GL, Prentice RL, et al. Risks and benefits of estrogen plus progestin in healthy postmenopausal women: principal results from the Women's Health Initiative randomized controlled trial. JAMA 2002;288(3):321–33.
67. Dennerstein G. Re: hormones down under: hormone therapy use after the women's health initiative. Aust N Z J Obstet Gynaecol 2006;47(1):80.
68. Modelska K, Cummings S. Female sexual dysfunction in postmenopausal women: systematic review of placebo-controlled trials. Am J Obstet Gynecol 2003;188(1):286–93.
69. Sherwin BB. The impact of different doses of estrogen and progestin on mood and sexual behavior in postmenopausal women. J Clin Endocrinol Metab 1991; 72:336–43.
70. Vestergaard P, Hermann AP, Stilgren L, et al. Effects of 5 years of hormonal replacement therapy on menopausal symptoms and blood pressure—a randomised controlled study. Maturitas 2003;46(2):123–32.
71. North American Menopause Society. The role of local vaginal estrogen for treatment of vaginal atrophy in postmenopausal women: 2007 position statement of The North American Menopause Society. Menopause 2007;14(3 Pt 1):355–69.
72. Shifren JL, Desindes S, McIlwain M, et al. A randomized, open-label, crossover study comparing the effects of oral versus transdermal estrogen therapy on serum androgens, thyroid hormones, and adrenal hormones in naturally menopausal women. Menopause 2007;14(6):985–94.

73. Braunstein GD, Sundwall DA, Katz M, et al. Safety and efficacy of a testosterone patch for the treatment of hypoactive sexual desire disorder in surgically meno-pausal women: a randomized, placebo-controlled trial. Arch Intern Med 2005; 165(14):1582–9.
74. Buster JE, Kingsberg SA, Aguirre O, et al. Testosterone patch for low sexual desire in surgically menopausal women: a randomized trial. Obstet Gynecol 2005;105:944–52.
75. Wu MH, Pan HA, Wang ST, et al. Quality of life and sexuality changes in postmen-opausal women receiving tibolone therapy. Climacteric 2001;4(4):314–9.
76. Nijland EA, Weijmar Schultz WC, Nathorst-Boos J, et al. Tibolone and transdermal E2/NETA for the treatment of female sexual dysfunction in naturally menopausal women: results of a randomized active-controlled trial. J Sex Med 2008;5(3): 646–56.

Substance Abuse in Women

Shelly F. Greenfield, MD, MPH[a],*, Sudie E. Back, PhD[b],
Katie Lawson, MA[b], Kathleen T. Brady, MD, PhD[b]

KEYWORDS

- Women • Gender • Addiction • Substance-use disorders
- Drug abuse • Alcohol

EPIDEMIOLOGY

Gender differences in rates of substance abuse have been consistently observed in the general population and treatment-seeking samples, with men exhibiting significantly higher rates of substance use, abuse, and dependence.[1–3] However, recent epidemiologic surveys suggest that this gap between men and women has narrowed in recent decades.[3,4] For example, surveys in the early 1980s estimated the male/female ratio of alcohol-use disorders as 5:1,[5] in contrast to more recent surveys that report a ratio of approximately 3:1.[6]

Data from the National Epidemiologic Survey on Alcohol and Related Conditions (NESARC; N = 43,093), the largest and most recent study of substance use and other psychiatric disorders, showed that men were 2.2 times more likely than women to have drug abuse, and 1.9 times more likely to have drug dependence.[1] Data regarding prescription drugs are less consistent. Although several studies indicate that rates of nonmedical prescription drug use are higher among women than men, particularly for narcotic analgesics and tranquilizers,[7] other studies report equivalent or higher rates among men.[8]

Telescoping

Telescoping is a term used to describe an accelerated progression from the initiation of substance use to the onset of dependence and first admission to treatment.[9–11] The phenomenon has been consistently observed in investigations of gender and

The authors would like to acknowledge support from grant K24DA019855 (SFG), K23DA021228 (SEB) and K24 DA00435 (KTB) from the NIH/NIDA, and P50 DA016511 (KTB) from NIAMS/ORWH.

[a] Alcohol and Drug Abuse Treatment Program, McLean Hospital, Harvard Medical School, 115 Mill Street, Belmont, MA 02478, USA

[b] Clinical Neuroscience Division, Department of Psychiatry, Medical University of South Carolina, 67 President Street/PO Box 250861, Charleston, SC 29425, USA

* Corresponding author.

E-mail address: sgreenfield@mclean.harvard.edu

substance-use disorders, with studies typically reporting an accelerated progression among women for opioids, cannabis, and alcohol.[9] Thus, when women enter substance abuse treatment they typically present with a more severe clinical profile (eg, more medical, behavioral, psychological, and social problems) than men, despite having used less of the substance and having used the substance for a shorter period of time compared with men.

BIOLOGICAL ISSUES
Neuroactive Gonadal Steroid Hormones

Ovarian steroid hormones (eg, estrogen, progesterone), metabolites of progesterone, and negative allosteric modulators of the γ-aminobutyric acid A (GABA-A) receptor, such as dehydroepiandrostenedione (DHEA), may influence the behavioral effects of drugs.[12,13] In human studies, the follicular phase of the menstrual cycle, in which estradiol levels are high and progesterone low, is associated with the greatest responsivity to stimulants.[14] A study investigating response to cocaine administration found that women in the luteal phase reported lower ratings of feeling high than women in the follicular phase or men.[14] Whether observed differences are accounted for by enhancing effects of estradiol or attenuating effects of progesterone remains unclear. However, one study found that progesterone attenuates the subjective response to smoked cocaine in women, but not men.[15] Studies of nicotine show a potential greater saliency in the luteal phase of the cycle,[12,16] although the effect of gonadal steroids on responses to alcohol is less clear than for other substances of abuse.[17]

Sex Differences in Stress Reactivity and Relapse to Substance Abuse

Sex differences in neuroendocrine adaptations to stress and reward systems may mediate women's susceptibility to drug abuse and relapse.[18] Several studies have examined sex differences in stress response (eg, subjective, autonomic) and relapse.[18,19] Among substance-dependent subjects, attenuated neuroendocrine stress response in women (ie, blunted adrenocorticotropic hormone and cortisol) has been shown following exposure to stress and drug cues.[20] This hypothalamic-pituitary-adrenocortical (HPA) dysregulation in women may be one key to enhanced vulnerability to relapse in response to negative affect, as it may be associated with greater emotional intensity at lower levels of HPA arousal.[21]

ROLE OF CO-OCCURRING DISORDERS
Mood and Anxiety Disorders

Lifetime rates of mood and anxiety disorders are significantly higher among women than men, with and without substance-use disorders.[22] A recent study by Goldstein[23] using the wave 1 NESARC (n = 24,575) found that the 12-month prevalence rates of mood and anxiety disorders among women with substance-use disorders were 29.7% and 26.2%, respectively. The most common mood disorder was major depressive disorder (15.4%) and the most common anxiety disorder was specific phobia (15.6%).

Given this high co-occurrence, a comprehensive psychiatric assessment is critical. Because chronic alcohol or drug use may enhance vulnerability for these disorders, or lead to organic changes that manifest as a mood or anxiety disorder, careful assessment is necessary to differentiate substance-induced, transient symptoms from a disorder that warrants treatment. One way to do this is to carefully monitor symptoms during a period of abstinence from alcohol or drugs. A family history of mood/anxiety disorders, onset of mood/anxiety symptoms before the onset of the substance-use disorder, and sustained mood/anxiety symptoms during periods of abstinence all point toward an independent mood or anxiety disorder.[24]

If an independent mood or anxiety disorder is diagnosed, evidence-based treatment that will adequately address both conditions is warranted. Few investigations have examined gender differences in response to psychotherapeutic or pharmacotherapeutic treatments for mood and anxiety disorders among individuals with co-occurring substance-use disorders, and studies examining agents targeting substance use, such as naltrexone or disulfiram, as add-on treatment of individuals with co-occurring mood or anxiety disorders is under explored. One study[25] examined gender differences among alcohol-dependent outpatients in the effectiveness of sertraline among type A and B alcoholics, of whom 57.9% had major depression. Type A alcoholic men, but not women, responded more favorably to sertraline than placebo (ie, longer time to relapse, fewer days drinking). No gender differences among type B alcoholics were observed.

Eating Disorders

Ninety percent of the cases of anorexia nervosa (AN) and bulimia nervosa (BN) are found in women. Eating disorders (EDs) are estimated to be 2 to 3 times higher in women than men.[26] Among women with substance-use disorders, high rates of EDs, in particular the purging subtypes of bulimia, have been reported. In their review of clinical populations, Holderness and colleagues[27] reported that lifetime ED behaviors co-occurred with substance-use disorders in up to 40% of women. Among women with BN or binge-eating disorder, rates of substance abuse are greater among those with, compared with without, a history of sexual or physical abuse.[28]

Treatment is complex and requires a multidisciplinary approach including, for example, nutritional counseling and medication supervision.[29] Evidence-based behavioral treatments for EDs include cognitive behavioral therapy and interpersonal therapy, and pharmacotherapy for EDs has focused on antidepressant medications. At present, no integrated, evidence-based treatments for EDs and substance-use disorders are available.[30] Like many co-occurring psychiatric conditions, individuals presenting to treatment with substance-use disorders and EDs typically receive treatment in programs specializing in substance-use disorders or EDs. They rarely receive services for both disorders. A recent national survey of screening and treatment practices at 351 addiction treatment programs revealed that only half (51%) screen for EDs at intake or assessment, and only 29% admit patients who screen positive for EDs.[30]

Posttraumatic Stress Disorder

The prevalence of posttraumatic stress disorder (PTSD) is 1.4 to 5 times higher among individuals with, compared to those without, co-occurring substance-use disorders.[31] Similarly, data from the Australian National Survey of Mental Health and Well-being found that 34.4% of respondents with PTSD also had at least 1 substance-use disorder.[32] Among treatment-seeking women with substance abuse, rates of physical or sexual abuse are high, ranging from 55% to 99%,[33] with many of these women manifesting trauma-related symptoms consistent with a diagnosis of PTSD.

Consensus is lacking regarding the best treatment approach for co-occurring PTSD and substance-use disorders; however, accumulating data confirm the efficacy (ie, significant before and after decreases in PTSD and substance-use symptoms) of integrated interventions that address both conditions simultaneously.[34–37] Addressing trauma-related symptoms early in treatment may provide the opportunity for improved likelihood of recovery from substance-use disorders, as many individuals report using alcohol or drugs in response to symptoms of PTSD (eg, sleep impairment, flashbacks, nightmares, avoidance of trauma reminders, hyperarousal). Selective serotonin reuptake inhibitors are the pharmacological treatments of choice for PTSD. However, only 3 published studies have examined their use among patients with co-occurring alcohol- or drug-use disorders, and all of these studies have examined the use of sertraline.[38–40] The findings suggest that the medication-responsive group tended to have onset of PTSD preceding the onset of the substance-use disorder (ie, primary PTSD), highlighting the potential relationship between temporal order of onset and treatment outcome.

SPECIFIC SUBSTANCES
Alcohol

Although men consume and misuse alcohol at significantly higher rates than women, this gender gap has decreased over time[3] and has been well documented in several large epidemiological studies. For example, the 2001 to 2002 NESARC, which sampled more than 42,000 individuals, found that sex differences in rates of alcohol use and abuse or dependence were smallest for younger cohorts (with cohorts ranging from 1913–1932 to 1968–1984).[3] In a similar vein, examination of changes in the age of initiation of alcohol use in the past 50 years shows significant narrowing of the gender gap.[3,41] In the 1950s, the male/female ratio of initiation in the 10- to 14-year-old age group was 4:1, and by the early 1990s it was 1:1.

Compared with men, women experience significantly shorter time intervals between the initiation of alcohol use and the onset of significant alcohol-related problems and treatment entry.[9] This accelerated course, known as telescoping, may be attributed to a variety of biological, socioeconomic, psychological, and cultural factors that affect women. For example, compared with men, women may be more adversely affected by alcohol because of the lower percentage of total body water, decreased first pass metabolism because of lower levels of alcohol dehydrogenase in the gastric mucosa, and slower rates of alcohol metabolism.[42,43]

Gender differences in motives for alcohol use have been observed, with women being more likely than men to consume alcohol in response to stress and negative emotions. In contrast, men seem more likely than women to consume alcohol to enhance positive emotions or to conform to a group.[44] Compared with men, women with alcohol-use disorders are significantly more likely to have co-occurring psychiatric disorders[22,23,27] that may serve to impede substance-use treatment efforts. Thus, prevention and treatment intervention efforts should incorporate these gender differences in motives and co-occurring psychiatric conditions to enhance effectiveness.[45]

Women are less likely than men to seek treatment, and more likely to face gender-specific treatment barriers.[46] Various factors, such as childcare responsibilities, transportation, financial status, and social stigma, may help explain this finding. To enhance treatment seeking and retention, programs should consider offering childcare, prenatal care, women-only treatment, and services specific for women's issues.[47] Interventions specifically designed for women-only groups show promise, indicating that women-only treatment is associated with fewer relapses and higher treatment satisfaction ratings.[48,49]

Stimulants

Although rates of stimulant use are similar among men and women,[50] preclinical and clinical studies suggest that women may be particularly vulnerable to the reinforcing effects of stimulant drugs.[51,52] Recent public health monitoring indicates that methamphetamine use is increasing, with an estimated 5.8% of individuals aged 12 years and older in the United States endorsing lifetime methamphetamine use.[53] According to the Treatment Episode Dataset (TEDS), admissions for methamphetamine between 1995 and 2005 more than doubled from 3.7% to 9.2%.[54] Increased use among pregnant women has also been observed. Among pregnant women admitted to federally funded substance abuse treatment centers in 1994, 8% were admitted for methamphetamine dependence; that proportion rose to 24% in 2006,[55] leading the study's investigators to conclude that methamphetamine is the primary substance of abuse for which pregnant women seek care.

The reinforcing effects of stimulants may be strongly influenced by women's hormonal milieu. Basic and clinical studies show that estrogen increases, and progesterone decreases, the reinforcing effects of stimulants for women.[14,15,51,56] In response to cocaine administration, women have been found to report increased subjective feelings of high and increased heart rate during the follicular phase, when levels of estrogen are high and progesterone levels are low.[14,15] Moreover, exogenous administration of progesterone among women has been shown to result in attenuated subjective responses to cocaine administration among women.[15]

Cognitive behavioral therapy has been shown to be as effective in treating stimulant-use disorders among women as among men.[57] Modified therapeutic community programs may also be effective for methamphetamine-using women.[58] At present, there are no approved pharmacotherapy treatments for cocaine dependence. However, preclinical studies suggest that baclofen, a GABAergic drug, may help reduce cocaine use among women, in particular.[59] In contrast, studies using naltrexone to reduce cocaine use,[60] and bupropion to decrease methamphetamine use,[61] indicate that these pharmacotherapies may be more effective for men than for women.

Opioids

Prescription opioids

The use of prescription opioids has soared in the past 2 decades. For example, from 1992 to 2003, a 141% increase in prescription opioid abuse was reported.[62] Two large epidemiological surveys found that women engage in the nonmedical use of prescription opioids more often than men.[7] In contrast, other studies suggest that rates of nonmedical use are similar for men and women,[53] or higher among men.[63] Gender differences in prescription opioid use may also occur within specific age groups. Regarding prescription opioid abuse or dependence, data from the 2002 to 2004 National Survey on Drug Use and Health (NSDUH) found that women aged 12 to 17 years had higher rates than men, but that men aged 18 to 25 years had higher rates than women.[64]

Gender differences in motives for use and aberrant drug-taking behaviors have also been observed. Among college students, McCabe and colleagues[65] found that men were significantly more likely than women to use prescription opioids for experimentation (35.3% vs 18.4%) or to get high (39.4% vs 24.4%). A recent study of 121 chronic pain patients found that women were significantly more likely than men to hoard unused medications and to use additional drugs (eg, sedatives) to enhance the effectiveness of prescription opioids.[66]

Heroin and intravenous drug abuse

Approximately 0.2% of the population of the United States aged 12 years and older endorses lifetime heroin use.[50] One study (N = 408) found that, compared with men, women use smaller amounts of heroin, use heroin for shorter periods of time, and are less likely to inject heroin.[67] A recent study of 111 individuals who were opioid-dependent and not in treatment found that women, compared with men, had more severe vocational impairment and used significantly more cocaine.[68]

Research indicates that women's injection of drugs may be particularly influenced by their sexual partner's injection risk behavior.[69] Powis and colleagues[67] found that women who injected heroin were significantly more likely than men to have a sexual partner who also injected heroin (96% vs 82%). In addition, women are also more likely than men to be introduced to injection by their sexual partners.[67] Powis and colleagues[67] reported that 51% of the female heroin users were first injected by their male sexual partner, whereas 90% of men were injected the first time by a friend. Compared with men who inject, women who inject report being more influenced by social pressure and by sexual partner encouragement.[70]

Risks of sharing needles or preparation equipment include enhanced vulnerability to numerous physical diseases, including hepatitis B and C, as well as human immunodeficiency virus (HIV).[70] To date, it is unclear whether there are significant sex differences in injection risk behaviors. Frajzyngier and colleagues[70] failed to observe sex differences in sharing needles during the first injection. However, women were significantly more likely than men to share preparation equipment. Other results suggest that, although women may be more likely to share needles,[71,72] women are also more likely than men to engage in risk-reducing behaviors such as carrying clean syringes.[72]

Treatment

Less than one-fourth of individuals with opioid-use disorders receive treatment.[73] Preliminary findings for a manual-based, 12-session group treatment of women using methadone suggests that this may be an effective way to treat opioid dependence in women.[74] Regarding opioid agonist therapies, Jones and colleagues[75] found that men and women remained in treatment for a significantly longer period of time when given methadone as opposed to L-α acetylmethadol (LAAM). Although buprenorphine, LAAM, and methadone reduced drug use for all participants, results suggest that sex differences may occur in the effectiveness of these pharmacologic agents. Specifically, buprenorphine was associated with significantly fewer positive urine samples and less self-reported opioid use than methadone among women. LAAM was associated with less drug use than buprenorphine among men.

Cannabis

Marijuana is the most commonly used illicit drug in the United States. According to the 2004 NSDUH, approximately 96.6 million Americans (40.2%) have tried marijuana.[76] Compared with women, men are more likely to use marijuana daily (2.0% vs 0.7%),[77] have more initial opportunities to use marijuana,[78] and initiate marijuana use at a younger age (16.4 years vs 17.6 years).[79]

Unlike other substances, such as stimulants, a relationship between the menstrual phase and women's use of,[80] or response to, marijuana (eg, mood, pulse rate)[81,82] has not been observed. However, marijuana use may be related to the menstrual cycle for women who have severe premenstrual syndrome or premenstrual dysphoric disorder.[82]

Attention processes and memory may be affected by marijuana use for up to 7 days following use.[83] The effects of marijuana use on neuropsychological processes may differ by sex. In a study of heavy versus light marijuana users, Pope and colleagues[84] reported that visual-spatial memory was impaired for women who smoked heavily, compared with women who were light smokers. However, no such difference was observed for men.

Research suggests that women enter treatment for marijuana-use disorder after significantly fewer years of use than men do (ie, telescoping effects).[9] Because of the low numbers of women in treatment, no studies have been published regarding gender differences in the effectiveness of treatment of marijuana-use disorders. However, research suggests that cognitive behavioral therapy, contingency management treatments, motivational enhancement therapies, and administering oral tetrahydrocannabinol (THC) and nefazodone are effective treatments for marijuana dependence.[85–88] However, a limitation of these studies is that they were predominately conducted with male participants.

Nicotine

In 2008, approximately 28.4% citizens of the United States reported being current nicotine users. Men use nicotine at higher rates than women (34.5% vs 22.5%),[50] but women may be at an increased risk for health problems caused by smoking. Women who smoke are twice as likely as men to have heart attacks,[89] women experience faster lung deterioration than men, and are at increased risk for chronic obstructive pulmonary disease[90] and lung cancer.[91] Smoking may also cause women to commence menopause earlier, experience increased menstrual bleeding, have difficulty becoming pregnant, or to experience spontaneous abortion.

Pharmacological and nonpharmacological factors influence nicotine use. Nonpharmacological factors are stimuli that are often paired with nicotine. Such stimuli can be proximal (eg, the smell of a cigarette) or distal (eg, people associated with smoking).[92] Compared with men, women seem to be less influenced by nicotine factors[93,94] and more influenced by proximal cues.[95] These gender differences in underlying motivations or triggers for use may help inform etiologic understanding of nicotine use and help improve the design of gender-sensitive treatment approaches.

Compared with men, women may have more difficulty quitting smoking. A study conducted by the Centers for Disease Control and Prevention,[96] which surveys more than 100,000 citizens of the United States, indicates that more than 1 million fewer women than men older than 35 years are able to quit smoking.[97] Gonadal steroid hormones may be associated with women's success at smoking cessation.[12,16] Women who attempt to quit during the first 14 days of their menstrual cycle (ie, the follicular phase) seem more likely to succeed than women who attempt to quit in the second half of the cycle (ie, the luteal phase).[12,16] Another obstacle to smoking cessation is women's concern about weight gain. Women worry twice as much about weight gain caused by smoking cessation than men,[98] and relapse 3 times more often than men because of weight gain.[99]

Sex differences in the efficacy of nicotine replacement therapy (NRT) may exist, but research to date is inconclusive. For example, a meta-analysis of 11 placebo-controlled NRT patch trials found that NRT is equally effective for men and women.[100] More recently, Perkins and Scott[101] added 3 placebo-controlled trials to this meta-analysis. The findings revealed that NRT is significantly more effective for men than women. Studies examining non-nicotine medication (eg, bupropion, varenicline) report equal effectiveness in men and women up to 12 weeks after treatment,[102,103] and bupropion may be a particularly effective method for women because it has been found to also help relieve depression.[103] Although medications are the standard treatment approach, therapy and counseling enhance the efficacy of medication treatment and may be more effective in women than men.[104] Interventions that teach women how to cope with cues and address co-occurring mood and anxiety disorders may be particularly helpful.

A pertinent nicotine-related concern for women is smoking during pregnancy.[105] Behavioral treatment approaches are particularly important for smoking cessation during this time, as many medications are contraindicated in pregnancy. Modifications may be made to therapy to tailor it for pregnant women (eg, incentives for cessation, such as vouchers that can be exchanged for baby supplies) while women are pregnant and after delivery. These modifications should continue after the baby has been delivered, because the majority (65%) of women who quit smoking during pregnancy relapse within 6 months of delivery.[106]

TREATMENT OUTCOME FOR WOMEN WITH SUBSTANCE-USE DISORDERS

Data from the TEDS, which captures data on national treatment admission rates, report that the overall proportion of men to women within the treatment system has remained fairly constant from 1995 to 2005 at 2:1.[107] A recent review of the literature between 1975 and 2005 concluded that women are less likely to enter substance abuse treatment than men.[46] However, once women enter treatment, gender itself is not a predictor of treatment retention, completion, or outcome.[46] Several gender-specific predictors of outcome, and patient characteristics and treatment approaches can affect outcomes differentially by gender.[46] Some characteristics have been shown to be associated with more favorable outcomes for men and women, such as greater financial resources, fewer mental health problems, and less severe drug problems.[46,108] Studies in women-only samples have found associations between certain characteristics and retention, including better psychological functioning, higher levels of personal stability and social support, lower levels of anger, treatment beliefs, and referral source.[46,109,110]

Gender differences in treatment referral sources have been documented, highlighting the differential pathways by which women and men enter substance abuse treatment facilities. For example, significantly more men than women are referred to treatment through the criminal justice system (40% men vs 28% women). Approximately twice as many women as men (15% women vs 6% men) are referred from other community agencies, such as welfare, mental health, and other health care providers.[107,111] The number of female prisoners in the United States is growing rapidly (eg, 53% since 1995), which means that the criminal justice system is increasingly becoming more relevant to the lives of women with substance-use disorders.[112] This increase in the number of female prisoners is largely the result of changes in sentencing for drug-related charges that have disproportionately affected women, particularly women of color.[112]

In treatment seeking for women, their relationship with and responsibility for children is particularly important. Most women who enter substance abuse treatment are mothers, and at least half have had contact with child welfare.[113,114] One study of methadone maintenance treatment found that women who were residing with their children were significantly more likely than women not residing with their children to enter treatment.[115] For some women, residing with their children may serve as an impediment to treatment entry if they fear they may lose custody of their children.[116] Once in treatment, women who are able to keep their children with them or retain custody of their children while in treatment are more likely to stay in treatment.[117]

Differences in the sources of payment for substance abuse treatment have also been reported. Significantly more men than women report self-pay (26% men vs 18% women) and more women than men report being dependent on public insurance (26% women vs 12% men).[107] This finding suggests that women may be more vulnerable to changes in insurance-related benefits and coverage because of their greater reliance on public insurance to pay for treatment. In addition to childcare and financial issues, other factors may present as impediments to women's treatment seeking and use. Social stigma, lack of awareness regarding treatment options, concerns about confrontational approaches that were pervasive in male-dominated traditional substance abuse treatment, co-occurring mental disorders or a history of trauma and victimization, as well as homelessness all present possible barriers for women.

Gender-specific Treatment of Women with Substance-use Disorders

To date, most substance abuse treatment models have been designed for men and based predominantly on male norms.[46,118] However, gender-specific interventions that are designed to deliver information and services tailored for women are beginning to emerge in response to mixed-gender programs, which often fail to address women's specific needs, such as childcare assistance, pregnancy, parenting, domestic violence, sexual trauma and victimization, psychiatric comorbidity, housing, income support, and social services.[46,118–120]

It is unclear at this point whether gender-specific treatments are superior.[46,47,121] However, this research is severely limited because only a few randomized clinical trials have examined the relative effectiveness of comparable women-only versus mixed-gender interventions.[49] In a meta-analysis examining single-gender substance abuse treatment of women, Orwin and colleagues[119] concluded that single-gender treatment was effective, but its strongest effect was on pregnancy outcomes, psychological well-being, attitudes/beliefs, and HIV risk reduction. One study that randomized women (N = 1573) to women-only versus mixed-gender treatment found no significant differences in retention.[122] In contrast, another study that randomized cocaine-dependent women to a women-only day treatment program or a mixed-gender outpatient program found that participants in the women-only program had significantly higher retention rates[123] (60.2% vs 46.1%). More recently, treatment outcomes and costs of women-only and mixed-gender day treatment programs were compared among 122 women randomized to a women-only program or 1 of 3 standard mixed-gender programs.[124] Compared with the hospital-based program, participants in the women-only program showed significantly lower total abstinence during the follow-up. Limitations included a small sample size and the focus on only day treatment programs.[46]

In a recent stage I behavioral development trial, Greenfield and colleagues[49] developed a manual-based, 12-session women's recovery group (WRG; n = 16) and compared WRG with mixed-gender group drug counseling (GDC; n = 7), an effective manual-based treatment of substance-use disorders. During the 12-week treatment phase, WRG and GDC were equally effective in reducing substance use, but WRG showed significantly greater improvement in reductions in drug and alcohol use during the 6-month follow-up phase. In addition, women were significantly more satisfied with WRG than GDC.[49] Secondary analyses revealed a 3-way interaction effect of treatment condition, time, and baseline Brief Symptom Inventory scores, indicating that women with greater baseline psychiatric severity had greater reductions in substance use during treatment and follow-up if they were in the WRG rather than the GDC condition.[125] Furthermore, women with low self-efficacy showed improved treatment outcomes if assigned to WRG compared with the GDC group.[126]

Behavioral Couples Treatment

For women, the risk of consuming alcohol secondary to marital discord, divorce, negative emotional states, and interpersonal conflict is higher than for men.[44,127] Similarly, having a partner who abuses alcohol or drugs is more strongly related to relapse for women than for men.[114] Because of this, treatment interventions designed specifically to address these dyadic issues may be particularly beneficial. Behavioral couples therapy (BCT) is founded on 2 fundamental assumptions: (1) family members, specifically spouses or other intimate partners, can reward abstinence; and (2) a reduction of relationship distress and conflict leads to improved substance-use outcomes by reducing possible antecedents to relapse and heavy use. Participation in BCT results in significantly less partner violence, higher rates of marital satisfaction, lower substance-use severity, greater improvements in psychosocial functioning of children living with parents, and better cost benefit and cost-effectiveness compared with traditional individual-based treatments (IBTs).[128] In one study of 138 married or cohabiting women, Fals-Stewart and colleagues[128] randomly assigned subjects to: (1) BCT, (2) IBT, or (3) a psychoeducational attention control treatment (PACT) condition. The findings showed that women who received BCT, compared with IBT or PACT, had significantly fewer days drinking and higher levels of dyadic adjustment during a 1-year follow-up period.[128]

CONCLUSIONS AND FUTURE DIRECTIONS

Gender differences in substance-use disorders and treatment outcomes for women with substance-use disorders have been a focus of research in the last 15 years. The initiation, use patterns, acceleration of disease course, and help-seeking patterns are affected by gender differences in biologic, psychological, cultural, and socioeconomic factors. Important gender-specific factors also predict women's substance abuse treatment entry, retention, and outcomes. Understanding the basic biological mechanisms that underlie these gender differences in vulnerability and responsiveness to substances will enhance the development of gender-specific treatments. Additional research is also necessary to elucidate gender differences in response to specific pharmacologic and behavioral treatments, to identify subgroups of women who can benefit from single-gender versus mixed-gender treatments, and to improve understanding of the effectiveness and cost-effectiveness of gender-specific versus standard treatments.

REFERENCES

1. Compton WM, Thomas YF, Stinson FS, et al. Prevalence, correlates, disability, and comorbidity of DSM-IV drug abuse and dependence in the United States: results from the National Epidemiologic Survey on Alcohol and Related Conditions. Arch Gen Psychiatry 2007;64:566–76.
2. Kessler RC, Chiu WT, Demler O, et al. Prevalence, severity, and comorbidity of 12-month DSM-IV disorders in the National Comorbidity Survey Replication. Arch Gen Psychiatry 2005;62(6):617–27.
3. Grucza RA, Norberg K, Bucholz KK, et al. Correspondence between secular changes in alcohol dependence and age of drinking onset among women in the United States. Alcohol Clin Exp Res 2008;32(8):1493–501.
4. Wagner FA, Anthony JC. Male-female differences in the risk of progression from first use to dependence upon cannabis, cocaine, and alcohol. Drug Alcohol Depend 2007;86:191–8.
5. Helzer JE, Burnam A, McEvoy LT. Alcohol abuse and dependence. In: Robins LN, Regier DA, editors. Psychiatric disorders in America: the epidemiological catchment area study. New York: The Free Press; 1991. p. 81–115.

6. Hasin DS, Stinson FS, Ogburn E, et al. Prevalence, correlates, disability, and comorbidity of DSM-IV alcohol abuse and dependence in the United States: results from the National Epidemiologic Survey on Alcohol and Related Conditions. Arch Gen Psychiatry 2007;64(7):830–42.

7. Simoni-Wastila L, Ritter G, Strickler G. Gender and other factors associated with the nonmedical use of abusable prescription drugs. Subst Use Misuse 2004; 39(1):1–23.

8. Blanco C, Alderson D, Ogburn E, et al. Changes in the prevalence of non-medical prescription drug use and drug use disorders in the United States: 1991–1992 and 2001–2002. Drug Alcohol Depend 2007;90(2–3):252–60.

9. Hernandez-Avila CA, Rounsaville BJ, Kranzler HR. Opioid-, cannabis-, and alcohol-dependent women show more rapid progression to substance abuse treatment. Drug Alcohol Depend 2004;74(3):265–72.

10. Hser YI, Anglin MD, Booth MW. Sex differences in addict careers: 3. Addiction. Am J Drug Alcohol Abuse 1987;13(3):231–51.

11. Randall CL, Roberts JS, Del Boca FK, et al. Telescoping of landmark events associated with drinking: a gender comparison. J Stud Alcohol 1999;60:252–60.

12. Newman JL, Mello NK. Neuroactive gonadal steroid hormones and drug addiction in women. In: Brady KT, Back SE, Greenfield SF, editors. Women and addiction: a comprehensive handbook. New York: Guilford Press; 2009. p. 35–64.

13. Doron R, Fridman L, Gispan-Herman I, et al. DHEA, a neurosteroid, decreases cocaine self-administration and reinstatement of cocaine-seeking behavior in rats. Neuropsychopharmacology 2006;31(10):2231–6.

14. Sofuoglu M, Dudish-Poulsen S, Nelson D, et al. Sex and menstrual cycle differences in the subjective effects from smoked cocaine in humans. Exp Clin Psychopharmacol 1999;7(3):274–83.

15. Evans SM, Foltin RW. Exogenous progesterone attenuates the subjective effects of smoked cocaine in women, but not in men. Neuropsychopharmacology 2006; 31(3):659–74.

16. Perkins KA, Levine M, Marcus M. Tobacco withdrawal in women and menstrual cycle phase. J Consult Clin Psychol 2000;68(1):176–80.

17. Holdstock L, de Wit H. Effects of ethanol at four phases of the menstrual cycle. Psychopharmacology 2000;150:374–82.

18. Sinha R. How does stress increase risk of drug abuse and relapse? Psychopharmacology 2001;142:343–51.

19. Sinha R, Fox H, Hong KI, et al. Sex steroid hormones, stress response, and drug craving in cocaine-dependent women: implications for relapse susceptibility. Exp Clin Psychopharmacol 2007;15(5):445–52.

20. Back SE, Waldrop AE, Saladin ME, et al. Effects of gender and cigarette smoking on reactivity to psychological and pharmacological stress provocation. Psychoneuroendocrinology 2008;33(5):560–8.

21. Fox HC, Hong KA, Paliwal P, et al. Altered levels of sex and stress steroid hormones assessed daily over a 28-day cycle in early abstinent cocaine-dependent females. Psychopharmacology 2008;195(4):527–36.

22. Conway KP, Compton W, Stinson FS, et al. Lifetime comorbidity of DSM-IV mood and anxiety disorders and specific drug use disorders: results from the National Epidemiologic Survey on Alcohol and Related Conditions. J Clin Psychiatry 2006;67:247–57.

23. Goldstein RB. Comorbidity of substance use with independent mood and anxiety disorders in women: results from the National Epidemiologic Survey on Alcohol and Related Conditions. In: Brady KT, Back SE, Greenfield SF,

editors. Women and addiction: a comprehensive handbook. New York: Guilford Press; 2009. p. 173–92.

24. Greenfield SF. Assessment of mood and substance use disorders. In: Westermeyer J, Weiss RD, Ziedonis D, editors. Integrated treatment for mood and substance use disorders. Baltimore (MD): Johns Hopkins University Press; 2003. p. 432–67.

25. Pettinati HM, Dundon W, Lipkin C. Gender differences in response to sertraline pharmacotherapy in type A alcohol dependence. Am J Addict 2004;13(3):236–47.

26. Hudson JI, Hiripi E, Pope HG, et al. The prevalence and correlated of eating disorders in the National Comorbidity Survey Replication Study. Biol Psychiatry 2007;61:348–58.

27. Holderness CC, Brooks-Gunn J, Warren MP. Co-morbidity of eating disorders and substance abuse: review of the literature. Int J Eat Disord 1994;16:1–34.

28. Dohm FA, Striegal-Moore R, Wilfley DE, et al. Self harm and substance use in a community sample of black and white women with binge eating disorders or bulimia nervosa. Intl J Eat Disord 2002;32:389–400.

29. Bowers WA, Andersen AE, Evans K. Management of eating disorders: inpatient and partial hospital programs. In: Brewerton TD, editor. Clinical handbook of eating disorders: an integrated approach. New York: Marcel Dekker; 2004. p. 349–76.

30. Gordon SM, Johnson JA, Greenfield SF, et al. Assessment and treatment of co-occurring eating disorders in publicly funded addiction treatment programs. Psychiatr Serv 2008;59:1056–9.

31. Cottler LB, Compton WM, Mager D, et al. Post-traumatic stress disorder among substance users from the general population. Am J Psychiatry 1992;149:664–70.

32. Mills KL, Teesson M, Ross J, et al. Trauma, PTSD, and substance use disorders: findings from the Australian National Survey on mental health and well-being. Am J Psychiatry 2006;163:652–8.

33. Najavits LM, Weiss R, Shaw S. The link between substance abuse and posttraumatic stress disorder in women: a research review. Am J Addict 1997;6(4):237–83.

34. Brady KT, Dansky BS, Back SE, et al. Exposure therapy in the treatment of PSTD among cocaine-dependent individuals: preliminary findings. J Subst Abuse Treat 2001;21:47–54.

35. Back SE, Dansky BS, Carroll KM, et al. Exposure therapy in the treatment of PTSD among cocaine-dependent individuals: description of procedures. J Subst Abuse Treat 2001;21(1):35–45.

36. Hien DA. Trauma, posttraumatic stress disorder and addiction among women. In: Brady KT, Back SE, Greenfield SF, editors. Women and addiction: a comprehensive handbook. New York: Guilford Press; 2009. p. 242–56.

37. Najavits LM. Seeking safety: a treatment manual for PTSD and substance abuse. New York: Guilford Press; 2002.

38. Brady KT, Sonne SC, Roberts JM. Sertraline treatment of comorbid posttraumatic stress disorder and alcohol dependence. J Clin Psychiatry 1995;56:502–5.

39. Brady KT, Sonne S, Anton RF, et al. Sertraline in the treatment of co-occurring alcohol dependence and posttraumatic stress disorder. Alcohol Clin Exp Res 2005;29(3):395–401.

40. Labbate LA, Sonne SC, Randal CL, et al. Does comorbid anxiety or depression affect clinical outcomes in patients with post-traumatic stress disorder and alcohol use disorders? Compr Psychiatry 2004;45(4):304–10.

41. Keyes KM, Grant BF, Hasin DS. Evidence for a closing gender gap in alcohol use, abuse, and dependence in the United States population. Drug Alcohol Depend 2008;93:21–9.
42. Brady KT, Randall CL. Gender differences in substance use disorders. Psychiatr Clin North Am 1999;22:241–52.
43. Frezza M, Pozzato G, Chiesa L, et al. Abnormal serum gamma-glutamyltrans-peptidase in alcoholics. Clues to its explanation. Neth J Med 1989;34(1–2):22–8.
44. Annis HM, Graham JM. Profile types on the Inventory of Drinking Situations: implications for relapse prevention counseling. Psychol Addict Behav 1995;9: 176–82.
45. Stewart SH, Gavric D, Collins P. Women, girls, and alcohol. In: Brady KT, Back SE, Greenfield SF, editors. Women & addiction. New York: Guilford Press; 2009. p. 341–59.
46. Greenfield SF, Brooks AJ, Gordon SM, et al. Substance abuse treatment entry, retention, and outcome in women: a review of the literature. Drug Alcohol Depend 2007;86:1–21.
47. Ashley OS, Marsden ME, Brady TM. Effectiveness of substance abuse treatment programming for women: a review. Am J Drug Alcohol Abuse 2003;29:19–53.
48. Dahlgren L, Willander A. Are special treatment facilities for female alcoholics needed? A controlled 2-year follow-up study from a specialized female unit (EWA) versus a mixed male/female treatment facility. Alcohol Clin Exp Res 1989;13:499–504.
49. Greenfield SF, Trucco EM, McHugh RK, et al. The Women's Recovery Group Study: a stage I trial of women-focused group therapy for substance use disorders versus mixed-gender group drug counseling. Drug Alcohol Depend 2007; 90:39–47.
50. Substance Abuse and Mental Health Services Administration (SAMHSA). Results from the 2008 National Survey on Drug Use and Health: national findings. (Office of Applied Studies, NSDUH Series H-36, HHS Publication No. SMA 09-4434). Rockville (MD): US Department of Health and Human Services; 2009.
51. Lynch WJ. Sex differences in vulnerability to drug self-administration. Exp Clin Psychopharmacol 2006;14(1):34–41.
52. Westermeyer J, Boedicker AE. Course, severity, and treatment of substance abuse among women versus men. Am J Drug Alcohol Abuse 2000;26(4):523–35.
53. Substance Abuse and Mental Health Services Administration. Methamphetamine use. In the NSDUH report. Rockville (MD): Office of Applied Studies; 2007.
54. Della Grotta S, LaGasse LL, Arria AM, et al. Patterns of methamphetamine use during pregnancy: results from the Infant Development, Environment, and Lifestyle (IDEAL) Study. Matern Child Health J 2009. Available at: http://www.springerlink.com/content/l70457522w85q525/fulltext.html. Accessed January 28, 2010.
55. Terplan M, Smith EJ, Kozoloski MJ, et al. Methamphetamine use among pregnant women. Obstet Gynecol 2009;113:1285–91.
56. Sofuoglu M, Mitchell E, Kosten TR. Effects of progesterone treatment on cocaine responses in male and female cocaine users. Pharmacol Biochem Behav 2004; 78(4):699–705.
57. Hser YI, Evans E, Huang YC. Treatment outcomes among women and men methamphetamine abusers in California. J Subst Abuse Treat 2005;28(1):77–85.
58. Rowan-Szal GA, Joe GW, Simpson DD, et al. During-treatment outcomes among female methamphetamine-using offenders in prison-based treatments. J Offender Rehabil 2009;8:388–401.

59. Campbell UC, Morgan AD, Carroll ME. Sex differences in the effects of baclofen on the acquisition of intravenous cocaine self-administration in rats. Drug Alcohol Depend 2002;66(1):61–9.

60. Pettinati HM, Kampman KM, Lynch KG, et al. Gender differences with high-dose naltrexone in patients with co-occurring cocaine and alcohol dependence. J Subst Abuse Treat 2008;34(4):378–90.

61. Elkashef AM, Rawson RA, Anderson AL, et al. Bupropion for the treatment of methamphetamine dependence. Neuropsychopharmacology 2008;33(5): 1162–70.

62. Center on Addiction and Substance Abuse at Columbia University (2005, July). Under the counter: the diversion and abuse of controlled prescription drugs in the U.S. Available at: http://www.casacolumbia.org/absolutenm/articlefiles/380-Under%20the%20Counter%20-%20Diversion.pdf. Accessed September 15, 2008.

63. Tetrault JM, Desai RA, Becker WC, et al. Gender and non-medical use of prescription opioids: results from a national US survey. Addiction 2008;103: 258–68.

64. Colliver JD, Kroutil LA, Dai L, et al. Misuse of prescription drugs: data from the 2002, 2003, and 2004 National Surveys on Drug Use and Health. (DHHS Publication No. SMA 06-4192, Analytic Series A-28). Rockville (MD): Substance Abuse and Mental Health Services Administration, Office of Applied Studies; 2006.

65. McCabe SE, Cranford JA, Boyd CJ, et al. Motives, diversion and routes of administration associated with nonmedical use of prescription opioids. Addict Behav 2007;32(3):562–75.

66. Back SE, Payne R, Waldrop AE, et al. Prescription opioid aberrant behaviors: a pilot study of gender differences. Clin J Pain 2009;25:477–84.

67. Powis B, Griffiths P, Gossop M, et al. The differences between male and female drug users: community samples of heroin and cocaine users compared. Subst Use Misuse 1996;31(5):529–43.

68. Kelly SM, Schwartz RP, O'Grady KE, et al. Gender differences among in- and out-of-treatment opioid-addicted individuals. Am J Drug Alcohol Abuse 2009; 35(1):38–42.

69. Bryant J, Treload C. The gendered context of initiation to injecting drug use: evidence for women as active initiates. Drug Alcohol Rev 2007;26:287–93.

70. Frajzyngier V, Neaigus A, Gyarmathy VA, et al. Gender differences in injection risk behaviors at the first injection episode. Drug Alcohol Depend 2007;89: 145–52.

71. Breen C, Roxburgh A, Degenhardt L. Gender differences among regular injecting drug users in Sydney, Australia, 1996–2003. Drug Alcohol Rev 2005;24: 353–8.

72. Montgomery SB, Hyde J, De Rosa CJ, et al. Gender differences in HIV risk behaviors among young injectors and their social network members. Am J Drug Alcohol Abuse 2002;28(3):453–75.

73. Grant BF, Moore TC, Shepard J, et al. Source and accuracy statement for Wave 1 of the 2001–2002 National Epidemiologic Survey on Alcohol and Related Conditions. Bethesda (MD): National Institute on Alcohol abuse and Alcoholism; 2003.

74. Najavits LM, Rosier M, Nolan AL, et al. A new gender-based model for women's recovery from substance abuse: results of a pilot outcome study. Am J Drug Alcohol Abuse 2007;33(1):5–11.

75. Jones HE, Fitzgerald H, Johnson RE. Males and females differ in response to opioid agonist medications. Am J Addict 2005;14:223–33.

76. Substance Abuse and Mental Health Services Administration (SAMHSA). National Survey of Substance Abuse Treatment Services (N-SSATS). Rockville (MD): Department of Health and Human Services; 2005.

77. Substance Abuse and Mental Health Services Administration. The NSDUH Report: daily marijuana users based on the 2003 National Survey on Drug Use and Health: national findings. (Office of Applied Studies, NSDUH Series H-25, DHHS Publication No. SMA 04-3964). Rockville (MD): U.S. Department of Health and Human Services; 2004.

78. Van Etten ML, Anthony JC. Comparative epidemiology of initial drug opportunities and transitions to first use: marijuana, cocaine, hallucinogens, and heroin. Drug Alcohol Depend 1999;54:117–25.

79. Gfroerer JC, Wu LT, Penne MA. Initiation of marijuana use: trends, patterns, and implications. (DHHS Publication No. SMA 02-3711, Analytic Series: A-17). Rockville (MD): Substance Abuse and Mental Health Administration, Office of Applied Studies; 2002.

80. Griffin ML, Mendelson JH, Mello NK, et al. Marijuana use across the menstrual cycle. Drug Alcohol Depend 1986;18:213–24.

81. Lex BW, Mendelson JH, Bavli S, et al. Effects of acute marijuana smoking on pulse rate and mood states in women. Psychopharmacology 1984;84:178–87.

82. Terner JM, de Wit H. Menstrual cycle phase and responses to drugs of abuse in humans. Drug Alcohol Depend 2006;84:1–13.

83. Pope HG, Gruber AJ, Hudson JI, et al. Neuropsychological performance in long-term cannabis users. Arch Gen Psychiatry 2001;58:909–15.

84. Pope HG, Jacobs A, Mialet JP, et al. Evidence for a sex-specific residual effect of cannabis on visuospatial memory. Psychother Psychosom 1997;66:179–84.

85. Budney AJ, Higgins ST, Radonovich PL, et al. Adding voucher-based incentives to coping skills and motivational enhancement improves outcomes during treatment for marijuana dependence. J Consult Clin Psychol 2000;68:1051–61.

86. Haney M, Hart CL, Ward AS, et al. Nefazodone decreases anxiety during marijuana withdrawal in humans. Psychopharmacology 2003;165:157–65.

87. Haney M, Hart CL, Vosburg SK, et al. Marijuana withdrawal in humans: effects of oral THC or divalproex. Neuropsychopharmacology 2004;29:158–70.

88. Marijuana Treatment Project Research Group. Brief treatments for cannabis dependence: findings from a randomized multisite trial. J Consult Clin Psychol 2004;72:455–66.

89. Prescott E, Hippe M, Schnohr P, et al. Smoking and risk of myocardial infarction in women and men: longitudinal population study. Br Med J 1998;316:1043–7.

90. Dransfield MT, Davis JJ, Gerald LB, et al. Racial and gender differences in susceptibility to tobacco smoke among patients with chronic obstructive pulmonary disease. Respir Med 2006;100:1110–6.

91. International Early Lung Cancer Action Program Investigators. Women's susceptibility to tobacco carcinogens and survival after diagnosis of lung cancer. JAMA 2006;296:180–4.

92. Conklin CA. Environments as cues to smoke: implication for human extinction-based research and treatment. Exp Clin Psychopharmacol 2006;14:12–9.

93. Perkins KA, Jacobs L, Sanders M, et al. Sex differences in the subjective and reinforcing effects of cigarette nicotine dose. Psychopharmacology 2002;163:194–201.

94. Perkins KA, Doyle T, Ciccocioppo M, et al. Sex differences in the influence of nicotine and dose instructions on subjective and reinforcing effects of smoking. Psychopharmacology 2006;184:600–7.

95. Perkins KA, Gerlach D, Vender J, et al. Sex differences in the subjective and re-inforcing effects of visual and olfactory cigarette smoke stimuli. Nicotine Tob Res 2001;3:141–50.

96. Centers for Disease Control and Prevention. Cigarette smoking among adults—United States, 2005. MMWR Morb Mortal Wkly Rep 2006;55:1145–8.

97. Rodu B, Cole P. Declining mortality from smoking in the United States. Nicotine Tob Res 2007;9:781–4.

98. Pirie PL, Murray DM, Luepker RV. Gender differences in cigarette smoking and quitting in a cohort of young adults. Am J Public Health 1991;81:324–7.

99. Swan GE, Ward MM, Carmelli D, et al. Differential rates of relapse in subgroups of male and female smokers. J Clin Epidemiol 1993;46:1041–53.

100. Munafo M, Bradburn M, Bowes L, et al. Are there sex differences in transdermal nicotine replacement therapy patch efficacy? A meta-analysis. Nicotine Tob Res 2004;6:769–76.

101. Perkins KA, Scott J. Sex differences in long-term smoking cessation rates due to nicotine patch. Nicotine Tob Res 2008;10:1245–51.

102. Gonzales D, Rennard SI, Nides M, et al. Varenicline, an a4b2 nicotinic acetyl-choline receptor partial agonist, vs. sustained-release bupropion and placebo for smoking cessation. J Am Med Assoc 2006;296:47–55.

103. Scharf D, Shiffman S. Are there gender differences in smoking cessation, with and without bupropion? Pooled and meta-analyses of clinical trials of Bupropion SR. Addiction 2004;99:1462–9.

104. Cepeda-Benito A, Reynoso JT, Erath S. Meta-analysis of the efficacy of nicotine replacement therapy for smoking cessation: differences between men and women. J Consult Clin Psychol 2004;72:712–22.

105. England LJ, Grauman A, Qian C, et al. Misclassification of maternal smoking status and effects on an epidemiologic study of pregnancy outcomes. Nicotine Tob Res 2007;9:1005–13.

106. McBride CM, Pirie PL. Postpartum smoking relapse. Addict Behav 1990;15:165–8.

107. Office of Applied Studies, Substance Abuse and Mental Health Services Admin-istration. Treatment Episode Data Set (TEDS) highlights-2005 national admis-sions to substance abuse treatment services: 1995–2005. Rockville (MD): SAMHSA; 2006. Available at: http://oas.samhsa.gov/teds2k5/TEDSHi2k5.htm. Accessed November 8, 2007.

108. Green CA, Polen MR, Dickinson DM, et al. Gender differences in predictors of initiation, retention, and completion in an HMO-based substance abuse treat-ment program. J Subst Abuse Treat 2002;23:285–95.

109. Kelly PJ, Blacksin B, Mason E. Factors affecting substance abuse treatment completion for women. Issues Ment Health Nurs 2001;22:287–304.

110. Loneck B, Garrett J, Banks SM. Engaging and retaining women in outpatient alcohol and other drug treatment: the effect of referral intensity. Health Soc Work 1997;22:38–46.

111. Schmidt L, Weisner C. The emergence of problem-drinking women as a special population in need of treatment. In: Galanter M, editor. Recent developments in alcoholism: alcoholism and women. New York: Plenum Press; 1995. p. 309–34.

112. Harrison PM, Beck AJ. 2005. Prisoners in 2004 (BJS Bulletin, NCJ 210677). Washington, DC: Bureau of Justice Statistics, US Department of Justice. Avail-able at: http://www.ojp.gov/bjs/abstract/p04.htm. Accessed October 10, 2006.

113. Conners NA, Bradley RH, Mansell LW, et al. Children of mothers with serious substance abuse problems: an accumulation of risks. Am J Drug Alcohol Abuse 2004;30(1):85–100.

114. Grella CE, Scott CK, Foss MA, et al. Gender differences in drug treatment outcomes among participants in the Chicago Target Cities Study. Eval Program Plann 2003;26:297–310.
115. Lundgren LM, Schilling RF, Fitzgerald T, et al. Parental status of women injection drug users and entry to methadone maintenance. Subst Use Misuse 2003;38(8):1109–31.
116. Haller DL, Miles DR, Dawson KS. Factors influencing treatment enrollment by pregnant substance abusers. Am J Drug Alcohol Abuse 2003;29(1):117–31.
117. Chen X, Burgdorf K, Dowell K, et al. Factors associated with retention of drug abusing women in long-term residential treatment. Eval Program Plann 2004;27:205–12.
118. Greenfield SF, Grella CE. Alcohol & drug abuse: what is "women-focused" treatment for substance use disorders? Psychiatr Serv 2009;60:880–2.
119. Orwin RG, Francisco L, Bernichon T. Effectiveness of women's substance abuse treatment programs: a meta-analysis. Center for Substance Abuse Treatment. Arlington, Virginia: SAMHSA; 2001.
120. Volpicelli J, Markman I, Monterosso J, et al. Psychosocially enhanced treatment for cocaine-dependent mothers: evidence of efficacy. J Subst Abuse Treat 2000;18:41–9.
121. Smith WB, Weisner C. Women and alcohol problems: a critical analysis of the literature and unanswered questions. Alcohol Clin Exp Res 2001;24:1320–1.
122. Condelli WS, Koch MA, Fletcher B. Treatment refusal/attrition among adults randomly assigned to programs at a drug treatment campus. The New Jersey Substance Abuse Treatment Campus, Seacaucus, NJ. J Subst Abuse Treat 2000;18:395–407.
123. Strantz IH, Welch SP. Postpartum women in outpatient drug abuse treatment: correlates of retention/completion. J Psychoactive Drugs 1995;27:357–73.
124. Kaskutas LA, Zhang L, French MT, et al. Women's programs versus mixed-gender day treatment: results from a randomized study. Addiction 2005;100:60–9.
125. Greenfield SF, Potter JS, Lincoln MF, et al. High psychiatric severity is a moderator of substance abuse treatment outcomes among women in single vs. mixed gender group treatment. Am J Drug Alcohol Abuse 2008;34:594–602.
126. Cummings A, Gallop R. Self-efficacy and substance use outcomes for women in single gender versus mixed-gender group treatment. J Groups Addict Recover 2010, in press.
127. Connors GJ, Maisto SA, Zywiak WH. Male and female alcoholics' attributions regarding the onset and termination of relapses and the maintenance of abstinence. J Subst Abuse 1998;10:27–42.
128. Fals-Stewart W, Birchler GR, Kelley ML. Learning sobriety together: a randomized clinical trial examining behavioral couples therapy with alcoholic female patients. J Consult Clin Psychol 2006;74:579–91.

Gender Differences in Attention-Deficit/ Hyperactivity Disorder

Julia J. Rucklidge, PhD

KEYWORDS

• Gender • ADHD • Treatment • Review • Sex differences

Attention-deficit/hyperactivity disorder (ADHD) is one of the most common childhood disorders, characterized by problems with inattention, hyperactivity, and impulsivity[1]; the worldwide pooled prevalence estimate for childhood ADHD is 5.29%.[2] Throughout its history, ADHD has been considered to be a childhood disorder that, in only a small minority of cases, persists into adulthood[3]; however, the longitudinal studies published in the mid-1980s recognized that ADHD persists in a significant proportion of cases.[4] It is now estimated that as many as 4% to 5% of adults may suffer from ADHD.[5,6] Follow-up studies of boys and girls with ADHD from preschool to adolescence confirm that significant levels of impairment continue through; only a minority of such children are well adjusted in adolescence.[7]

In addition to the shift in conceptualization of ADHD as a disorder present across the lifespan, in the last 2 decades there has been a slowly growing body of research that has clearly identified that ADHD is not a predominantly male disorder, although estimates indicate that boys out-represent girls by 2:1 to 9:1 depending on the subtype and the setting (clinic-referred children are more likely to be male).[1,8–12] However, in adult samples, one study found a higher prevalence of ADHD in women than in men in a psychiatric outpatient service.[5] Staller and Faraone[13] estimated that 32 million females worldwide have ADHD, based on current information on prevalence and sex ratios, making the diagnosis of ADHD in females a major public health concern. Research suggests that referral bias continues to underidentify ADHD in females, particularly the younger ones.[14] Furthermore, research has challenged the

Author note: This review represents an update of a previous review: Rucklidge JJ. Review of gender differences in ADHD: implications for psychosocial treatments. Expert Rev Neurother 2008;8(4):643–55.

There are no financial disclosures.

Department of Psychology, University of Canterbury, Private Bag 4800, Christchurch 8140, New Zealand

E-mail address: julia.rucklidge@canterbury.ac.nz

earlier perceptions that females with ADHD are not as impaired by ADHD as their male counterparts. Studies have now convincingly shown that females with ADHD struggle significantly compared with females without ADHD in all areas of functioning, including academically, cognitively, psychosocially, and psychiatrically, with similar rates of problems as males with ADHD (see later discussion for an extensive review of this literature). However, concerns have been raised that only girls with substantial impairments are referred to clinics, complicating the interpretation of results in that clinic samples may mask true gender differences in the expression of ADHD across the sexes.[15] Therefore, it is important to be aware of the differential effect of ADHD on gender across these areas of functioning to optimize the effectiveness of psychosocial treatments for both sexes. This article addresses each of these areas of functioning in turn to inform how treatments may need to be modified depending on the gender and the developmental age of the individual being treated. If the information is available, specific groups are referred to directly and precisely (such as adolescent boys or women); however, if age is unknown or a statement applies to all age groups of a gender, the terms males and females are used. The terms gender and sex are used interchangeably. **Table 1** summarizes gender differences across these areas of functioning. This review is an update of a previous review.[16]

Table 1
Summary of sex differences across psychosocial, cognitive, and psychiatric variables (the reader is referred to the text for references used to develop this table)

Variable	Boys vs Girls	Men vs Women
Hyperactivity/impulsivity	M>F	M>F
Inattention	F>M	F>M
Tactile defensiveness (sensory processing)	F>M	?
Low self-esteem	F>M	F = M?
Poorer coping skills	F>M	F = M
Deficit in IQ	F>M	?
Deficit in executive functioning	F = M[a]	F = M
Motor function deficits	M>F	?
Anxiety	F>M (SAD only?)	=
Depression	F>M?	=
ODD/CD	M>F	M>F (criminal offenses and psychopathy)
Substance abuse	F>M	M>F
Treatment response to psychosocial interventions	F = M?	?
Adult psychiatric admissions	—	F>M
Rates of school suspensions	M>F	—
Childhood history of sexual abuse	—	F>M

Abbreviations: CD, conduct disorder; F, female; M, male; ODD, oppositional defiant disorder; SAD, separation anxiety disorder. ? indicates unknown, tentative (as based on only a limited number of studies), or inconclusive (eg, some studies report greater in males, others lower in males).
   [a] Processing speed may be slower in boys with ADHD and inhibition, vocabulary skills, and visual-spatial reasoning may be poorer in girls with ADHD; no other neuropsychological differences noted across gender.

GENDER DIFFERENCES IN PSYCHIATRIC FUNCTIONING

Research has consistently confirmed that when girls are diagnosed with ADHD they are more likely to be diagnosed with the predominantly inattentive type than boys,[17,18] although this finding was not found in a Puerto Rican community sample.[8] Parents and teachers of children with ADHD are more likely to rate boys as being more hyperactive than girls, and girls to be more inattentive than boys.[19] Gershon's[14] 2002 meta-analysis revealed some interesting findings on gender differences in psychiatric conditions. He found that depression and anxiety may be more problematic in girls with ADHD, with higher ratings of internalizing problems being rated in this group. This finding has been confirmed by more recent studies. For example, girls with ADHD who have been followed to adulthood are 2.4 times more likely to have a psychiatric admission in adulthood compared with boys with ADHD who have been followed to adulthood.[20] Of significant alarm are rates of self-reported self-harm and suicidal ideation. Both are significantly higher for adolescent boys and girls with ADHD compared with their non-ADHD peers, with one study reporting rates of current suicidal ideation for adolescent girls with ADHD at 17.9% and that of adolescent boys with ADHD at 5.7% compared with none of the adolescent boys without ADHD and 3.7% of the adolescent girls without ADHD.[21] The gender difference within the ADHD sample was not significant. However, although this same study found, like Gershon's[14] meta-analysis, that girls with ADHD self-report more symptoms of depression than boys with ADHD, there were no gender differences on psychiatric diagnoses. In contrast, Bauermeister and colleagues[8] found that when they analyzed their data with consideration of subtypes, the boys with ADHD combined type had higher rates of depressive disorders than the girls with ADHD combined type, even though, overall, there were no gender differences in rates of depression across the larger ADHD sample. They wondered whether this difference was due to more demoralizing experiences for the boys compared with the girls. This study also found that the girls with ADHD predominantly inattentive type had higher rates of separation anxiety disorder compared with the boys with ADHD predominantly inattentive type.

European,[22] Puerto Rican,[8] and American[17] data have found that girls and boys with ADHD had similar levels of coexisting psychiatric disorders in pediatric samples. All 3 of these studies involved nonreferred samples. Although overall it seems that gender differences in psychiatric comorbidities in ADHD samples may be small, the range of co-occurring psychiatric diagnoses is large in ADHD samples and percentage affected is important when considering treatment options. For example, rates of anxiety range from 18% to 29%, depression 8% to 65%, oppositional defiant disorder and conduct disorder 7% to 43%, learning disorders 20% to 55%, eating disorders 12% to 16%, substance use disorder 14% to 50%, and coordination problems 30% to 33%.[8,21–27]

Prospective studies of girls with ADHD confirm these cross-sectional data, showing that, in adolescence, ADHD was associated with a significantly increased lifetime risk for major depression, multiple anxiety disorders, bipolar disorder, oppositional defiant disorder, conduct disorder, tics, enuresis, language disorder, nicotine dependence, and substance dependence.[23,24] Other research from this same team found that the presence of an eating disorder in adolescent girls with ADHD further increased the risk of developing co-occurring mood and anxiety disorders and disruptive behavioral disorders (DBDs).[28] Other longitudinal research indicates that the impulsive symptoms of ADHD in adolescent girls are the best predictors of eating pathology, compared with the other symptoms.[29] Prospective studies indicate that childhood ADHD may predict more steeply rising symptoms of anxiety and depression during adolescence in girls than in boys with ADHD.[30] Studies of clinic samples of adults with ADHD confirm that women with ADHD were more likely to be diagnosed with an affective disorder compared with men with ADHD, 49% versus 28% respectively.[27] Rates and sex differences vary depending on whether the sample is from a community or a clinic. Based on a nationally representative sample of Australian youth, Graetz and colleagues[31] determined that case identification (ie, how the diagnosis was made), and not sample source, may be responsible for discrepant ADHD patterns between clinic- and community-based studies. Once this and other variables are controlled for, it seems that, with the possible exception of depression, co-occurring psychiatric diagnoses are similar across the sexes.

An area of particular concern relates to the high overlap between ADHD and post-traumatic stress disorder (PTSD). The psychological sequelae of childhood abuse are well documented to include depression, anxiety, behavioral problems, sleep and somatic complaints, aggression, and ADHD (see Ref.[32] for a review of this topic). This review highlighted the high degree of overlap between the symptoms of ADHD and PTSD, including inattention, restlessness, irritability, and impulsivity, but also raised the significant concern that assessments of ADHD do not systematically include an assessment of trauma; indeed, the Diagnostic and Statistical Manual IV (DSM-IV) does not include PTSD as a differential diagnosis. However, consider that inattention, one of the cardinal symptoms of ADHD, may result from reexperiencing hypervigilance, trauma, or avoidance of stimuli as a result of trauma.[32] Similarly, hyperarousal could be misconstrued as hyperactivity.[33] A recent study of children who experienced severe early deprivation shows that ADHD symptoms feature prominently as a characteristic outcome.[34]

Those studies that have investigated the prevalence of ADHD in a population of abused children have found a high overlap between ADHD and PTSD,[35] with one study reporting that 46% of their sample of children with a history of sexual abuse met ADHD criteria.[36] A recent study of men and women identified with ADHD in adulthood confirmed these findings. Rucklidge and colleagues[37] determined that 23.1% of the women with ADHD and 12.5% of the men with ADHD reported moderate to severe sexual abuse as children, compared with 2% to 5% in the controls. This 2:1 gender ratio of sexual abuse mirrors the ratio found in the controls, and the women with ADHD reported significantly more sexual abuse than the other 3 groups. For the entire ADHD sample, 56% reported moderate to severe abuse and neglect of some form during childhood. More research needs to investigate whether ADHD places a child at higher risk of abuse or whether the sequelae of abuse mimics the symptoms of ADHD; or perhaps, more likely, that the relationship is bidirectional. Regardless, it is an area that has been under-investigated to date.

It has been consistently reported that boys with ADHD tend to be more disruptive, engage in more rule breaking, and are more likely to have comorbid DBDs,[38–40] a difference that has contributed to the later referral and diagnosis of ADHD in girls.[38] Furthermore, those with DBD are more likely to have more severe ADHD. However, some studies show that this sex differences is more likely to be present based on teacher reports than parental reports,[41] and other research finds no differences between the sexes on comorbid conduct problems.[8,30,42] However, although Bauermeister and colleagues[8] did not find gender differences in their community sample of children with ADHD on rates of DBD, they did find that boys were more likely to be suspended from school than girls with ADHD, hypothesizing that boys with ADHD present with higher rates of annoyance and distress to teachers. Other researchers have determined that covert symptoms of conduct disorder are more likely to be found in families of girls with ADHD.[43] Rates of criminality, violent crimes, and prison sentences have been found to be higher in men with ADHD compared with women with ADHD.[27] Studies of psychopathic traits in nonincarcerated adults shows that men with ADHD have higher scores of psychopathy compared with men without ADHD; these differences do not exist when women with ADHD are compared with women without ADHD.[44]

Substance abuse is also of significant concern in ADHD populations, with some research showing higher rates in girls versus boys with ADHD,[25] although it does seem that the connection between ADHD and substance abuse disorders is largely driven by the presence of comorbid conduct disorder. However, a study investigating alcohol and drug abuse in adults found that the frequency of both problems was significantly higher in men with ADHD than in women with ADHD.[27] A recent study suggested that women with ADHD symptoms may underestimate hangovers and that this underestimation was related to increased drinking compared with women with fewer ADHD symptoms.[45] This relationship was not studied in men.

GENDER DIFFERENCES IN PSYCHOSOCIAL FUNCTIONING

There have been hundreds of studies investigating the psychosocial effect of ADHD, but far fewer have considered gender as a moderator of outcome. In general, ADHD greatly affects all areas of psychosocial functioning but, for the most part, ADHD expresses itself similarly in males and females. The meta-analyses[14,46] have found few differences in social functioning of boys with ADHD compared with girls with ADHD, with the exception that the boys have been found to be more aggressive with peers than the girls. Studies of adolescents have found that adolescent girls with ADHD feel more ineffective, have lower self-esteem, and are more affected by negative life events compared with adolescent boys with ADHD,[21] although these differences are no longer evident in adult gender-comparison studies,[47] with men and women with ADHD reporting significant and similar psychosocial problems compared with controls. Rucklidge and colleagues[47] investigated the effect of a late diagnosis in adults with ADHD, determining that men and women identified with ADHD as adults struggle in all areas of functioning including negative attributions about themselves, poorer coping strategies, significantly lower self-esteem, and hopelessness for the future compared with their non-ADHD counterparts; however, it is unknown whether similar problems would be reported, and to what degree, in adults with ADHD who were identified with ADHD in childhood and who had received adequate treatment of their condition.

Those studies that have focused on girls with ADHD can inform us about specific issues relevant to this population compared with girls without ADHD; however, the differences identified could equally apply to boys. Findings of relevance to treatment include high rates of adoption in the girls with ADHD,[15] higher anticipation of negative peer responses,[48] and high rates of aggression and documented histories of child abuse in the girls with combined type, as well as more social isolation being reported in the girls with inattentive type.[15] Studies that have investigated sex and subtype effects within the same study indicate that subtype is a more powerful contributor to ADHD phenomenology than sex.[26,49] Similar findings have been found when considering comorbid profiles and their effect on personality.[50]

Attributions have been an interest of several research groups, and general findings indicate that individuals with ADHD (regardless of gender) typically hold a more positive illusory self-perception than controls, regardless of who the rater is and regardless of the deficits present in the children.[51,52] These children typically inflate their self-perceptions of behaviors and achievements and do so to an even greater extent in domains of greatest deficit. For example, Hoza and colleagues[51] found that children with ADHD who had conduct problems were even more likely to exhibit the greatest positive illusory thinking of their conduct behavior. One exception was noted: when a teacher criterion was used; girls in general (ADHD and non-ADHD) had less inflated self-perceptions regarding their behavior and were more likely than boys to have derogatory perceptions of their own physical appearance. Knowing that the typical children in this study were fairly accurate in their self-perceptions, it followed that the self-perceptions of children with ADHD were likely to be maladaptive.[51]

Some interesting findings have come from Abikoff and colleagues[38] who, through observational studies in the classroom, found that, although girls with ADHD are generally less physically aggressive than boys with ADHD, they are verbally aggressive (teasing, taunting, name calling) compared with girls without ADHD, a behavior that will likely result in increased rates of peer rejection. A longitudinal study of girls with and without ADHD showed that, although the adolescent girls with ADHD were reported to have more overt and relational aggression compared with the adolescent girls without ADHD,[53] these behaviors were not related to measures of social information-processing (SIP) measures 4.5 years earlier.[54] SIP (one of the strong predictors of aggression) was not found to be a good predictor in this sample. Other problems that may be more specific to girls with ADHD include poor self-efficacy, ineffective coping strategies, disrupted social support structures, a lack of confidence in social relationships,[21,55,56] and greater disturbance in sensory processing.[57] There is also some evidence to suggest that divorce in families may have a greater effect on girls than on boys with ADHD.[58]

GENDER DIFFERENCES IN COGNITIVE FUNCTIONING

Several studies have confirmed that girls with ADHD are more impaired in cognitive functioning compared with girls without ADHD.[59–61] Furthermore, this impairment has been confirmed to persist for at least a 5-year span, based on 2 longitudinal studies of girls with and without ADHD tested 5 years apart.[62,63] Two meta-analyses have been conducted to date on gender differences within ADHD,[14,46] and these have indicated that girls with ADHD display higher rates of speech and language disorders and delays, and may also have more compromised cognitive and intellectual abilities compared with boys with ADHD. Other gender differences noted in adolescent samples include poorer processing speed in adolescent boys with ADHD, and lower vocabulary scores in adolescent girls with ADHD[21] and more impaired inhibition.[59] Lower scores on block design, a measure of perceptual and visual-spatial reasoning, have been noted in girls with ADHD compared with boys with ADHD; performance on all other measures of cognitive functioning were similar across genders.[64] Results from the Multimodal Treatment Study of ADHD (MTA) found that girls with ADHD made fewer errors on the Conners Continuous Performance Test than did boys with ADHD.[65] A recent study investigating motor function indicated greater difficulties in motor control and dysrhythmia in boys compared with girls with ADHD, consistent with neuroimaging studies suggesting more neurological anomalies in boys compared with girls.[66]

However, most studies have found few or no cognitive differences across the sexes in ADHD populations,[41,49] with significant cognitive impairments across most areas of functioning (planning, set-shifting, working memory, attention, response inhibition, executive function, naming speed, and so forth) evident in males and females with ADHD across the lifespan compared with individuals without ADHD.[59,61,67–70] Type I errors could explain the few differences that have been noted given the large number of analyses typically reported in these studies. Stimulant medications have been known to influence outcomes of some studies (eg, Ref.[60]), emphasizing the importance of considering the mitigating effect that medications can have on cognitive test results. Nevertheless, similar cognitive profiles can generally be expected in individuals with ADHD, regardless of the sex of the individual concerned.

One potential caveat is noted. A recent study that divided the girls and boys with ADHD according to subtype found that although there were no overall differences between the sexes in cognitive functioning, when ADHD combined type girls were compared with ADHD combined type boys, the boys performed better on verbal fluency.[71] In contrast, the girls with predominantly inattentive type ADHD were compared with the boys with predominantly inattentive type ADHD. The girls performed better than the boys on verbal fluency, suggesting that the children with the ADHD subtype less common for their sex may have more relative deficits.[71]

GENDER DIFFERENCES IN TREATMENT

ADHD is a heterogeneous disorder that has led to the development of more homogeneous subtypes based on the inattentive and hyperactive/impulsive symptoms. These subtypes can be further conceptualized as those with and without comorbid disorders and, even further, the specific type of comorbidity (ie, anxiety versus disruptive behavioral problems). Is there a need to consider whether females with ADHD should receive a different form of treatment or specific considerations that would not normally apply to males? Can the treatments described be equally implemented with all individuals affected by ADHD, regardless of gender?

Generally, the literature has not provided a clear answer to this question, as gender by treatment effects, the moderating role of sex, and sex comparisons have largely been ignored in the treatment literature. However, the trend seems to indicate that males with ADHD are more similar to than different from females with ADHD, that they struggle with many of the same issues, and, therefore, treatments should be similarly effective. One study that did look at treatment adherence did not find a gender difference.[72] It is probably more pertinent to consider co-occurring problems and the developmental age of the individual being treated than the specific sex. There is no evidence of a treatment by gender interaction when all other variables are equal.

Pharmacological treatments for ADHD typically enhance dopamine or noradrenaline release presynaptically. In studies that have looked at gender differences in response to pharmacological (eg, methylphenidate, dexamphetamine) treatments, gender differences have not been observed[73,74] in pediatric and adult samples. There is some indication that females may need higher doses of methylphenidate compared with males because of more extensive first-pass metabolism.[75] Quinn[76] recommends, based on clinical experience, that cyclical variations in the menstrual cycle should be considered when deciding the optimal dose of medication for postpubescent girls and women. Studies confirm that estragon may enhance the response to stimulants, but that this effect may be dampened by the presence of progesterone.[77] Overall, although not directly assessed, these treatments seem equally safe for both genders.[13] However, there are no controlled studies on the use of these treatments while pregnant or lactating, and therefore prescribing physicians need to be cautious about using these medications with female patients who might be pregnant or breastfeeding. Quinn[78] emphasizes the importance of considering the high rate of eating problems in girls with ADHD and reports on cases in which treating the ADHD with medicines reduces impulsive eating.

To the best of the author's knowledge, only 1 study has had a sample large enough to investigate the moderating effect that gender may have on treatment response to psychosocial interventions.[79,80] The MTA study determined that gender did not moderate outcome and effect sizes confirmed this finding; however, 80% of that sample were male, somewhat limiting the generalizability of this finding. No other studies have investigated gender differences in response to nonmedical (psychosocial) treatments, most studies simply not having enough power to do such analyses, leaving it largely unknown whether gender differences exist in treatment response. Nangle and colleagues[81] challenged researchers to consider gender as a moderator of outcome to social skills training, arguing that boys show more overt forms of aggression, such as hitting and pushing, than girls, and therefore treatment approaches may need to be modified depending on the sex of the child being treated. However, no one to date, other than the MTA group, has taken up this challenge. de Boo and Prins,[82] in their recent review of social-skills training in ADHD, confirmed that, for those treatment studies that have included boys and girls, gender differences have not been included in treatment results. Even if these comparisons were included, power would likely severely limit any conclusions that could be drawn, given that samples are typically predominantly male. Furthermore, it is unknown whether women with ADHD respond differently to psychosocial treatments compared with men with ADHD. One recent longitudinal study of the relationship between SIP and later reports of aggression suggested that practitioners who are considering conducting interventions that target SIP, based on literature that shows that it may be helpful in boys to reduce aggression, need to be aware that it may be less relevant when targeting relational aggression in adolescent girls with ADHD.[54] More studies with larger samples and equal representation across gender are urgently needed.

Others emphasize the gender-appropriateness hypothesis when treating children with ADHD.[83] Although Diamantopoulou and colleagues[83] did not find recorded differences in self-perceptions of children with high levels of ADHD, their peers were more likely to be tolerant of higher levels of ADHD symptoms among boys than among girls; the investigators suggested that educators be aware of the influence that gender biasing may have in peer relations in girls with ADHD and the differential effect that ADHD symptoms may have on perceptions of peers.[83]

Of further relevance to treatment are the findings that adolescent girls with ADHD may have difficulty modifying their social behavior in response to shifting social demands, and may also be slow to recognize social cues, giving rise to misunderstandings. As such, interventions may need to include modules of social recognition, skills, and behavior.[55] Furthermore, given that these girls may tend to misjudge situations because their impulsive nature leads them to make fast decisive solutions based on less information than their peers, interventions could also target accurate appraisals of events, the inhibition of rapid but maladaptive responding, and the selection of more appropriate coping strategies such that they better deal with stressful situations.[55]

In contrast, adults with ADHD seem not to hold these positive illusory biases,[47] and therefore it will be important to assist such clients with developing a sense of personal control over life events to mitigate the feelings of helplessness often seen in these adults. Particularly if ADHD went undiagnosed for an extended period of time (which may be more likely for women than for men), corrections in interpretations of symptoms are important given that some adults with ADHD impairments attribute their problems to a character or moral flaw within themselves, compounding feelings of guilt and low self-esteem.[84] Furthermore, spouses or partners of people with attentional impairments can compound these feelings of inadequacy and blame, resulting in substantial interpersonal problems in relationships. Consider also the research literature that indicates that adults with ADHD report being victims of child abuse to a greater extent than adults without ADHD.[37] Given these high rates of reports of being victims of child abuse, it is vital that clinicians ask about histories of child abuse when working with adult clients with ADHD to incorporate this information in case conceptualization and treatment planning. Histories of sexual abuse are particularly relevant when working with women with ADHD.[37]

As the research consistently shows that girls, and particularly women, when diagnosed with ADHD, are more likely to be identified as inattentive compared with boys and men diagnosed with ADHD, the psychological struggles they face could be different from those of boys and men with ADHD. For example, the inattentive type is known to be slower to be identified than the hyperactive/impulsive type or combined type, and, therefore, with every year that goes by without a diagnosis, the more likely it is that there will be the development of secondary emotional problems and a longer history of failure, misattributions, relationship problems, and feelings of under achievement. Cognitive-behavioral therapy would be most useful in such cases as it takes into account the individual's unique circumstances, longstanding frustrations, and associated negative belief systems and developmental experiences, and focuses on assisting the individual to more effectively manage ADHD.[85] Other investigators wonder whether high IQ in girls masks ADHD so that they only come to clinical attention when there are symptoms of depression or anxiety.[86] Even then, ADHD may be overlooked.

Similarly, some co-occurring problems seem to be more common in girls with ADHD than boys with ADHD (eg, depression, anxiety), but these disorders should nevertheless be targeted in treatment with boys. Although not as common as in girls, it is possible that these comorbidities may still present as problematic in boys with ADHD and may need to be considered as increased, particularly in comparison with same-sex peers without ADHD.

Although treatments could be similar for both genders, a referral bias to treatment does exist, in that boys are more likely to be referred for treatment compared with girls with ADHD. The differing rates are substantial. One study found that only 6% of girls with ADHD were prescribed medication and 8% received counseling. In contrast, 47% of boys with ADHD received medication and 38% received counseling.[42] These researchers found that it was an over reporting of problems by teachers in the boys that accounted for this discrepancy. Another study found that, in adults, the men with ADHD were more likely to have received stimulant treatment of their symptoms in childhood compared with the women with ADHD, 25% versus 12% respectively.[27] Ultimately, despite the likelihood that females will respond to treatments equally to males, it is a public health concern that they are being under treated. Hyperactivity is often identified as the reason why boys are more likely to be referred for treatment compared with girls. A recent study, using clinical vignettes, found that it was not the presence of hyperactivity that influenced whether a teacher or parent referred a child for treatment; they identified that they felt girls with ADHD were less likely to benefit from educational treatments compared with boys with ADHD.[87] Further work is required in educating parents and teachers about the effectiveness of treatments, regardless of gender, to reduce the gender gaps in referral rates.

SUMMARY AND FUTURE DIRECTIONS

ADHD is a complex neurodevelopmental syndrome of impaired executive functioning that significantly affects, particularly over time, an individual's ability to successfully negotiate the world. Treatments need to be integrative, multimodal, and the case conceptualized with consideration of all the individual variables present. Although not all cases of ADHD need treatment beyond medication, many do, and the more complex presentations need to be identified so that these clients can be offered a combination of treatments with good empirical base, such that they can make informed decisions on treatment choices.

With queries related to the long-term effectiveness of front-line medications for the treatment of ADHD,[79] there is the challenge of investigating alternative treatment options. Psychosocial treatments have a solid grounding in empirically based research. Part of a clinician's role is to assist individuals with ADHD to find a good fit between their symptoms and their environment. Adults with ADHD are particularly likely to hold core beliefs of inadequacy and display concomitant behaviors, such as avoidance, that exacerbate the core symptoms of inattention, hyperactivity, and impulsivity.[88] Psychosocial treatments, regardless of gender, target these secondary problems. Particularly for those identified in adulthood with ADHD, instilling hope and reframing the past may be some of the more important foci of the early stages of therapy. However, to date, whether psychosocial treatments are equally effective for the treatment of ADHD across the sexes is largely unknown. Moreover, knowing that girls with ADHD may be less likely to be referred for treatment,[89,90] better ways must be found to reach this under served group of our population.

ADHD is the most commonly studied childhood psychiatric disorder and, as such, a significant amount is known of how it presents and what impairments are likely to coexist alongside it. Nevertheless, until recently, few researchers considered female profiles of ADHD, and so less is known about gender differences. Although there has been an impressive surge in research in the last decade, with more researchers considering sex effects and sex differences, it should be a standard comparison in studies in which samples are large enough to study such differences. However, small numbers of females and referral bias continue to hamper our ability to make good predictions about how the sexes may differ in various assessment and treatment approaches to ADHD. Most treatment studies are simply underpowered for anything other than main effect analyses.

In the future, continued emphasis on the development of separate standards for measurement for separate groups (ie, boys, girls; men, women) is needed. Although there has been an increasing appreciation of the importance of using separate standards when rating ADHD behaviors[91] (eg, Conners Scales have different norms for males and females across age groups), the DSM-IV uses cut-offs that are irrespective of gender. Research needs to focus on the development of gender-appropriate diagnostic criteria and diagnostic tools. Indeed, the current diagnostic criteria impede our ability to have a fresh look at gender differences. Attempts have been made to identify how ADHD symptoms might be better described to pick up the expression of these symptoms in girls,[92,93] given that research is finding that DSM-IV items may be better descriptors of ADHD in boys than in girls.[93] For example, Ohan and Johnston[93] suggested female-sensitive items for ADHD would include "giggles or talks excessively," "writes or passes notes instead of completing homework," and "changes friends impulsively or without thinking." Initial studies validating such items look promising; it will be intriguing to see whether this research has any effect on rating scales and DSM-V. Along a similar line, researchers are increasingly conscious of assessing impairment, such as family functioning, peer relationships, academic functioning, and how these variables may influence treatment outcome.[94,95] Future research will highlight whether gender differences are noted in the extent to which impairment affects developmental trajectories for boys and girls with ADHD.

Prospective studies, like the recently published study by Lahey and colleagues[30] that investigated sex differences in the predictive validity of DSM-IV symptoms, are likely to shed light on the role that development plays on the course of ADHD across genders, as well as expand on the role that sex differences in neurophysiological correlates of ADHD (eg, Ref.[96]) may play in prognosis, impairment, and clinical correlates. Lahey and colleagues[30] were the first to document the homotypic continuity (ie, childhood ADHD predicting future ADHD) and the heterotypic continuity (ie, childhood ADHD predicting future symptoms of other mental disorders) of ADHD for both sexes over a 9-year period, finding that girls with ADHD may have more steeply rising rates of depression and anxiety over time compared with boys with ADHD. Ongoing follow-ups of such carefully selected samples over time will be vital to the overall understanding of how different variables (eg, genetic factors, environmental factors, presence of other disorders) interact and influence the lifetime progression of this disorder. Collaborations across multiple sites, cultures, and countries will be essential to increase the sample sizes, as well as provide greater validity to any differences found.

There are ongoing debates about whether those individuals with inattentive ADHD are different from those with hyperactivity/impulsivity. Should these distinctions become more apparent with research, then treatments will need to be adjusted according to the subtype being presented. Barkley[97] speculated whether those with inattentive ADHD have a sluggish cognitive tempo and whether specific studies that divide ADHD groups into this subtype versus the more classic subtype will influence treatment outcomes. More studies investigating the influence of subtypes on treatment outcomes for males and females are required.

ADHD continues to go unidentified in adult populations, often because mental health professionals who primarily work with adult populations believe that ADHD is not a psychiatric disorder that affects adults. Continuing education on how this disorder manifests in adults is essential. Furthermore, because women may present with different histories from men, including less hyperactivity, more abuse, and perhaps greater problems with mood instability, those working in general psychiatry need to be alert to the more subtle expressions of the disorder in women, even though these are no less impairing than the more hyperactive and impulsive presentations. Consideration of the high prevalence of ADHD in prison populations[98] has yet to be fully appreciated, particularly in terms of which treatments will work and how prisoners can have better access to psychiatric and psychological treatments. With greater education of the public and professionals alike comes hope that those affected with ADHD will be recognized, understood within the complexities of their individual difficulties, life histories, and deficits, and offered treatments that have been empirically shown to be effective for females and males alike.

SUMMARY

- ADHD in males and females is more similar than different
- Boys with ADHD have more comorbid externalizing problems and girls with ADHD (especially adolescents) have more comorbid internalizing problems such as depression and anxiety (although nonreferred samples do not find gender differences in rates of coexisting psychiatric disorders in pediatric samples)
- Early recognition is vital to attempt to prevent the trajectory of increased morbidity associated with ADHD for both genders
- Treatment should be tailored according to subtype, level and type of impairment, and comorbid profiles rather than based on gender

- Consideration of subtype is important, as it may flag specific areas of concern and identify areas that may need to be directly targeted (such as improving attention or addressing hyperactive behaviors)
- Diagnostic criteria for ADHD should be adjusted according to gender, and possibly lowered or adapted for girls; alternative assessment methods that include descriptions of ADHD symptoms adapted to girls could be considered
- It is important to consider the timing of the diagnosis, as the longer it has gone undiagnosed, the more likely there will be psychosocial problems related to negative attributional styles and self-blame
- Routine inquiries about childhood abuse in cases of adult ADHD are strongly recommended
- The early diagnosis of ADHD may facilitate the early identification of girls who are at high risk for future mental disorders
- Although ADHD seems more similar than different in males and females and therefore psychosocial treatments should be equally effective across genders, gender has not typically been considered as a moderator of treatment outcome. Consequently, gender-by-treatment effects are largely unknown.

REFERENCES

1. American Psychiatric Association. Diagnostic and statistical manual of mental disorders. DSM-IV-TR, 4th edition, Text revision. Washington, DC: American Psychiatric Association; 2000.
2. Polanczyk G, de Lima MS, Horta BL, et al. The worldwide prevalence of ADHD: a systematic review and metaregression analysis. Am J Psychiatry 2007;164(6): 942–8.
3. American Psychiatric Association. Diagnostic and statistical manual of mental disorders. 3rd edition. Washington: American Psychiatric Association; 1980.
4. Gittelman R, Mannuzza S, Shenker R, et al. Hyperactive boys almost grown up: I. Psychiatric status. Arch Gen Psychiatry 1985;42(10):937–47.
5. Almeida Montes LG, Hernandez Garca AO, Ricardo-Garcell J. ADHD prevalence in adult outpatients with nonpsychotic psychiatric illnesses. J Atten Disord 2007; 11(2):150–6.
6. Kessler RC, Adler L, Barkley R, et al. The prevalence and correlates of adult ADHD in the United States: results from the National Comorbidity Survey Replication. Am J Psychiatry 2006;163(4):716–23.
7. Lee SS, Lahey BB, Owens EB, et al. Few preschool boys and girls with ADHD are well-adjusted during adolescence. J Abnorm Child Psychol 2008;36(3):373–83.
8. Bauermeister JJ, Shrout PE, Chávez L, et al. ADHD and gender: are risks and sequela of ADHD the same for boys and girls? J Child Psychol Psychiatry 2007;48(8):831–9.
9. Huss M, Holling H, Kurth BM, et al. How often are German children and adolescents diagnosed with ADHD? Prevalence based on the judgment of health care professionals: results of the German health and examination survey (KiGGS). Eur Child Adolesc Psychiatry 2008;17(1):52–8.
10. MTA Cooperative Group. A 14-month randomized clinical trial of treatment strategies for attention-deficit/hyperactivity disorder. Arch Gen Psychiatry 1999; 56(12):1073–86.
11. Robison LM, Skaer TL, Sclar DA, et al. Is attention deficit hyperactivity disorder increasing among girls in the US? Trends in diagnosis and the prescribing of stimulants. CNS Drugs 2002;16(2):129–37.

12. Szatmari P, Offord DR, Boyle MH. Correlates, associated impairments and patterns of service utilization of children with attention deficit disorder: findings from the Ontario Child Health Study. J Child Psychol Psychiatry 1989;30(2):205–17.
13. Staller J, Faraone SV. Attention-deficit hyperactivity disorder in girls: epidemiology and management. CNS Drugs 2006;20(2):107–23.
14. Gershon J. A meta-analytic review of gender differences in ADHD. J Atten Disord 2002;5(3):143–54.
15. Hinshaw SP. Preadolescent girls with attention-deficit/hyperactivity disorder: I. Background characteristics, comorbidity, cognitive and social functioning, and parenting practices. J Consult Clin Psychol 2002;70(5):1086–98.
16. Rucklidge JJ. Gender differences in ADHD: implications for psychosocial treatments. Expert Rev Neurother 2008;8(4):643–55.
17. Biederman J, Kwon A, Aleardi M, et al. Absence of gender effects on attention deficit hyperactivity disorder: findings in nonreferred subjects. Am J Psychiatry 2005;162(6):1083–9.
18. Weiss MD, Worling DE, Wasdell MB. A chart review study of the Inattentive and Combined Types of ADHD. J Atten Disord 2003;7(1):1–9.
19. Papageorgiou V, Kalyva E, Dafoulis V, et al. Differences in parents' and teachers' ratings of ADHD symptoms and other mental health problems. Eur J Psychiatr 2008;22(4):200–10.
20. Dalsgaard S, Mortensen PB, Frydenberg M, et al. Conduct problems, gender and adult psychiatric outcome of children with attention-deficit hyperactivity disorder. Br J Psychiatry 2002;181(5):416–21.
21. Rucklidge JJ, Tannock R. Psychiatric, psychosocial, and cognitive functioning of female adolescents with ADHD. J Am Acad Child Adolesc Psychiatry 2001;40(5):530–40.
22. Novik TS, Hervas A, Ralston SJ, et al. Influence of gender on attention-deficit/hyperactivity disorder in Europe - ADORE. Eur Child Adolesc Psychiatry 2006;15(Suppl1):5–24.
23. Biederman J, Ball SW, Monuteaux MC, et al. New insights into the comorbidity between ADHD and major depression in adolescent and young adult females. J Am Acad Child Adolesc Psychiatry 2008;47(4):426–34.
24. Biederman J, Monuteaux MC, Mick E, et al. Psychopathology in females with attention-deficit/hyperactivity disorder: a controlled, five-year prospective study. Biol Psychiatry 2006;60(10):1098–105.
25. Disney ER, Elkins IJ, McGue M, et al. Effects of ADHD, conduct disorder, and gender of substance use and abuse in adolescence. Am J Psychiatry 1999;156(10):1515–21.
26. Levy F, Hay DA, Bennett KS, et al. Gender differences in ADHD subtype comorbidity. J Am Acad Child Adolesc Psychiatry 2005;44(4):368–76.
27. Rasmussen K, Levander S. Untreated ADHD in adults: are there sex differences in symptoms, comorbidity, and impairment? J Atten Disord 2009;12(4):353–60.
28. Biederman J, Ball SW, Monuteaux MC, et al. Are girls with ADHD at risk for eating disorders? Results from a controlled, five-year prospective study. J Dev Behav Pediatr 2007;28(4):302–7.
29. Mikami AY, Hinshaw SP, Patterson KA, et al. Eating pathology among adolescent girls with attention-deficit/hyperactivity disorder. J Abnorm Psychol 2008;117(1):225–35.
30. Lahey BB, Hartung CM, Loney J, et al. Are there sex differences in the predictive validity of DSM-IV ADHD among younger children? J Clin Child Adolesc Psychol 2007;36(2):113–26.

31. Graetz BW, Sawyer MG, Baghurst P, et al. Are ADHD gender patterns moderated by sample source? J Atten Disord 2006;10(1):36–43.

32. Weinstein D, Staffelbach D, Biaggio M. Attention-deficit hyperactivity disorder and posttraumatic stress disorder: differential diagnosis in childhood sexual abuse. Clin Psychol Rev 2000;20:359–78.

33. Glod CA, Teicher MH. Relationship between early abuse, posttraumatic stress disorder, and activity levels in prepubertal children. J Am Acad Child Adolesc Psychiatry 1996;35:1384–93.

34. Sonuga-Barke EJ, Rubia K. Inattentive/overactive children with histories of profound institutional deprivation compared with standard ADHD cases: a brief report. Child Care Health Dev 2008;34(5):596–602.

35. Merry SN, Andrews LK. Psychiatric status of sexually abused children 12 months after disclosure of abuse. J Am Acad Child Adolesc Psychiatry 1994;33:939–46.

36. McLeer SV, Callaghan M, Henry D, et al. Psychiatric disorders in sexually abused children. J Am Acad Child Adolesc Psychiatry 1994;35:313–7.

37. Rucklidge JJ, Brown DL, Crawford S, et al. Retrospective reports of childhood trauma in adults with ADHD. J Atten Disord 2006;9:631–41.

38. Abikoff HB, Jensen PS, Arnold LLE, et al. Observed classroom behavior of children with ADHD: relationship to gender and comorbidity. J Abnorm Child Psychol 2002;30(4):349–59.

39. Gaub M, Carlson CL. Gender differences in ADHD: a meta-analysis and critical review. J Am Acad Child Adolesc Psychiatry 1997;36(8):1036–45.

40. Ruchkin V, Lorberg B, Koposov R, et al. ADHD symptoms and associated psychopathology in a community sample of adolescents from the European north of Russia. J Atten Disord 2008;12(1):54–63.

41. Hartung CM, Willcutt EG, Lahey BB, et al. Sex differences in young children who meet criteria for attention deficit hyperactivity disorder. J Clin Child Adolesc Psychol 2002;31(4):453–64.

42. Derks EM, Hudziak JJ, Boomsma DI. Why more boys than girls with ADHD receive treatment: a study of Dutch twins. Twin Res Hum Genet 2007;10(5):765–70.

43. Monuteaux MC, Fitzmaurice G, Blacker D, et al. Specificity in the familial aggregation of overt and covert conduct disorder symptoms in a referred attention-deficit hyperactivity disorder sample. Psychol Med 2004;34(6):1113–27.

44. Eisenbarth H, Alpers GW, Conzelmann A, et al. Psychopathic traits in adult ADHD patients. Pers Individ Dif 2008;45(6):468–72.

45. Rodriguez CA, Span SA. ADHD symptoms, anticipated hangover symptoms, and drinking habits in female college students. Addict Behav 2008;33(8):1031–8.

46. Carlson CL, Tamm L, Gaub M. Gender differences in children with ADHD, ODD, and co-occurring ADHD/ODD identified in a school population. J Am Acad Child Adolesc Psychiatry 1997;36(12):1706–14.

47. Rucklidge JJ, Brown D, Crawford S, et al. Attributional styles and psychosocial functioning of adults with ADHD. J Atten Disord 2007;10(3):288–98.

48. Thurber JR, Heller TL, Hinshaw SP. The social behaviors and peer expectation of girls with attention deficit hyperactivity disorder and comparison girls. J Clin Child Adolesc Psychol 2002;31(4):443–52.

49. Gross-Tsur V, Goldzweig G, Landau YE, et al. The impact of sex and subtypes on cognitive and psychosocial aspects of ADHD. Dev Med Child Neurol 2006;48(11):901–5.

50. Cukrowicz KC, Taylor J, Schatschneider C, et al. Personality differences in children and adolescents with attention-deficit/hyperactivity disorder, conduct disorder, and controls. J Child Psychol Psychiatry 2006;47(2):151–9.
51. Hoza B, Gerdes AC, Hinshaw SP, et al. Self-perceptions of competence in children with ADHD and comparison children. J Consult Clin Psychol 2004;72(3): 382–91.
52. Hoza B, Pelham WE, Milich R, et al. The self-perceptions and attributions of attention deficit hyperactivity disordered and nonreferred boys. J Abnorm Child Psychol 1993;21(3):271–86.
53. Zalecki CA, Hinshaw SP. Overt and relational aggression in girls with attention deficit hyperactivity disorder. J Clin Child Adolesc Psychol 2004;33(1):125–37.
54. Mikami AY, Lee SS, Hinshaw SP, et al. Relationships between social information processing and aggression among adolescent girls with and without ADHD. J Youth Adolesc 2008;37(7):761–71.
55. Young S, Chadwick O, Heptinstall E, et al. The adolescent outcome of hyperactive girls: self-reported interpersonal relationships and coping mechanism. Eur Child Adolesc Psychiatry 2005;14(5):245–53.
56. Young S, Heptinstall E, Sonuga-Barke EJS, et al. The adolescent outcome of hyperactive girls: self-report of psychosocial status. J Child Psychol Psychiatry 2005;46(3):255–62.
57. Broring T, Rommelse N, Sergeant J, et al. Sex differences in tactile defensiveness in children with ADHD and their siblings. Dev Med Child Neurol 2008;50(2): 129–33.
58. Heckel L, Clarke A, Barry R, et al. The relationship between divorce and the psychological well-being of children with ADHD: differences in age, gender, and subtype. Emotional and Behavioural Difficulties 2009;14(1):49–68.
59. Rucklidge JJ. Gender differences in neuropsychological functioning of New Zealand adolescents with and without attention deficit hyperactivity disorder. Int J Disabil Dev Educ 2006;53(1):47–66.
60. Seidman LJ, Biederman J, Faraone SV, et al. A pilot study of neuropsychological function in girls with ADHD. J Am Acad Child Adolesc Psychiatry 1997;36(3): 366–73.
61. Seidman LJ, Biederman J, Monuteaux MC, et al. Impact of gender and age on executive functioning: do girls and boys with and without attention deficit hyperactivity disorder differ neuropsychologically in preteen and teenage years? Dev Neuropsychol 2005;27(1):79–105.
62. Biederman J, Petty CR, Doyle AE, et al. Stability of executive function deficits in girls with ADHD: a prospective longitudinal followup study into adolescence. Dev Neuropsychol 2008;33(1):44–61.
63. Hinshaw SP, Carte ET, Fan C, et al. Neuropsychological functioning of girls with attention-deficit/hyperactivity disorder followed prospectively into adolescence: evidence for continuing deficits? Neuropsychology 2007;21(2): 263–73.
64. Yang P, Jong Y-J, Chung L-C, et al. Gender differences in a clinic-referred sample of Taiwanese attention-deficit/hyperactivity disorder children. Psychiatry Clin Neurosci 2004;58(6):619–23.
65. Newcorn J, Halperin JM, Jensen P, et al. Symptom profiles in children with ADHD: effects of comorbidity and gender. J Am Acad Child Adolesc Psychiatry 2001; 40(2):137–46.
66. Cole WR, Mostofsky SH, Larson JCG, et al. Age-related changes in motor subtle signs among girls and boys with ADHD. Neurology 2008;71(19):1514–20.

67. Biederman J, Faraone S, Monuteaux M, et al. Gender effects on attention-deficit/hyperactivity disorder in adults, revisited. Biol Psychiatry 2004;55: 692–700.
68. Castellanos FX, Marvasti FF, Ducharme JL, et al. Executive function oculomotor tasks in girls with ADHD. J Am Acad Child Adolesc Psychiatry 2000;39(5): 644–50.
69. Liotti M, Pliszka SR, Perez R III, et al. Electrophysiological correlates of response inhibition in children and adolescents with ADHD: influence of gender, age, and previous treatment history. Psychophysiology 2007;44(6):936–48.
70. Rucklidge JJ, Tannock R. Neuropsychological profiles of adolescents with ADHD: effects of reading difficulties and gender. J Child Psychol Psychiatry 2002;43(8): 988–1003.
71. Wodka EL, Mostofsky SH, Prahme C, et al. Process examination of executive function in ADHD: sex and subtype effects. Clin Neuropsychol 2008;22(5): 826–41.
72. Kandel RA. Predicting adherence to treatment recommendations for children with ADHD. Dissertation Abstracts International: Section B: The Sciences and Engineering 2006;66(12-B):6926.
73. Sharp WS, Walter JM, Marsh WL, et al. ADHD in girls: clinical comparability of a research sample. J Am Acad Child Adolesc Psychiatry 1999;38(1):40–7.
74. Spencer T, Biederman J, Wilens T, et al. A large, double-blind, randomized clinical trial of methylphenidate in the treatment of adults with attention-deficit/hyperactivity disorder. Biol Psychiatry 2005;57(5):456–63.
75. Markowitz JS, Straughn AB, Patrick KS. Advances in the pharmacotherapy of attention-deficit/hyperactivity disorder: focus on methylphenidate formulations. Pharmacotherapy 2003;23(10):1281–99.
76. Quinn PO. Treating adolescent girls and women with ADHD: gender-specific issues. J Clin Psychol 2005;61(5):579–87.
77. Justice AJ, deWit H. Acute effects of estradiol pretreatment on the response to D-amphetamine in women. Neuroendocrinology 2000;71:51–9.
78. Quinn P. Attention-deficit/hyperactivity disorder and its comorbidities in women and girls: An evolving picture. Curr Psychiatry Rep 2008;10(5):419–23.
79. Jensen PS, Arnold LE, Swanson JM, et al. 3-year follow-up of the NIMH MTA study. J Am Acad Child Adolesc Psychiatry 2007;46(8):989–1002.
80. Owens EB, Hinshaw SP, Kraemer HC, et al. Which treatment for whom for ADHD? Moderators of treatment response in the MTA. J Consult Clin Psychol 2003;71(3): 540–52.
81. Nangle DW, Erdley CA, Carpenter EM, et al. Social skills training as a treatment for aggressive children and adolescents: a developmental-clinical integration. Aggress Violent Behav 2002;7(2):169–99.
82. de Boo GM, Prins PJM. Social incompetence in children with ADHD: possible moderators and mediators in social-skills training. Clin Psychol Rev 2007;27(1): 78–97.
83. Diamantopoulou S, Henricsson L, Rydell A-M. ADHD symptoms and peer relations of children in a community sample: examining associated problems, self-perceptions, and gender differences. Int J Behav Dev 2005;29(5):388–98.
84. Kelley SDM, English W, Schwallie-Giddis P, et al. Exemplary counseling strategies for developmental transitions of young women with attention deficit/hyperactivity disorder. J Couns Dev 2007;85:173–81.
85. Waite R. Women and attention deficit disorders: a great burden overlooked. J Am Acad Nurse Pract 2007;19(3):116–25.

86. Taylor EW, Keltner NL. Messy purse girls: adult females and ADHD. Perspect Psychiatr Care 2002;38(2):69–72.
87. Ohan JL, Visser TA. Why is there a gender gap in children presenting for attention-deficit/hyperactivity disorder (ADHD) services? J Clin Child Adolesc Psychology 2009;38(5):650–60.
88. Ramsay JR, Rostain AL. Girl, repeatedly interrupted: the case of a young adult woman with ADHD. Clin Case Stud 2005;4(4):329–46.
89. Bussing R, Koro-Ljungberg ME, Gary F, et al. Exploring help-seeking for ADHD symptoms: a mixed-methods approach. Harv Rev Psychiatry 2005;13(2):85–101.
90. Robison LM, Sclar DA, Skaer TL, et al. Treatment modalities among US children diagnosed with attention-deficit hyperactivity disorder: 1995–99. Int Clin Psychopharmacol 2004;19(1):17–22.
91. Reid R, Riccio CA, Kessler RH, et al. Gender and ethnic differences in ADHD as assessed by behavior ratings. J Emot Behav Disord 2000;8(1):38–48.
92. Nadeau KG, Quinn PO. Women's AD/HD self assessment symptom inventory. In: Nadeau KG, Quinn PO, editors. Understanding women with AD/HD. Silver Spring (MD): Advantage Books; 2002. p. 24–43.
93. Ohan JL, Johnston C. Gender appropriateness of symptom criteria for attention-deficit/hyperactivity disorder, oppositional-defiant disorder, and conduct disorder. Child Psychiatry Hum Dev 2005;35(4):359–81.
94. Healey DM, Miller CJ, Castelli KL, et al. The impact of impairment criteria on rates of ADHD diagnoses in preschoolers. J Abnorm Child Psychol 2008;36:771–8.
95. Pelham J, William E, Fabiano GA, et al. Evidence-based assessment of attention deficit hyperactivity disorder in children and adolescents. J Clin Child Adolesc Psychol 2005;34(3):449–76.
96. Barry RJ, Clarke AR, McCarthy R, et al. Age and gender effects in EEG coherence: III. Girls with attention-deficit/hyperactivity disorder. Clin Neurophysiol 2006;117(2):243–51.
97. Barkley RA. A theory of ADHD. In: Barkley RA, editor. Attention-deficit hyperactivity disorder: a handbook for diagnosis and treatment. 3rd edition. New York: The Guilford Press; 2006. p. 297–394.
98. Rosler M, Retz W, Retz-Junginger P, et al. Prevalence of attention deficit-/hyperactivity disorder (ADHD) and comorbid disorders in young male prison inmates. Eur Arch Psychiatry Clin Neurosci 2004;254(6):365–71.

The Pathophysiology, Diagnosis and Treatment of Fibromyalgia

Lesley M. Arnold, MD

KEYWORDS

• Fibromyalgia • Diagnosis • Treatment • Comorbidity

In 1904, Gowers first coined the term "fibrositis" to describe a chronic painful condition of muscles believed to be caused by inflammation. However, pathologic inflammatory changes in the muscles were never discovered,[1] and in 1990, the multicenter criteria committee of the American College of Rheumatology (ACR) adopted the term fibromyalgia (FM), rather than fibrositis, because of the lack of inflammatory changes in the muscles of affected individuals.[2] The establishment of the ACR classification criteria has stimulated research in FM, which has improved our understanding of the possible causes and treatment of this chronic pain disorder.

DIAGNOSIS AND CLINICAL PRESENTATION OF FM
Diagnostic Criteria

The criteria for the ACR classification of FM include widespread pain of at least 3 months duration and pain on palpation of 11 or more of 18 specific tender point sites on the body (**Box 1**).[2] To assess the tender points, pressure is applied with the dominant thumb pad perpendicularly to each site and the force increased by approximately 1 kg per second until 4 kg of pressure is achieved, which usually leads to whitening of the thumb nail bed.

    Although the ACR classification criteria are the standard for identifying patients for participation in research studies, there are several problems with the ACR criteria. First, although there have been attempts to standardize the finger tender point palpation pressure at 4 kg, as recommended by the ACR criteria, the amount of pressure actually applied remains variable and not subject to measurement. Thus the classification of 1 individual with 11 tender points as having FM and another with only 10 tender points may represent an artificial division. Second, because women have lower pain thresholds than men, ACR diagnostic criteria may be biased toward the

Women's Health Research Program, Department of Psychiatry, University of Cincinnati College of Medicine, 222 Piedmont Avenue, Suite 8200, Cincinnati, OH 45219, USA
E-mail address: Lesley.Arnold@uc.edu

Psychiatr Clin N Am 33 (2010) 375–408
doi:10.1016/j.psc.2010.01.001
0193-953X/10/$ – see front matter © 2010 Elsevier Inc. All rights reserved.

Box 1
American College of Rheumatology 1990 criteria for fibromyalgia

1. History of widespread pain

    Definition: Pain in the right and left side of the body, pain above and below the waist, axial skeletal pain (cervical spine or anterior chest or thoracic spine or low back). In this definition, shoulder and buttock pain is considered as pain for each involved side. Low back pain is considered lower segment pain.

2. Pain in 11 of 18 tender point sites on digital palpation

    Definition: Pain, on digital palpation, must be present in at least 11 of the following 18 tender point sites:

    Occiput: bilateral, at the suboccipital muscle insertion

    Low cervical: bilateral, at the anterior aspects of the intertransverse spaces at C5 to C7

    Trapezius: bilateral, at the midpoint of the upper border

    Supraspinatus: bilateral, at origins, above the scapula spine near the medial border

    Second rib: bilateral, at the second costochondral junctions, just lateral to the junctions on upper surfaces

    Lateral epicondyle: bilateral, 2 cm distal to the epicondyles

    Gluteal: bilateral, in upper outer quadrants of buttocks in anterior fold of muscle

    Greater trochanter: bilateral, posterior to the trochanteric prominence

    Knee: bilateral, at the medial fat pad proximal to the joint line

Digital palpation should be performed with an approximate force of 4 kg. For a tender point to be considered positive the patient must state that the palpation was painful. Tender is not to be considered painful.

Adapted from Wolfe F, Smythe HA, Yunus MB, et al. The American College of Rheumatology 1990 criteria for the classification of fibromyalgia. Report of the multicenter criteria committee. Arthritis Rheum 1990;33:160–72; with permission.

---

identification of women rather than men because of this pain threshold difference.[3] Third, although the ACR criteria are based on detecting 11 of 18 tender points, increased sensitivity to pressure extends beyond these specific sites and involves the entire body.[4] There is no evidence of specific pathology at the tender point sites, and the focus on specific musculoskeletal sites conveys a false impression that FM is a disorder of the muscles. Fourth, the ACR digital tender point examination is significantly influenced by various measures of psychological distress and is vulnerable to psychophysical biases. Thus, the tender point ACR examination is not an adequate measure of pain sensitivity.[4] Fifth, the ACR classification of widespread pain may be too loose to define a group of patients whose pain is truly widespread. An alternative, more restrictive definition of widespread pain requires the presence of more diffuse limb pain.[5] Defining FM only by pain and tenderness does not account for the presence of other common symptoms. In the study that established the ACR criteria, 73% to 85% of patients with FM reported fatigue, sleep disturbance (nonrestorative sleep or insomnia), and morning stiffness. Pain all over, paresthesias, headache, history of depression, and anxiety were experienced by 45% to 69% of patients, and co-occurring irritable bowel syndrome, sicca (dryness) symptoms, and Raynaud phenomenon were less common (<35%).[2] Many patients with FM also report weakness, forgetfulness, concentration difficulties, urinary frequency, dysmennorrhea history, subjective swelling, and restless legs. Revision of the ACR criteria may become necessary in the future as more is learned about the neurobiological and genetic basis of FM, improved measures of sensory function are developed, and possible biomarkers of FM are identified.

Pope and Hudson[6] developed alternative diagnostic criteria for FM that include some of the characteristic symptoms of FM in addition to pain and tender points (**Box 2**). The Pope and Hudson criteria were derived from the preliminary criteria proposed by Yunus and colleagues[7] that closely approached the diagnostic accuracy of the ACR criteria.[2] Using the format of the Structured Clinical Interview for DSM-IV (SCID),[8] Pope and Hudson incorporated their criteria for FM into a structured interview, which has been used in family studies and clinical trials.[9–11]

Other diagnostic criteria that are more practical for use in clinical settings than the ACR classification criteria have also been proposed recently.[12] These criteria combine a self-administered regional pain score and a 0 to 10 visual analog scale (VAS) for fatigue. The regional pain score is a count of the number of painful nonarticular regions of the body with a score range of 0 to 19. FM is diagnosed when the regional pain score is 8 or more and the VAS score for fatigue is 6 or more. These proposed diagnostic criteria had moderate level of concordance with the ACR criteria.

Gender Differences

The clinical presentation of FM differs between women and men. In a study of FM in a general population in the United States, fatigue and sleep disturbance were about threefold more common in women than men. Pain all over and irritable bowel syndrome were also more common in women.[3] In a study of community cases of FM in Canada, women and men had similar symptoms but women rated more symptoms of FM as being major problems and were older.[13] Gender differences in FM were also found in a US rheumatology clinic; women had more symptoms and tender points and more

---

Box 2
Pope and Hudson criteria for fibromyalgia

A. Generalized pain affecting the axial, plus upper and lower segments, plus left and right sides of the body

Either B or C:

B. At least 11 of 18 reproducible tender points

C. At least 4 of the following symptoms:

1. Generalized fatigue

2. Generalized headache (of a type, severity, or pattern that is different from headaches the patient may have had in the premorbid state)

3. Sleep disturbance (hypersomnia or insomnia)

4. Neuropsychiatric complaints (1 or more of the following: forgetfulness, excessive irritability, confusion, difficulty thinking, inability to concentrate, depression)

5. Numbness, tingling sensations

6. Symptoms of irritable bowel syndrome (periodically altered bowel habits with lower abdominal pain or distension usually relieved or aggravated by bowel movements; no blood)

D. It cannot be established that the disturbance was caused by another systemic condition

Adapted from Pope HG Jr, Hudson JI. A supplemental interview for forms of "affective spectrum disorder." Int J Psychiatry Med 1991;21:205–32; with permission.

common pain all over, fatigue, morning fatigue, and irritable bowel syndrome compared with men.[14,15] The number of tender points was the most powerful discriminator between women and men with FM.[14] In contrast, a study of rheumatology outpatients in Israel found that men with FM had greater pain, fatigue, functional disability, and worse quality of life than women.[16] The disparate results in the Israeli study suggest that sociocultural factors might play a role in determining gender differences in FM.[15]

Differential Diagnosis

The ACR criteria allow for the diagnosis of FM irrespective of the presence of other disorders, and exclusionary laboratory, imaging, or other tests are not required in the ACR criteria for FM. The distinction between primary and secondary FM (FM occurring in the presence of another rheumatic disorder) was eliminated in the criteria because the clinical presentations were indistinguishable.[2] However, most of the research in FM has focused on primary FM. Furthermore, it is important for clinicians to identify other illnesses that have similar symptoms and require different treatment.[17] **Table 1** lists some of the important medical disorders that might present with widespread musculoskeletal pain and other symptoms that mimic FM or are comorbid with FM.[18–21] Complicating the differential diagnosis of FM, as many as 25% of patients with rheumatic conditions such as systemic lupus erythematosis, rheumatoid arthritis, and spondyloarthropathies such as ankylosing spondylitis have secondary FM.[17] To avoid over treatment with antirheumatic regimens, it is important to determine whether symptoms associated with these rheumatic disorders might be attributable to concomitant FM.[19]

EPIDEMIOLOGY

FM is common in the United States, with an estimated prevalence of 2% in the adult (18 years of age or older) general population. FM affects women disproportionately, with a prevalence of 3.4% in women compared with 0.5% in men.[22] The community prevalence of FM in Europe, South Africa, and Canada varies from 0.7% to 4.5%, with a greater prevalence in women compared with men.[23–29] It is unclear why there are international differences in the community prevalence of FM, but differences in case detection strategies might be one explanation.[28] The prevalence of FM in adults increases with age, rising sharply in middle age (50–59 years) and then dropping off in the oldest age groups (80+ years).[22] The average age of onset is between 30 and 50 years. In the general population, FM is most common in women aged 50 years and older.[22]

Demographic and social factors associated with FM in the general population include female sex, failure to complete high school, low household income, and divorce.[22,28] Female sex remains a predictor of FM after controlling for age and clinical factors.[22] Widespread pain occurs in women about 1.5 times more often than in men, but women are 10 times more likely than men to have 11 out of 18 positive tender points.[3] FM occurs in 5% to 6% of patients presenting to general medical and family practice clinics, and 15% to 20% of patients presenting to rheumatologists, making it one of the most common diagnosis in office-based rheumatology practices,[30] particularly among women.[31,32] In a survey of Canadian rheumatologists, FM was the only disorder perceived by the majority to have increased in frequency in their practices in the previous 5 years,[33] which might reflect increasing awareness and recognition of FM among physicians and patients.[34]

There is one published population study of the incidence of FM in a sample of women between the ages of 20 and 49 years who were followed for 5.5 years in

Norway.[35] The incidence of FM among women who began the observation period without any complaints of musculoskeletal pain was 3.2%, which corresponds to an average annual incidence of 583 cases/100,000 women between 20 and 49 years of age.[35] As part of this population study, women with any self-reported pain at the beginning of the observation period were followed for 5.5 years for the development of FM.[36] The incidence of FM was high (25%), and risk factors for the development of FM included pain for 6 years or more, self-assessed depression, lack of professional education, and the presence of 4 or more associated symptoms. A subgroup of these symptoms, namely, disturbed bowel function, not feeling refreshed in the morning, paresthesias, and subjective swelling, were also separately associated with the development of FM. Extensive (chronic multifocal or chronic widespread) and limited (recurrent, nonchronic, or chronic regional) pain predicted the development of FM, although the risk was higher in women with extensive pain. Age, age of onset of pain, and number of tender points did not predict the development of FM. Within the age group studied (20–49 years), there were no differences in the risk of developing FM in younger or older women, when controlling for pain duration. These results suggest that the higher prevalence of FM in older age groups[22] is because of pain duration rather than age.[36]

COMORBIDITY
Psychiatric Comorbidity

In clinic and community groups, FM was strongly associated with multiple somatic complaints, depressive and anxiety symptoms as well as a personal and family history of depression and subsequent antidepressant treatment.[22] Depressive and anxiety symptoms are common and frequently severe, even among community cases of FM.[37] Consistent with previous controlled studies of psychiatric comorbidity in FM,[38,39] a recent study reported a high lifetime prevalence of mood and anxiety disorders in patients with FM (**Table 2**).[40] The co-occurrence odds ratio (OR) for lifetime major mood disorder in individuals with versus those without FM was 6.2 (95% confidence interval [CI] 2.9–14); the OR for any lifetime anxiety disorder was 6.7 (95% CI 2.3–20).[40]

Medical Comorbidity

Studies that have assessed the comorbidity of FM with other medical disorders have found high rates of tension and migraine headaches, irritable bowel syndrome, chronic fatigue syndrome, temporomandibular disorder, interstitial cystitis, chronic pelvic pain, and multiple chemical sensitivities.[41,42] Some of these disorders, like FM, are associated with high lifetime rates of comorbid mood and anxiety disorders.[40,41,43,44] There are other similarities between FM and some of these disorders, including overlaps in case definition and symptoms, and female predominance.[45] This raises the possibility that these disorders are less distinct than previously believed[45,46] and that they, along with mood and anxiety disorders, might be related by a common central nervous system pathophysiology.[40,44]

Patients with FM report more general medical conditions and medically unexplained symptoms compared with medical controls such as patients with rheumatoid arthritis or osteoarthritis.[39,43,47] Medical conditions commonly reported by patients with FM include hypertension, allergy, asthma, gastrointestinal, pulmonary, thyroid, fractures, cancer, genitourinary, and gall bladder disorders.[47] Obesity is common in patients with FM[48] and contributes to dysfunction related to FM.[49] Comorbid disorders that may contribute to sleep disturbances in these patients include periodic involuntary

Table 1
Medical disorders that mimic symptoms of FM or are comorbid with FM

Medical Disorder	Differentiating Signs and Symptoms	Laboratory Tests
Rheumatoid arthritis	Predominate joint pain, joint swelling and joint line tenderness	Positive rheumatoid factor in 80%–90% of patients, radiographic evidence of joint erosion
Systemic lupus erythematosus	Multisystem involvement, commonly arthritis, arthralgia, and rash	Antinuclear antibody test, other autoantibodies
Polyarticular osteoarthritis	Multiple painful joints	Radiographic evidence of joint degeneration
Polymyalgia rheumatica	Proximal shoulder and hip girdle pain, more common in the elderly	Increased erythrocyte sedimentation rate in about 80% of patients
Polymyositis or other myopathies	Symmetric proximal muscle weakness	Increased serum muscle enzyme levels (creatinine kinase, aldolase), abnormal electromyography, abnormal muscle biopsy
Spondyloarthropathy	Localization of spinal pain to specific sites in the neck, mid-thoracic, anterior chest wall, or lumbar regions, objective limitation of spinal mobility because of pain and stiffness	Radiographic sacroiliitis, vertebral body radiographic changes
Osteomalacia	Diffuse bone pain, fractures, proximal myopathy with muscle weakness	Low 25-hydroxyvitamin D levels, low phosphate levels, dual-energy X-ray absorptiometry (DEXA) scan abnormalities
Lyme disease	Rash, arthritis or arthralgia, occurs in areas of endemic disease	Positive Lyme serologies (enzyme-linked immunosorbent assay [ELISA], Western blot)
Hypothyroidism	Cold intolerance, mental slowing, constipation, weight gain, hair loss	Increased TSH level

Sleep apnea	Interrupted breathing during sleep, heavy snoring, excessive sleepiness during the day	Polysomnography abnormalities
Hepatitis C	Right upper quadrant pain, nausea, decreased appetite	Increased liver enzymes (alanine aminotransferase), hepatitis C antibody, hepatitis C RNA
Hyperparathyroidism	Increased thirst and urination, kidney stones, nausea/vomiting, decreased appetite, thinning bones, constipation	Increased serum calcium and parathyroid levels
Cushing syndrome	Hypertension, diabetes, hirsutism, moon facies, weight gain	Increased 24-hour urinary free cortisol level
Addison disease	Postural hypotension, nausea, vomiting, skin pigmentation, weight loss	Blunted corticotropin stimulation test
Multiple sclerosis	Visual changes (unilateral partial or complete loss, double vision), ascending numbness in a leg or bandlike truncal numbness, slurred speech (dysarthria)	Magnetic resonance imaging of brain/spinal cord, cerebrospinal fluid for immunoglobulins, visual evoked potentials
Neuropathy	Shooting or burning pain; tingling; numbness	Tests to identify underlying cause (eg, diabetes, herniated disc), electromyography (EMG), nerve conduction study, nerve biopsy

Table 2 Lifetime prevalence of mood and anxiety disorders in FM	
Disorder	FM (N = 108), n (%)
Mood Disorders	
Bipolar disorder	12 (11.1)
Major depressive disorder	67 (62.0)
Major mood disorder[a]	79 (73.1)
Anxiety Disorders	
Generalized anxiety disorder	5 (4.6)
Obsessive-compulsive disorder	7 (6.5)
Panic disorder	31 (28.7)
Posttraumatic stress disorder	23 (21.3)
Social phobia	21 (19.4)
Specific phobia	17 (15.7)
Agoraphobia without panic disorder	1 (0.9)
Any anxiety disorder	60 (55.6)

[a] Major depressive disorder or bipolar disorder.
    Data from Arnold LM, Hudson JI, Keck Jr. PE, et al. Comorbidity of fibromyalgia and psychiatric disorders. J Clin Psychiatry 2006;67:1219–25.

limb movements and restless leg syndrome,[50] sleep apnea,[50,51] and inspiratory airflow limitation with arousal.[52] In a recent study of the prevalence of comorbidities among FM patients compared with age- and sex-matched non-FM patients from a US health insurance database, patients with FM were more likely to have comorbidities, including painful neuropathies, circulatory disorders, depression, diabetes, sleep disorders, gastroesophageal reflux disorder, irritable bowel disorder, and anxiety.[53]

COURSE OF FM

In one of the longest follow-up studies of rheumatology outpatients with FM, all 29 patients, who were surveyed by telephone 10 years after the original evaluation, had persistence of some FM symptoms, with moderate to severe pain or stiffness in 16 (55%), moderate to severe sleep difficulties in 14 (48%), and moderate to severe fatigue in 17 (59%). However, despite persistent symptoms, 19 (66%) of 29 felt better overall than when first diagnosed with FM. The only baseline variables that correlated with doing well were younger age and shorter duration of symptoms at diagnosis.[54] In a large multicenter outcome study of 538 patients followed in rheumatology centers, measures of pain, global severity, fatigue, sleep disturbance, anxiety, depression, and health status were unchanged throughout the 7-year study period, functional disability worsened slightly, and health satisfaction improved slightly.[55] Other outcome studies of FM outpatients have also documented persistence of FM symptoms over time,[56,57] although there is some evidence that patients adapt to the symptoms.[58] Two studies reported more favorable outcomes for FM patients in rheumatology settings. In the first study, remission of FM in a 2-year period was identified in 24% of 44 rheumatology outpatients.[59] In a recent 3-year outcome study, 47% of 70 outpatients with FM reported moderate to marked improvement.[60]

Individuals in the community with chronic pain, including those with FM, have a better outcome than patients in rheumatology clinics.[61] In a prospective study of persons with chronic pain in the community, only 12 of 34 subjects (35%) with chronic widespread pain at baseline still had this symptom at the 27-month follow-up. However, the presence of at least 11 of 18 tender points with widespread pain, consistent with the ACR diagnosis of FM, increased 5-fold the odds of persistent pain. Other predictors of persistent pain in those with FM were female sex, older age, low educational achievement, psychological disturbance, fatigue, micturition problems, abdominal pain, sleep disturbance, and headaches.[62]

FM is associated with substantial compromise in the quality of life, self-reported loss of function, work disability and increased work absenteeism, and higher than expected health care use.[53,63,64] The symptoms of pain, fatigue, and weakness are most often reported to interfere with work performance.[65] In a multicenter survey of 1604 patients with FM, 26.5% reported receiving disability payments.[66] Patients with FM also report disabilities in activities of daily living that are comparable with those reported by patients with rheumatoid arthritis.[67] FM patients also rate their quality of life as worse and report lower quality of well-being than patients with rheumatoid arthritis and other chronic medical illnesses.[68,69] The effect of comorbid psychiatric symptoms on the course of FM is illustrated by the finding that mood and anxiety disorders are associated with functional disability in patients with FM.[39,70]

CAUSE OF FM
Genetic Factors

The cause of FM is unknown, although genetic and environmental factors probably contribute to the liability to FM. Early small, uncontrolled family studies provided evidence for familial aggregation of FM.[71–73] A recent, large, controlled study confirmed that FM aggregates strongly in families. In this study, the OR measuring the odds of FM in a first-degree relative of a patient with FM versus the odds of FM in a relative of a patient with the control condition, rheumatoid arthritis, was 8.5 (95% CI 2.8–26, $P = .0002$).[11] Using dolorimeter measures, tender point count and total myalgic scores were strongly associated with FM in families, suggesting that inherited factors may be involved in pain sensitivity. FM co-aggregated in families with major mood disorder, a finding that replicated results from previous family history studies.[38,44] FM also co-aggregated with mood disorder, anxiety disorder, eating disorders, irritable bowel syndrome, and migraine, taken collectively.[74] These results suggest that FM may share a common physiologic abnormality with some psychiatric and medical disorders.

Recent preliminary genetic studies of FM revealed possible association of FM with genetic polymorphisms in monoamine-related genes, including the serotonin-2A receptor gene (HTR2A),[75,76] the serotonin transporter gene (HTTLPR) regulatory region,[77,78] and the dopamine D4 receptor gene.[79] A functional val158met polymorphism, in which substitution of val to met at codon 158 results in reduction in the activity of the catechol-O-methyltransferase (COMT) enzyme that metabolizes catecholamines, is associated with human pain sensitivity.[80] The COMT gene may play a role in pain sensitivity across several pain conditions, including FM,[81] temporomandibular disorder,[82] osteoarthritis,[83] dyspepsia,[84] and shoulder pain.[85] COMT activity is decreased by estrogen,[86] which may help to explain why women may be more susceptible to developing several chronic pain disorders, including FM.

Stress

Environmental stressors have been associated with the development of FM, and patients with FM often report the onset of their symptoms after a period of substantial stress. Patients with FM report higher levels of stress as measured by daily hassles than patients with rheumatoid arthritis,[87] and experience more stressful, negative lifetime events than healthy controls.[88] FM patients have significantly higher prevalence rates of all forms of childhood and adult victimization than patients with rheumatoid arthritis.[89] Childhood maltreatment, including emotional abuse, physical abuse, sexual abuse, emotional neglect, and physical neglect, is associated with FM, but particular forms of maltreatment (eg, sexual abuse per se) do not have specific effects on the risk of FM.[89] The evidence suggests that, when an event of abuse occurs in childhood, it happens in the context of other psychosocial childhood adversities, including insufficiently supportive relationships with the primary caretakers, poor emotional relationships and a low-level feeling of security, poor physical care, as well as experiences of physical and sexual violence.[90] Patients with FM are also likely to experience repeated abuse in adulthood, and adult physical abuse has a strong and specific relationship with FM.[89] Therefore, many patients with FM have lifelong victimization that contributes to the experience of chronic stress.[91]

Stress-response Systems

Chronic stress might promote disturbances in the stress-response system that could lead to the development of symptoms of FM. Patients with FM have disturbances in the 2 major interacting stress-response systems: the autonomic nervous system and the hypothalamic-pituitary-adrenal (HPA) axis.[92] Although the interpretation of these disturbances is still debated, some of the available data on neuroendocrine function in patients with FM suggest that there is mild to moderate reduction in the activities of the HPA axis.[93–96] Some studies suggest that FM is associated with decreased hypothalamic corticotropin-releasing hormone (CRH) secretion, an impaired ability to activate the hypothalamic CRH-pituitary corticotropin axis in response to stress, and possibly, a decreased cortisol response to stress.[94,97–99] CRH is a key mediator of the HPA axis and a behaviorally active peptide that leads to physiologic and behavioral arousal,[100] and decreased pain perception through opioid peptide secretion.[101] Chronically decreased CRH secretion could therefore contribute to the clinical features of FM either through a direct effect or indirectly by causing a relative glucocorticoid deficiency that results in the characteristic symptoms of FM including fatigue, arthralgias, myalgias, immunologic disturbances, and disruption in mood and sleep.[102,103] Atypical depression and chronic fatigue syndrome, which share symptoms of FM, including lethargy and fatigue, are also associated with reduced activation of the HPA axis and a functional deficit in the release of hypothalamic CRH.[104] Hypofunctioning of the HPA axis may be one of the common pathophysiologic features of certain forms of major depressive disorder, chronic fatigue syndrome, and FM.

However, other evidence suggests that FM is associated with hyperactivity of CRH neurons, including studies showing increased cortisol levels associated with a flattened diurnal pattern[105] and increase in cortisol level in the late evening quiescent period, consistent with a loss of HPA axis resiliency.[106] In recent studies of the HPA axis in patients with FM, pain symptoms, but not fatigue, were strongly associated with CRH concentration in cerebrospinal fluid (CSF)[107] and increased cortisol levels,[108] supporting the hypothesis that HPA axis hyperactivity is linked specifically to FM pain.[107] Women with FM who had a history of physical or sexual abuse had significantly lower levels of CSF CRH than those without abuse histories.[107] Therefore, the inconsistencies of HPA findings in FM may be related to several factors, including failure to adjust for comorbidities, symptom variability (eg, the presence of prominent fatigue, sleep disturbances, or depressed mood), duration of FM, and the confounding influence of abuse and other stressors.

Alterations in HPA axis function may also provide an explanation for the observation of subnormal growth hormone secretion in some patients with FM, which might contribute to the development of impaired cognition, fatigue, muscle weakness, and decreased exercise tolerance.[94] The impairment of growth hormone secretion results in a low level of insulin-like growth factor-1 (IGF-1), which is produced in the liver in response to stimulation by growth hormone, and significantly lower IGF-1 levels were found in women with FM compared with controls.[109] The changes in growth hormone seem to be caused by changes in the hypothalamic regulation of growth hormone, but could also be secondary to the development of other symptoms of FM including disturbed sleep and decreased physical conditioning.[94] Thyroid function is also affected by HPA activity, and studies of thyroid function in patients with FM show a reduced increase in thyroid-stimulating hormone (TSH) following administration of thyrotropin-releasing hormone (TRH).[99,110]

A consistent finding in studies of the autonomic nervous system in FM patients is impairment in the sympathetic response to stressors.[101,111] For example, patients with FM have reduced vasoconstrictor responses to acoustic and cold stressors, reduced heart rate response to exercise, and reduced epinephrine response to hypoglycemia stress.[93,94,112,113] There is also evidence that FM patients have an altered sympathetic response to upright posture and tilt table testing[114-116] and abnormal heart rate variability, suggesting a persistently hyperactive sympathetic nervous system that is hyporeactive to stress.[117] The decreased sympathetic response to exercise and the evidence for a paradoxical decrease rather than increase in cortisol levels after exercise[113] might explain the postexertional pain and fatigue reported by many patients with FM.[101]

The cause of the changes in the responsiveness of the stress-response systems in FM is unknown. It is also unclear whether the disturbances of neuroendocrine and autonomic function are primary causes of FM or secondary to the development of FM.[94] Evidence suggests that early adverse experiences result in persistent changes in the HPA axis and autonomic nervous system that could contribute to the development of stress-related conditions.[118] Animal studies have also shown that early-life stressors have a permanent and profound effect on the activity of the stress-response system.[101] Trauma and chronic stress may promote dysfunction of the stress systems that leads to the development of disorders like FM.[118] In a recent, population-based, prospective study of individuals at risk for chronic widespread pain based on high levels of distress and other somatic symptoms, high levels of serum cortisol after dexamethasone, low levels of morning salivary cortisol, and high levels in evening salivary cortisol were all associated with the development of chronic widespread pain.[119] These results support the possible role of abnormalities of HPA axis function in FM and suggest that HPA dysfunction precedes the onset of widespread pain. Genetic differences in the activity of the stress-response system could also predispose individuals to FM, and genetic variation in HPA axis genes has been found to be associated with musculoskeletal pain in preliminary studies.[120]

Reproductive Axis

Although FM is far more common in women than men, there are remarkably little data on the reproductive axis and FM. Levels of estradiol, progesterone, follicle-stimulating hormone, and luteinizing hormone in premenopausal women with FM were found to be similar to healthy women.[121-124] Furthermore, hormonal fluctuations during the menstrual cycle do not significantly influence pain sensitivity in women with FM.[124] Estrogen-responsive elements have been discovered in the promoter area of the CRH gene, and there are direct stimulatory estrogen effects on CRH gene expression,[125] implicating the CRH gene as a potentially important target of ovarian steroids and mediator of sex differences in the stress response and potentially in the development of FM.[126] Some women develop FM after menopause,[127] suggesting that for these women, alterations in estrogen may contribute to decreased responsiveness to CRH and increased risk of symptoms of FM. Low androgen levels might also constitute a risk factor for FM, but more study is needed.[128]

Central Nervous System Processing of Pain

There is evidence that FM is associated with aberrant central nervous system (CNS) processing of pain.[92,129–131] Although the ACR criteria for FM require tenderness in 11 out of 18 discrete regions, patients with FM have increased sensitivity to pain throughout the body. FM patients often develop an increased response to painful stimuli (hyperalgesia) and experience pain from normally nonnoxious stimuli (allodynia).[130] Both hyperalgesia and allodynia reflect an enhanced CNS processing of painful stimuli that is characteristic of central sensitization, which develops as a result of the plasticity of neuronal synapses.[132–134]

Painful stimuli, such as occurs after an injury, may initiate the process that leads to central sensitization in susceptible individuals. Indeed, many patients with FM report the onset of symptoms after physical trauma or repetitive injuries.[135] Various injuries, including trauma and infections, or other stressors may also induce a CNS immune response that leads to subsequent production of proinflammatory cytokines that have been implicated in the generation of chronic pain states.[131,136,137]

The level of substance P, an important nociceptive neurotransmitter, was found to be increased in the CSF of individuals with FM compared with healthy controls.[138,139] Substance P, along with pronociceptive excitatory amino acids acting at the N-methyl-D-aspartate (NMDA) receptor, and other neuropeptides may play a role in neuronal hyperactivity and the generation of central pain sensitization.[140] Substance P levels might be influenced by serotonin activity as shown by a recent study that found a strong negative correlation between serum concentrations of the primary serotonin metabolite, 5-hydroxyindoleacetic acid and substance P, pain, and insomnia.[141] Substance P is also a potent inhibitor of CRH and may contribute to the low activity of CRH found in some patients with FM, as discussed earlier.[92] There is also evidence for increased levels of nerve growth factor (NGF), brain-derived neurotrophic factor (BDNF), and glutamate in the CSF of patients with FM. These results suggest that NGF might indirectly enhance glutamatergic transmission via BDNF, which could account for the sustained central sensitization in FM.[142] Changes in glutamate levels in the insula of the brain were associated with changes in multiple pain domains in patients with FM, underscoring the importance of glutamate as a major excitatory neurotransmitter involved in pain transmission and in FM.[143]

Another pain mechanism that is likely to be important in the development of FM is disinhibition, which can also lead to increased excitability and pain.[133] Patients with FM have been shown to have a deficit in diffuse noxious inhibitory control, one of the principal endogenous inhibitory pain systems.[144] There is evidence of a functional reduction in serotonergic activity in patients with FM and reduced concentrations of the primary norepinephrine metabolite, 3-methoxy-4-hydroxyphenethylene, in the CSF of FM patients.[141,145–147] Norepinephrine and serotonin are involved in the descending inhibitory pain pathways in the brain and spinal cord that act to diminish pain.[148,149] A reduction of serotonin- and norepinephrine-mediated descending pain inhibitory pathways is a possible mechanism for the development of pain in FM. In addition, a reduction in serotonin, which normally activates the HPA axis and increases CRH expression,[150] may contribute to the blunted hypothalamic CRH activity and development of FM symptoms as discussed previously.

Central serotonergic neurotransmission was postulated to mediate a qualitative abnormality of sleep in patients with FM.[151] This sleep abnormality consists of inappropriate intrusion of alpha waves (normally seen during wakefulness or rapid eye movement sleep) into deep sleep (characterized by delta waves).[152] Alpha-delta sleep intrusion was believed to contribute to the musculoskeletal pain and fatigue of FM.[151] However, the sleep abnormality is not specific to FM and is found in other disorders.

Abnormalities in serotonin and norepinephrine neurotransmission are also involved in the pathophysiology of major depressive disorder and could be a common etiologic link between major depressive disorder and FM. Using positron emission tomography, the rate of serotonin synthesis in the brain was found to be 52% higher in normal men compared with normal women.[153] A lower rate of serotonin synthesis in women provides a possible explanation for the increased vulnerability of women to disorders in which low serotonin activity might play a pathogenic role, such as FM and major depressive disorder.

Neuroimaging studies of patients with FM have provided evidence for central augmentation of pain sensitivity in FM. In a study using functional magnetic resonance imaging, the pattern of cerebral activation during the application of painful pressure was assessed in FM patients compared with controls.[154] The results showed an overlap between activations in patients and activations evoked by greater stimulus pressures in controls. In addition, application of mild pressure to FM patients and controls resulted in a greater number of activated regions in the patients. Both of these findings provide evidence that pain sensitivity is augmented in FM.[154] Studies using single photon emission computed tomography imaging found that patients with FM compared with healthy controls exhibited significantly lower levels of cerebral blood flow (rCBF), a marker for brain synaptic activity, in the thalamus and caudate nucleus.[155] Hypoperfusion of the caudate and thalamus could be a marker for the presence of centrally mediated abnormalities in pain sensitivity in FM and other chronic pain conditions.[155]

Summary

Since the publication of the ACR criteria, increased research has expanded our understanding of the possible genetic and environmental factors that could be involved in the etiology of FM. Environmental stressors and genetic vulnerability could act alone or together to initiate a series of biological events in individuals that eventually lead to the development of FM. There is now substantial evidence for augmentation of central pain processing in FM. Although the causal nature of the findings discussed earlier is unclear, it seems that disturbances in the stress-response system may play a key role in the process that leads to FM. These same CNS changes could also be involved in the development of symptoms of depression and other comorbid conditions. FM, like melancholic and atypical forms of major depressive disorder, may be heterogeneous in its presentation and underlying pathophysiology.

TREATMENT OF FM

Because the clinical presentation of FM is heterogeneous, the treatment should be individualized for each patient, depending on the severity of the patient's pain, the presence of other symptoms or comorbidities, and the degree of functional impairment. The management of FM includes the identification and treatment of all symptoms or disorders that commonly occur in patients with FM, such as pain, fatigue, sleep disturbances, cognitive impairment, stiffness, and mood or anxiety disorders. The treatment should strive to improve the patient's function and global health status.

The management of FM usually includes pharmacologic and nonpharmacologic treatments.

Pharmacological Treatment

Antidepressants

The rationale for using antidepressants to treat FM is based on several lines of evidence. First, antidepressants are effective in the treatment of other chronic pain conditions.[156] Second, antidepressants are effective for the treatment of depressive and anxiety disorders, which are frequently comorbid with FM and possibly share a physiologic abnormality with FM.[40,44] Third, antidepressants might enhance serotonin and norepinephrine neurotransmission in the descending inhibitory pain pathways, resulting in a reduction of pain perception.[148] In preclinical and clinical studies, it seems that medications with combined effects on serotonin and norepinephrine have more antinociceptive activity than those with effects on serotonin alone.[156] Fourth, the antinociceptive activity of medications that enhance serotonin and norepinephrine neurotransmission are largely independent of their effects on mood, making them potentially efficacious for patients with or without depressive or anxiety symptoms.[157] Finally, some antidepressants have other pharmacological properties, including NMDA antagonism and ion-channel blocking activity, that may mediate their antinociceptive effects.[95,158]

Cyclic antidepressants A meta-analysis assessed 9 placebo-controlled trials of cyclic drugs that inhibit the reuptake of serotonin and norepinephrine.[159] Seven outcome measures were assessed, including the patient's self-ratings of pain, stiffness, fatigue, and sleep; the patient's and the physician's global assessment of improvement; and tender points. The largest effect was found in measures of sleep quality, with more modest changes in tender point measures and stiffness. In another meta-analysis of randomized, placebo-controlled studies of another cyclic medication, cyclobenzaprine, in FM, there was moderate improvement in sleep, modest improvement in pain, and no improvement in fatigue or tender points.[160]

Although the meta-analyses indicate that the overall effect of the cyclic drugs on most symptoms of FM was moderate, possibly related to the low doses that were typically used in the studies, cyclic medications continue to be recommended for the treatment of patients with FM, usually as a nighttime medication.[161] However, even at low doses (eg, amitriptyline 25 mg/d), many patients experience problems with the safety and tolerability of these medications related to their anticholinergic, antiadrenergic, antihistaminergic, and quinidinelike effects.[162]

Selective serotonin reuptake inhibitors Selective serotonin reuptake inhibitors (SSRIs), although generally better tolerated than tricyclics, have been studied in only 6 double-blind, placebo-controlled trials in FM: 2 with citalopram,[163,164] 3 with fluoxetine,[165–167] and 1 with paroxetine CR.[168] The results with the SSRIs have been inconsistent, with insignificant reduction in pain in studies of citalopram and paroxetine and mixed results for fluoxetine. In the most recent study of fluoxetine, a randomized, placebo-controlled, parallel-group, flexible-dose, 12-week trial, patients receiving fluoxetine (mean ± SD dose of 45 ± 25 mg/d) displayed significantly greater reduction in pain as well as fatigue and depressed mood compared with subjects receiving placebo. The effect of fluoxetine on pain was still significant after adjustment for change in depressed mood.[167]

The inconsistent results for SSRIs suggests that medications with selective serotonin effects are less consistent in relieving pain and other symptoms associated with FM. There is evidence that serotonin has pro- and antinociceptive actions in the descending pain modulatory pathways in the brain and spinal cord.[169] Therefore, although there may be a synergistic effect of serotonin and norepinephrine that mediates the antinociceptive effects of the serotonin and norepinephrine reuptake inhibitors (SNRIs), medications that effect only serotonin may be more weakly antinociceptive.[170]

Selective SNRIs Venlafaxine sequentially engages serotonin uptake inhibition at low doses (75 mg/d) and norepinephrine uptake inhibition at higher doses (375 mg/d).[171] In a pilot, 8-week, open-label, flexible-dose study in FM, venlafaxine at a mean dose of 167 ± 76 mg/d significantly improved pain and other symptoms.[9] By contrast, a low, fixed dose of venlafaxine (75 mg/d) in a 6-week, randomized, placebo-controlled, double-blind trial did not significantly improve the primary measures of pain.[172] Venlafaxine at this low dose may have selective serotonergic activity, which makes it less antinociceptive than higher doses of venlafaxine that have dual activity on serotonin and norepinephrine.

Duloxetine, a potent SNRI with dual reuptake inhibition of serotonin and norepinephrine over the entire clinically relevant dose range,[173] is currently indicated by the US Food and Drug Administration (FDA) for acute and maintenance treatment of major depressive disorder in adults, acute treatment of generalized anxiety disorder in adults, the management of neuropathic pain associated with diabetic peripheral neuropathy in adults, and in 2008, duloxetine was approved by the FDA for the management of FM in adults.[174] **Table 3** summarizes randomized controlled trials of duloxetine in FM.[175–177] The most commonly reported treatment-emergent adverse events in placebo-controlled FM studies that were reported at a rate of 5% or more and at least twice the rate of placebo were nausea, dry mouth, constipation, somnolence, decreased appetite, increased sweating, and agitation.[174] A pooled analysis of almost 24,000 duloxetine patients from 64 studies found that most of the commonly reported adverse effects occurred early in treatment and were mild to moderate in severity.[178] In addition, an analysis of 8 pooled double-blind studies showed that nausea, the most frequently reported side effect, occurred in the first few weeks of treatment with duloxetine, and resolved for most patients within a few days to a week.[179] Furthermore, an evaluation of more than 8500 patients treated with duloxetine from 42 placebo-controlled studies found no increased cardiovascular risk associated with duloxetine.[180] In summary, the results of randomized, controlled trials of duloxetine in FM show that duloxetine monotherapy at doses of 60 mg once daily and 120 mg once daily reduces pain and improves other key symptoms of FM, such as mental fatigue, and is associated with improvement in function, health-related quality of life, and global assessments. Duloxetine is efficacious in FM patients with or without current depression, and the effect of duloxetine on reduction in pain seems to be independent of its effect on mood.

Milnacipran is another SNRI that has been approved for treatment of depression since 1997 in parts of Europe, Asia, and elsewhere. In the United States, milnacipran has been studied for the treatment of FM and received FDA approval for the management of FM in 2009.[181] Milnacipran is a dual serotonin and norepinephrine reuptake inhibitor within its therapeutic dose range and also exerts mild inhibition of NMDA.[95] Like duloxetine and venlafaxine, milnacipran lacks the side effects of tricyclics associated with antagonism of adrenergic, cholinergic, and histaminergic receptors. **Table 4** summarizes randomized controlled trials of milnacipran in FM.[182–184] Adverse events occurring in at least 5% of patients in the milnacipran treatment group at an incidence of at least 2 times that of patients in the placebo group included constipation, increased sweating, hot flush, vomiting, heart rate increase, dry mouth,

Table 3
Results from clinical trials of duloxetine in FM

Duloxetine Study	Duloxetine (Dosage, mg/d)	Study Design (No. of Patients)	Duration (Weeks)	Significant Efficacy Outcomes, Treatment Versus Placebo
Arnold et al (2004)[175]	Duloxetine (120)	Duloxetine vs placebo, parallel (207)	12	Reduction in total impact of FM, pain severity, stiffness, interference from pain, tender points. Improvement in measures of quality of life, function, and vitality. Improvement in clinician assessment of severity and patient global impression of improvement
Arnold et al (2005)[176]	Duloxetine (60 and 120)	Duloxetine vs placebo, parallel (354)	12	Reduction in total impact of FM, pain severity, interference from pain, tender points (120 mg). Improvement in measures of quality of life, function, and vitality. Improvement in clinician assessment of severity and patient global impression of improvement
Russell et al (2008)[177]	Duloxetine (20, 60, 120)	Duloxetine vs placebo, parallel (520)	15 (primary endpoint), 28 (secondary endpoint)	At 15 weeks: reduction in pain severity (60 mg, 120 mg), and total impact of FM. Improvement in motivation (60 mg, 120 mg), mental fatigue (60 mg), reduced activity (20 mg, 120 mg), clinician assessment of severity (60 mg, 120 mg); patient impression of improvement, and measures of function. At 28 weeks: reduction in pain severity. Improvement in patient global impression of improvement (20 mg, 120 mg), mental fatigue; physical fatigue (120 mg); reduced motivation (120 mg); reduced activity (120 mg); clinician assessment of severity, and measures of function (20 mg, 120 mg)

Table 4
Results from clinical trials of milnacipran in FM

Milnacipran Study	Milnacipran (Dosage, mg/d)	Study Design (No. of Patients)	Duration (Weeks)	Significant Efficacy Outcomes, Treatment Versus Placebo
Gendreau et al (2005)[182]	Milnacipran (up to 200)	Milnacipran vs placebo, parallel (125)	12	Reduction in pain severity Improvement in patient global impression of change, measures of physical function, fatigue, and morning stiffness
Clauw et al (2008)[183]	Milnacipran (100 and 200)	Milnacipran vs placebo, parallel (1196)	15	FM composite responder ($\geq$30% reduction in pain, much or very much improved on the patient global impression of change, and clinically significant improvement in physical function measure) FM pain composite responder ($\geq$30% reduction in pain, and much or very much improved on the patient global impression of change) Reduction in pain severity and total impact of FM Improvement in measures of function, self-perceived cognitive function (200 mg), fatigue (100 mg)
Mease et al (2009)[184]	Milnacipran (100 and 200)	Milnacipran vs placebo, parallel (888)	15 (primary endpoint), 27 (secondary endpoint)	At 15 weeks: FM composite responder; FM pain composite responder (200 mg) Reduction in pain severity; improvement in measures of function (200 mg), self-perceived cognitive function (200 mg), fatigue At 27 weeks: FM pain composite responder (200 mg) Reduction in pain severity; improvement in measures of function, self-perceived cognitive function (200 mg), fatigue (200 mg)

palpitations, and hypertension. The most common adverse event in all treatment groups was nausea, which tended to be dose related, mild to moderate in severity, and typically resolved in 2 to 4 weeks with continued therapy. In summary, the results of randomized controlled trials of milnacipran in FM show that milnacipran monotherapy at doses of 50 mg twice daily and 100 mg twice daily reduces pain and improves global assessments, function, and quality of life as well as other key symptoms of FM, such as fatigue and cognition.

Anticonvulsants

Pregabalin and gabapentin are alpha-2-delta ligands that have analgesic, anxiolytic, and anticonvulsant activity. The analgesic action of both drugs is believed to be mediated through binding to the alpha-2-delta (α-2-δ) protein, an auxiliary subunit of voltage-dependent calcium channels, and modulating the influx of calcium ions into hyperexcited neurons, and thereby reducing the synaptic release of several neurotransmitters believed to play a role in pain processing, including glutamate and substance P.[185–187]

Pregabalin is approved by the FDA for neuropathic pain associated with diabetic peripheral neuropathy, postherpetic neuralgia, adjunctive therapy for adults with partial onset seizures, and in 2007, was approved for the management of FM.[188] **Table 5** summarizes randomized controlled trials of pregabalin in FM.[189–192] Dizziness and somnolence were the most common adverse events associated with pregabalin treatment. Other events reported by at least 5% of patients in any of the treatment groups and more common in the combined pregabalin groups included increased weight, peripheral edema, fatigue, blurred vision, constipation, disturbance in attention, balance disorder, euphoric mood, sinusitis, back pain, dry mouth, increased appetite, and memory impairment. In summary, the results of randomized controlled trials of pregabalin in FM show that pregabalin monotherapy reduces pain and improves other key symptom domains of FM, such as sleep, and is associated with improvement in function, health-related quality of life, and global assessments. Pregabalin dosed at 150 mg twice a day, 225 mg twice a day, and 300 mg twice a day, has a durable effect for maintaining patient's improvement in pain associated with FM as well as in measures of global assessment, sleep, fatigue, and functional status in those who respond to pregabalin.

Another alpha-2-delta ligand, gabapentin, is indicated by the FDA for adjunct therapy in adults with partial seizures and for postherpetic neuralgia.[193] A multicenter, randomized, placebo-controlled, 12-week monotherapy trial tested the safety and efficacy of gabapentin 1200 mg/d to 2400 mg/d, administered 3 times daily, in 150 patients with FM.[194] The outcomes that responded significantly to gabapentin (median dose 1800 mg/d) compared with placebo were the primary outcome of reduction of pain, as well as secondary outcomes including the reduction in interference from pain, reduction in the total impact of FM, the clinician-rated impression of overall severity, the patient global impression of improvement, and improvement in measures of sleep and vitality. Significantly more patients treated with gabapentin compared with patients treated with placebo experienced a response to treatment, defined as a reduction of 30% or more in pain from baseline to end point. Most adverse events were mild to moderate in severity. The side effects reported by at least 5% of the patient treated with gabapentin and were more common in the gabapentin group were headache, dizziness, sedation, somnolence, edema, lightheadedness, insomnia, diarrhea, asthenia, depression, flatulence, nervousness, weight gain, amblyopia, anxiety, and dry mouth.

Table 5
Results from clinical trials of pregabalin in FM

Pregabalin Study	Pregabalin (Dosage, mg/d)	Study Design (No. of Patients)	Duration (Weeks)	Significant Efficacy Outcomes, Treatment Versus Placebo
Crofford et al (2005)[189]	Pregabalin (150, 300, 450)	Pregabalin vs placebo, parallel (529)	8	Reduction in pain severity (450 mg) Improvement in sleep quality (300 mg, 450 mg), sleep problems, fatigue (300 mg, 450 mg), patient and clinician global impression of change (300 mg, 450 mg), measures of function
Mease et al (2008)[190]	Pregabalin (300, 450, 600)	Pregabalin vs placebo, parallel (748)	13	Reduction in pain severity Improvement in patient global impression of change, sleep quality, sleep problems
Arnold et al (2008)[191]	Pregabalin (300, 450, 600)	Pregabalin vs placebo, parallel (750)	14	Reduction in pain severity; total impact of FM (450 mg, 600 mg) Improvement in patient global impression of change, sleep quality, sleep problems, anxiety (600 mg), vitality (450 mg, 600 mg), measures of function (450 mg, 600 mg)
Crofford et al (2008)[192]	Pregabalin (300, 450, 600)	Open-label phase to identify pregabalin responders, followed by randomization to placebo or pregabalin (1051)	6-week open-label, 26-week double-blind phase	Time to loss of therapeutic response (LTR) on pain (or clinical worsening) significantly longer for pregabalin group than for patients on placebo Time to LTR significantly longer for pregabalin group than placebo patients on patient global impression of change, total impact of FM, sleep problems, fatigue, and measures of function

Other pharmacological agents

Patients with FM frequently use nonsteroidal antiinflammatory drugs (NSAIDs), although there is no evidence from clinical trials that NSAIDs are effective when used alone in the treatment of FM.[195] However, studies have documented some benefit of ibuprofen and naproxen when combined with another medication (eg, amitriptyline, cyclobenzaprine).[196,197] The corticosteroid, prednisone, was found to be ineffective in FM, and corticosteroids are not recommended in the treatment of FM.[198]

Tramadol is a centrally acting opiate receptor agonist and a monoamine reuptake inhibitor that may exert antinociceptive effects within the ascending and descending pain pathways.[95] A multicenter, double-blind, randomized, placebo-controlled, 91-day study examined the efficacy of the combination of tramadol (37.5 mg) and acetaminophen (325 mg) in 315 patients with FM. Patients taking tramadol and acetaminophen (4 ± 1.8 tablets/d) were significantly more likely than placebo-treated subjects to continue treatment and experience an improvement in pain and physical function.[199] Although tramadol is marketed as an analgesic without scheduling under the Drug Enforcement Administration (DEA) Controlled Substances Act, it should be used with caution because of reports of classic opioid withdrawal with discontinuation and dose reduction, and some reports of abuse and dependence.[200] Other opioid agents have not been assessed in controlled trials of FM. A 4-year nonrandomized study found that patients with taking opiates did not report significant reduction in pain at the 4-year follow-up, and experienced increased depression in the last 2 years of the study.[201] Despite the lack of data supporting the use of opiates in FM, a survey of US academic medical centers found that about 14% of FM patients are treated with opiates,[202] and an Internet survey of more than 2500 self-identified patients with FM found that opioids were among the most commonly used treatments for FM.[203] The use of opiates in FM continues to be controversial, not only because of the lack of supportive efficacy data but also because of the abuse potential of opiates, and the emerging evidence of opioid-induced hyperalgesia.[204,205] The risk of opioid-induced hyperalgesia might limit the usefulness of opioids in controlling chronic pain associated with FM.

The short-acting nonbenzodiazepine sedatives, zolpidem and zopiclone, improved sleep in patients with FM but did not improve pain, limiting their usefulness in FM.[206–208] Although the combination of alprazolam and ibuprofen was somewhat beneficial in a pilot trial of FM,[209] another study found no significant benefit of another benzodiazepine, bromazepan, over placebo in the treatment of FM.[210]

Sodium oxybate, the sodium salt of γ-hydroxybutyrate (GHB), is a metabolite of the neurotransmitter, γ-aminobutyric acid (GABA), and has marked sedative properties. An 8-week study of sodium oxybate monotherapy evaluated 4.5 g or 6 g per day taken in 2 equally divided doses (bedtime and 2.5–4 hours later) in 188 patients with FM.[211] The primary outcome, a composite of changes from baseline in 3 coprimary measures including pain from electronic diaries, the total impact of fibromyalgia, and the patient global assessment of change, improved significantly with both dosages of sodium oxybate compared with placebo. Both dosages were also significantly superior to placebo in improvement in sleep quality, but the tender point count improved only in the higher sodium oxybate dose compared with placebo. The most common side effects were nausea and dizziness. GHB is associated with a high likelihood of abuse, cases of date rape, and, along with pentobarbital and methaqualone, is more likely to be lethal at supratherapeutic doses than other hypnotics.[212,213]

Nonpharmacological Treatment of FM

Exercise

Patients with FM may become sedentary because of symptoms such as pain and fatigue, and the deconditioning that results from lack of physical activity can make the symptoms of FM worse.[49] Exercise may help to reverse the effects of deconditioning and improve fitness, but the exact mechanism by which exercise improves FM symptoms is still unclear. A Cochrane review of exercise in the treatment of FM[214] concluded that moderate-intensity aerobic training for 12 weeks may improve overall well-being and physical function, but probably leads to little or no difference in pain or tender points. Strength training for 12 weeks may result in reductions in pain, tender points, and depression, and improvement in overall well-being, but may not improve physical function. Another recent review of exercise studies in FM[215] concluded that a gradual increase in exercise to reach a goal of 30 to 60 minutes of low- to moderate-intensity aerobic exercise (eg, walking, running, stationary bike, full-body exercise, aerobic sports, pool-based exercises in warm water) at least 2 to 3 times a week for more than 10 weeks seems to be associated with positive short-term benefits, with maintenance of those effects with ongoing exercise. Supervised group exercise interventions may be preferable to home-based exercise regimens, especially in helping patients initiate an exercise program and improving adherence. The use of exercise in patients with FM must be carefully prescribed and supervised to reduce muscle microtrauma induced by over training, which could lead to an exacerbation of FM pain and poor compliance.[216] Furthermore, aerobic exercise is a physiologic stressor to which FM patients often respond poorly because of the decreased sympathetic response to exercise and the evidence for a paradoxical decrease rather than increase in cortisol levels after exercise, as discussed previously. Therefore, it is important to carefully pace the patients' activities and prescribe an exercise program to fit the individual's level of fitness. A general rule is to recommend that patients initially do less than they think they can accomplish and slowly build endurance.[216] An additional benefit of exercise is weight loss, which could possibly improve neuroendocrine function.[128]

Cognitive behavioral therapy

Cognitive behavioral therapy (CBT) may help patients improve the way they think about and cope with FM. CBT that is targeted to a specific outcome such as function might be efficacious in patients with FM. For example, significantly more patients who attended CBT group sessions (6 sessions in 4 weeks) that were specifically aimed at improving physical function achieved a clinically meaningful and sustained improvement in physical function compared with the control group of patients receiving standard medical care.[217] Despite these positive results, there was a low level of adherence to the CBT, with only 15% of the patients consistently achieving their stated monthly cognitive behavioral goals.

There may be important patient characteristics that predict responsiveness to different psychological treatment approaches of patients with FM. One study evaluated CBT and operant behavioral therapy (based on the principles of operant conditioning and antecedents and consequences of behavior) compared with attention control.[218] At the 12-month follow-up, patients in the 2 therapy groups experienced significant reduction in pain intensity and physical impairment. Patients who responded to operant behavioral therapy had more pain behaviors, physical impairment, physician visits, solicitous spouse behaviors, and level of catastrophizing before treatment compared with nonresponders. The CBT responders, compared with nonresponders, had higher levels of affective distress, lower coping, less solicitous spouse behaviors, and lower pain behaviors before treatment. The study results suggest that it may be important to match treatments to patient characteristics to improve outcomes.

Education

Studies suggest that education about FM is an important component of overall FM management. In one study, patients with FM who participated in a social support and education group experienced significantly less helplessness, compared with a social support control group and a no-treatment control group.[219] Another 12-week study evaluated a supervised aerobic exercise program, a self-management education program, and the combination of exercise and education in women with FM.[220] For patients who complied with the protocol (only about half of the group), the combination of supervised exercise and group education improved self-efficacy for coping with some symptoms compared with the control group. A recent study evaluated the potential effect of 4 common self-management interventions in women with FM who were randomly assigned to 16 weeks of (1) group aerobic and flexibility exercise, (2) strength training, aerobic, and flexibility exercise, (3) the Arthritis Foundation's Fibromyalgia Self-Help Course, or (4) a combination of strength training, aerobic, flexibility exercises and the Fibromyalgia Self-Help Course.[221] The study found the beneficial effects of exercise were enhanced with the addition of the group-based self-management education.

Other nonpharmacological treatment

A review of studies conducted between 1975 and 2002[222] evaluating the use of complementary and alternative medicine in FM found that no single treatment approach was consistently effective. Among all of the treatments tested, acupuncture had the strongest evidence for efficacy, and there was moderate support for magnesium supplementation, S-adenosyl-L-methionine supplementation, and massage therapy. A more recent systematic review of randomized clinical trials of acupuncture in ACR-defined FM that included 5 trials, each with a sham treatment control group, concluded that there was no evidence that acupuncture is an effective treatment of FM symptoms.[223]

In conclusion, nonpharmacologic treatments have an important role in the management of FM. There is a need for improved access to treatment centers that offer these types of interventions. In addition, future studies should focus on ways to improve the adherence to nonpharmacologic therapies. Further studies are also needed to assess the efficacy of the combination of pharmacologic and nonpharmacologic strategies in the management of FM.

SUMMARY AND RECOMMENDATIONS FOR TREATMENT OF FM

Because the clinical presentation of FM is heterogeneous, treatment recommendations must be individualized for each patient. The rapid growth of trials in FM in recent years has resulted in new evidence-based approaches to pharmacological treatment.[215] Recent evidence suggests that comorbidity and the presence and severity of symptom domains are important when selecting initial medication treatments for FM. Until recently, a trial of tricyclic antidepressants or cyclobenzaprine was the first-line approach to the medication treatment of FM.[161] However, these medications are often poorly tolerated and are not effective at low doses for the treatment of mood or anxiety disorders, two common comorbid conditions. An alternative approach would be to recommend one of the new selective SNRIs as a first-line treatment of pain in patients with or without depression or anxiety. One caveat related to the use of SNRIs or other medications with antidepressant effects in FM is that they should not be used as monotherapy in patients with bipolar disorder, another frequently reported comorbid condition,[40] because of the risk of increased mood instability. An alternative first-line medication approach is an alpha-2-delta ligand, which may be particularly helpful in patients with prominent sleep disturbances or anxiety. For those patients who do not respond completely to monotherapy with either an SNRI or an alpha-2-delta ligand, a combination of these medications should be considered, although studies of this and other combination pharmacotherapies are still limited.[215] More recent work will likely expand the pharmacological treatment options for patients with FM.

Cardiovascular fitness training has been shown to be beneficial for some patients with FM. However, many patients report difficulty getting an exercise program started because of pain and fatigue, and are at risk of exercise-induced exacerbation of FM. Pharmacological treatment may help patients experience enough relief of symptoms to begin an adjunctive exercise program. Patients should be instructed to begin a program slowly and to pace themselves based on their level of fitness. Integration of psychoeducational approaches, including education about the disorder, support groups, and CBT, may also be helpful in improving patients' ability to cope with FM.

REFERENCES

1. Reynolds MD. The development of the concept of fibrositis. J Hist Med Allied Sci 1983;38:5–35.
2. Wolfe F, Smythe HA, Yunus MB, et al. The American College of Rheumatology 1990 criteria for the classification of fibromyalgia. Report of the multicenter criteria committee. Arthritis Rheum 1990;33:160–72.
3. Wolfe F, Ross K, Anderson J, et al. Aspects of fibromyalgia in the general population: sex, pain threshold, and fibromyalgia symptoms. J Rheumatol 1995;22: 151–6.
4. Gracely RH, Grant MAB, Giesecke T. Evoked pain measures in fibromyalgia. Best Pract Res Clin Rheumatol 2003;17:593–609.
5. MacFarlane GJ, Croft PR, Schollum J, et al. Widespread pain: is an improved classification possible? J Rheumatol 1996;23:1628–32.
6. Pope HG Jr, Hudson JI. A supplemental interview for forms of "affective spectrum disorder". Int J Psychiatry Med 1991;21:205–32.
7. Yunus MB, Masi AT, Aldag JC. Preliminary criteria for primary fibromyalgia syndrome (PFS): multivariate analysis of a consecutive series of PFS, other pain patients, and normal subjects. Clin Exp Rheumatol 1989;7:63–9.
8. First MB, Spitzer RL, Gibbon M, et al. Structured interview for the DSM-IV axis I disorders-patient edition (SCID-I/P). Version 2.0. New York: Biometrics Research Department, New York State Psychiatric Institute; 1995.
9. Dwight MM, Arnold LM, O'Brien H, et al. An open clinical trial of venlafaxine treatment of fibromyalgia. Psychosomatics 1998;39:14–7.
10. Hudson JI, Mangweth B, Pope HG Jr, et al. Family study of affective spectrum disorder. Arch Gen Psychiatry 2003;60:170–7.
11. Arnold LM, Hudson JI, Hess EV, et al. Family study of fibromyalgia. Arthritis Rheum 2004;50:944–52.
12. Katz RS, Wolfe F, Michaud K. Fibromyalgia diagnosis. A comparison of clinical, survey, and American College of Rheumatology Criteria. Arthritis Rheum 2006; 54:169–76.

13. White KP, Speechley M, Harth M, et al. The London fibromyalgia epidemiology study: comparing the demographic and clinical characteristics in 100 random community cases of fibromyalgia versus controls. J Rheumatol 1999;26: 1577–85.
14. Yunus MB, Inanici F, Aldag JC, et al. Fibromyalgia in men: comparison of clinical features with women. J Rheumatol 2000;27:485–90.
15. Yunus MB. Gender differences in fibromyalgia and other related syndromes. J Gend Specif Med 2002;5:42–7.
16. Buskila D, Neumann L, Alhoashle A, et al. Fibromyalgia syndrome in men. Semin Arthritis Rheum 2000;30:47–51.
17. Clauw DJ. Fibromyalgia syndrome: an update on current understanding and medical management. Rheumatol Grand Rounds 2000;3:1–9.
18. Fitzcharles MA, Esdaile JM. The overdiagnosis of fibromyalgia syndrome. Am J Med 1997;103:44–50.
19. Reilly PA. The differential diagnosis of generalized pain. Baillieres Clin Rheumatol 1999;13:391–401.
20. Daoud KF, Barkhuizen A. Rheumatic mimics and selected triggers of fibromyalgia. Curr Pain Headache Rep 2002;6:284–8.
21. Leventhal LJ, Bouali H. Fibromyalgia: 20 clinical pearls. J Musculoskel Med 2003;20:59–65.
22. Wolfe F, Ross K, Anderson J, et al. The prevalence and characteristics of fibromyalgia in the general population. Arthritis Rheum 1995;38:19–28.
23. Makela M, Heliovaara M. Prevalence of primary fibromyalgia in the Finnish population. BMJ 1991;303:216–9.
24. Lyddell C, Meyers OL. The prevalence of fibromyalgia in a South African community. Scand J Rheumatol 1992;21:8.
25. Raspe H, Baumgartner CH. The epidemiology of fibromyalgia syndrome (FMS) in a German town. Scand J Rheumatol 1992;21:8.
26. Prescott E, Kjoller M, Jacobsen S, et al. Fibromyalgia in the adult Danish population: I. A prevalence study. Scand J Rheumatol 1993;22:233–7.
27. Schochat T, Croft P, Raspe H. The epidemiology of fibromyalgia. Workshop of the standing committee on Epidemiology European League Against Rheumatism (EULAR), Bad Sackingen 19–21, November 1992. Br J Rheumatol 1994;33:783–6.
28. White KP, Speechley M, Harth M, et al. The London fibromyalgia epidemiology study: the prevalence of fibromyalgia syndrome in London, Ontario. J Rheumatol 1999;26:1570–6.
29. Lindell L, Bergman S, Petersson IF, et al. Prevalence of fibromyalgia and chronic widespread pain. Scand J Prim Health Care 2000;18:149–53.
30. Goldenberg DL, Simmus RW, Geiger A, et al. High frequency of fibromyalgia patients with chronic fatigue seen in primary care practice. Arthritis Rheum 1990;33:381–7.
31. Yunus M, Masi AT, Calabro JJ, et al. Primary fibromyalgia (fibrositis): clinical study of 50 patients with matched normal controls. Semin Arthritis Rheum 1981;11:151–71.
32. Yunus MB, Masi AT, Aldag JC. A controlled study of primary fibromyalgia syndrome: clinical features and association with other functional syndromes. J Rheumatol 1989;16:62–71.
33. White KP, Harth M, Speechley M, et al. Fibromyalgia in rheumatology practice. A survey of Canadian rheumatologists. J Rheumatol 1995;22:722–6.
34. White KP, Harth M. Classification, epidemiology, and natural history of fibromyalgia. Curr Pain Headache Rep 2001;5:320–9.

35. Forseth KO, Gran JT, Husby G. A population study of the incidence of fibromyalgia among women aged 26–55 yr. Br J Rheumatol 1997;36:1318–23.
36. Forseth KO, Husby G, Gran JT, et al. Prognostic factors for the development of fibromyalgia in women with self-reported musculoskeletal pain. A prospective study. J Rheumatol 1999;26:2458–67.
37. White KP, Nielson WR, Harth M, et al. Chronic widespread musculoskeletal pain with or without fibromyalgia: psychological distress in a representative community adult sample. J Rheumatol 2002;29:588–94.
38. Hudson JI, Hudson MS, Pliner LF, et al. Fibromyalgia and major affective disorder: a controlled phenomenology and family history study. Am J Psychiatry 1985;142:441–6.
39. Walker EA, Keegan D, Gardner G, et al. Psychosocial factors in fibromyalgia compared with rheumatoid arthritis: I. Psychiatric diagnoses and functional disability. Psychosom Med 1997;59:565–71.
40. Arnold LM, Hudson JI, Keck PE Jr, et al. Comorbidity of fibromyalgia and psychiatric disorders. J Clin Psychiatry 2006;67:1219–25.
41. Hudson JI, Pope HG Jr. The relationship between fibromyalgia and major depressive disorder. Rheum Dis Clin North Am 1996;22:285–303.
42. Aaron LA, Buchwald D. Chronic diffuse musculoskeletal pain, fibromyalgia, and co-morbid unexplained clinical conditions. Best Pract Res Clin Rheumatol 2003; 17:563–74.
43. Katon W, Sullivan M, Walker E. Medical symptoms without identified pathology: relationship to psychiatric disorders, childhood and adult trauma, and personality traits. Ann Intern Med 2001;134:917–25.
44. Hudson JI, Goldenberg DL, Pope HG Jr, et al. Comorbidity of fibromyalgia with medical and psychiatric disorders. Am J Med 1992;92:363–7.
45. Wessely S, Nimnuan C, Sharpe M. Functional somatic syndromes: one or many? Lancet 1999;354:936–9.
46. Sullivan PF, Smith W, Buchwald D. Latent class analysis of symptoms associated with chronic fatigue syndrome and fibromyalgia. Psychol Med 2002;32:881–8.
47. Wolfe F, Hawley D. Evidence of disordered symptom appraisal in fibromyalgia: increased rates of reported comorbidity and comorbidity severity. Clin Exp Rheumatol 1999;17:297–303.
48. Wolfe F, Hawley DJ. Psychosocial factors and the fibromyalgia syndrome. Z Rheumatol 1998;57:88–91.
49. Okifuji A, Bradshaw DH, Olson C. Evaluating obesity in fibromyalgia: neuroendocrine biomarkers, symptoms, and functions. Clin Rheumatol 2009;28:475–8.
50. Moldofsky H. Management of sleep disorders in fibromyalgia. Rheum Dis Clin North Am 2002;28:353–65.
51. May KP, West SG, Baker MR, et al. Sleep apnea in male patients with the fibromyalgia syndrome. Am J Med 1993;94:505–8.
52. Gold AR, Dipalo F, Gold MS, et al. Inspiratory airflow dynamics during sleep in women with fibromyalgia. Sleep 2004;27:459–66.
53. Berger A, Dukes E, Martin S, et al. Characteristics and healthcare costs of patients with fibromyalgia syndrome. Int J Clin Pract 2007;61:1498–508.
54. Kennedy M, Felson DT. A prospective long-term study of fibromyalgia syndrome. Arthritis Rheum 1996;39:682–5.
55. Wolfe F, Anderson J, Harkness D, et al. Health status and disease severity in fibromyalgia. Arthritis Rheum 1997;40:1571–9.
56. Ledingham J, Doherty S, Doherty M. Primary fibromyalgia syndrome—an outcome study. Br J Rheumatol 1993;32:139–42.

57. Henriksson CM. Longterm effects of fibromyalgia on everyday life: a study of 58 patients. Scand J Rheumatol 1994;23:36–41.
58. Baumgartner E, Finckh A, Cedraschi C, et al. A six year prospective study of a cohort of patients with fibromyalgia. Ann Rheum Dis 2002;61:644–5.
59. Granges G, Zilko P, Littlejohn GO. Fibromyalgia syndrome: assessment of the severity of the condition 2 years after diagnosis. J Rheumatol 1994;21:523–9.
60. Fitzcharles MA, Da Costa D, Poyhia R. A study of standard care in fibromyalgia syndrome: a favorable outcome. J Rheumatol 2003;30:154–9.
61. Goldenberg DL. Fibromyalgia syndrome a decade later: what have we learned? Arch Intern Med 1999;159:777–85.
62. MacFarlane GJ, Thomas E, Papageorgiou AC, et al. The natural history of chronic pain in the community: a better prognosis than in the clinic? J Rheumatol 1996;23:1617–20.
63. Hoffman DL, Dukes EM. The health status burden of people with fibromyalgia: a review of studies that assessed health status with the SF-36 or the SF-12. Int J Clin Pract 2008;62:115–26.
64. White LA, Birnbaum HG, Kaltenboeck A, et al. Employees with fibromyalgia: medical comorbidity, healthcare costs, and work loss. J Occup Environ Med 2008;50:13–24.
65. White KP, Speechley M, Harth M, et al. Comparing self-reported function and work disability in 100 community cases of fibromyalgia syndrome versus controls in London, Ontario. Arthritis Rheum 1999;42:76–83.
66. Wolfe F, Anderson J, Harkness D, et al. Work and disability status of persons with fibromyalgia. J Rheumatol 1997;24:1171–8.
67. Hawley DJ, Wolfe F. Pain, disability, and pain/disability relationships in seven rheumatic disorders: a study of 1,522 patients. J Rheumatol 1991;18:1552–7.
68. Burckhardt CS, Clark SR, Bennett RM. Fibromyalgia and quality of life: a comparative analysis. J Rheumatol 1993;20:475–9.
69. Kaplan RM, Schmidt SM, Cronan TA. Quality of well being in patients with fibromyalgia. J Rheumatol 2000;27:785–9.
70. Epstein SA, Kay G, Clauw D, et al. Psychiatric disorders in patients with fibromyalgia. Psychosomatics 1999;40:57–63.
71. Pellegrino MJ, Waylonis GW, Sommer A. Familial occurrence of primary fibromyalgia. Arch Phys Med Rehabil 1989;70:61–3.
72. Buskila D, Neumann L, Hazanov I, et al. Familial aggregation in the fibromyalgia syndrome. Semin Arthritis Rheum 1996;26:605–11.
73. Buskila D, Neumann L. Fibromyalgia syndrome (FM) and nonarticular tenderness in relatives of patients with FM. J Rheumatol 1997;24:941–4.
74. Hudson JI, Arnold LM, Keck PE Jr, et al. Family study of fibromyalgia and affective spectrum disorder. Biol Psychiatry 2004;56:884–91.
75. Bondy B, Spaeth M, Offenbaecher M, et al. The T102C polymorphism of the 5-HT2A-receptor gene in fibromyalgia. Neurobiol Dis 1999;6:433–9.
76. Gursoy S, Erdal E, Herken H, et al. Association of T102C polymorphism of the 5-HT2A receptor gene with psychiatric status in fibromyalgia syndrome. Rheumatol Int 2001;21:58–61.
77. Offenbaecher M, Bondy B, de Jonge S, et al. Possible association of fibromyalgia with a polymorphism in the serotonin transporter gene regulatory region. Arthritis Rheum 1999;42:2482–8.
78. Gursoy S. Absence of association of the serotonin transporter gene polymorphism with the mentally healthy subset of fibromyalgia patients. Clin Rheumatol 2002;21:194–7.

79. Buskila D, Cohen H, Neumann L, et al. An association between fibromyalgia and the dopamine D4 receptor exon III repeat polymorphism and relationship to novelty seeking personality traits. Mol Psychiatry 2004;9:730–1.

80. Zubieta JK, Heitzeg MM, Smith YR, et al. COMT val158met genotype affects mu-opioid neurotransmitter responses to a pain stressor. Science 2003;299:1240–3.

81. Gursoy S, Erdal E, Herken H, et al. Significance of catechol-O-methyltransferase gene polymorphism in fibromyalgia syndrome. Rheumatol Int 2003;23:104–7.

82. Diatchenko L, Slade GD, Nackley AG, et al. Genetic basis for individual variations in pain perception and the development of a chronic pain condition. Hum Mol Genet 2005;14:135–43.

83. van Meurs JB, Uitterlinden AG, Stolk L, et al. A functional polymorphism in the catechol-O-methyltransferase gene is associated with osteoarthritis-related pain. Arthritis Rheum 2009;60:628–9.

84. Tahara T, Arisawa T, Shibata T, et al. COMT gene val158met polymorphism in patients with dyspeptic symptoms. Hepatogastroenterology 2008;55:979–82.

85. George SZ, Wallace MR, Wright TW, et al. Evidence for a biopsychosocial influence on shoulder pain: pain catastrophizing and catechol-O-methyltransferase (COMT) diplotype predict clinical pain ratings. Pain 2008;136:53–61.

86. Harrison PJ, Tunbridge EM. Catechol-O-methyltransferase (COMT): a gene contributing to sex differences in brain function, and to sexual dimorphism in the predisposition to psychiatric disorders. Neuropsychopharmacology 2008;33:3037–45.

87. Dailey PA, Bishop GD, Russell IJ, et al. Psychological stress and the fibrositis/fibromyalgia syndrome. J Rheumatol 1990;17:1380–5.

88. Anderberg UM, Marteinsdottir I, Theorell T, et al. The impact of life events in female patients with fibromyalgia and in female healthy controls. Eur Psychiatry 2000;15:295–301.

89. Walker EA, Keegan D, Gardner G, et al. Psychosocial factors in fibromyalgia compared with rheumatoid arthritis: II. Sexual, physical and emotional abuse and neglect. Psychosom Med 1997;59:572–7.

90. Imbierowicz K, Egle UT. Childhood adversities in patients with fibromyalgia and somatoform pain disorder. Eur J Pain 2003;7:113–9.

91. Van Houdenhove B, Neerinckx E, Lysens R, et al. Victimization in chronic fatigue syndrome and fibromyalgia in tertiary care. Psychosomatics 2001;42:21–8.

92. Pillemer SR, Bradley LA, Crofford LJ, et al. The neuroscience and endocrinology of fibromyalgia. Arthritis Rheum 1997;40:1928–39.

93. Adler GK, Kinsley BT, Hurwitz S, et al. Reduced hypothalamic-pituitary and sympathoadrenal responses to hypoglycemia in women with fibromyalgia syndrome. Am J Med 1999;106:534–43.

94. Adler GK, Manfredsdottir VF, Creskoff KW. Neuroendocrine abnormalities in fibromyalgia. Curr Pain Headache Rep 2002;6:289–98.

95. Kranzler JD, Gendreau JF, Rao SG. The psychopharmacology of fibromyalgia: a drug development perspective. Psychopharmacol Bull 2002;36:165–213.

96. Torpy DJ, Dapanicolaou DA, Lotsikas AJ, et al. Responses of the sympathetic nervous system and the hypothalamic-pituitary-adrenal axis to interleukin-6: a pilot study in fibromyalgia. Arthritis Rheum 2000;43:872–80.

97. Griep EN, Boersma JW, de Kloet ER. Altered reactivity of the hypothalamic-pituitary-adrenal axis in the primary fibromyalgia syndrome. J Rheumatol 1993;20:469–74.

98. Griep EN, Boersma JW, Lentjes EG, et al. Function of the hypothalamic-pituitary-adrenal axis in patients with fibromyalgia and low back pain. J Rheumatol 1998;25:1374–81.
99. Riedel W, Kayka H, Neeck G. Secretory pattern of GH, TSH, thyroid hormones, ACTH, cortisol, FSH and LH in patients with fibromyalgia syndrome following systemic injection of the relevant hypothalamic-releasing hormones. Z Rheumatol 1998;57:81–7.
100. Chrousos GP, Gold PW. The concepts of stress and stress system disorders. JAMA 1992;267:1244–52.
101. Clauw DJ, Chrousos GP. Chronic pain and fatigue syndromes: overlapping clinical and neuroendocrine features and potential pathogenic mechanisms. Neuroimmunomodulation 1997;4:134–53.
102. Demitrack MA, Crofford LJ. Evidence for and pathophysiologic implications of hypothalamic-pituitary-adrenal axis dysregulation in fibromyalgia and chronic fatigue syndrome. Ann N Y Acad Sci 1998;840:684–97.
103. Heim C, Ehlert U, Hellhammer DH. The potential role of hypocortisolism in the pathophysiology of stress-related bodily disorders. Psychoneuroendocrinology 2000;25:1–35.
104. Gold PW, Chrousos GP. The endocrinology of melancholic and atypical depression: relation to neurocircuitry and somatic consequences. Proc Assoc Am Physicians 1999;111:22–34.
105. Neeck G, Crofford LJ. Neuroendocrine perturbations in fibromyalgia and chronic fatigue syndrome. Rheum Dis Clin North Am 2000;26:989–1002.
106. Crofford LJ, Young EA, Engleberg NC, et al. Basal circadian and pulsatile ACTH and cortisol secretion in patients with fibromyalgia and/or chronic fatigue syndrome. Brain Behav Immun 2004;18:314–25.
107. McClean SA, Williams DA, Stein PK, et al. Cerebrospinal fluid corticotrophin-releasing factor concentration is associated with pain but not fatigue symptoms in patients with fibromyalgia. Neuropsychopharmacology 2006;31:2776–82.
108. McClean SA, Williams DA, Harris RE, et al. Momentary relationship between cortisol secretion and symptoms in patients with fibromyalgia. Arthritis Rheum 2005;52:3660–9.
109. Bennett RM, Clark SR, Burckhardt CS, et al. Hypothalamic-pituitary-insulin-like growth factor-I axis dysfunction in patients with fibromyalgia. J Rheumatol 1997;24:1384–9.
110. Neeck G, Riedel W. Thyroid function in patients with fibromyalgia syndrome. J Rheumatol 1992;19:1120–2.
111. Petzke F, Clauw DJ. Sympathetic nervous system function in fibromyalgia. Curr Rheumatol Rep 2000;2:116–23.
112. Qiao ZG, Vaeroy H, Morkrid L. Electrodermal and microcirculatory activity in patients with fibromyalgia during baseline, acoustic stimulation, and cold pressor tests. J Rheumatol 1991;18:1383–9.
113. Van Denderen JC, Boersma JW, Zeinstra P, et al. Physiological effects of exhaustive physical exercise in primary fibromyalgia syndrome (PFS): is PFS a disorder of neuroendocrine reactivity? Scand J Rheumatol 1992;21:35–7.
114. Bou-Holaigah I, Calkins H, Flynn JA, et al. Provocation of hypotension and pain during upright tilt table testing in adults with fibromyalgia. Clin Exp Rheumatol 1997;15:239–46.
115. Martinez-Lavin M, Hermosillo AG, Mendoza C, et al. Orthostatic sympathetic derangement in subjects with fibromyalgia. J Rheumatol 1997;24:714–8.

116. Raj SR, Brouillard D, Simpson CS, et al. Dysautonomia among patients with fibromyalgia: a noninvasive assessment. J Rheumatol 2000;27:2660–5.
117. Martinez-Lavin M. Biology and therapy of fibromyalgia. Stress, the stress response system, and fibromyalgia. Arthritis Res Ther 2007;9:216.
118. Heim C, Newport DJ, Heit S, et al. Pituitary-adrenal and autonomic responses to stress in women after sexual and physical abuse in childhood. JAMA 2000;284: 592–7.
119. McBeth J, Silman AJ, Gupta A, et al. Moderation of psychosocial risk factors through dysfunction of the hypothalamic-pituitary-adrenal stress axis in the onset of chronic widespread musculoskeletal pain. Findings of a population-based prospective cohort study. Arthritis Rheum 2007;56:360–71.
120. Holliday KL, Nicholl BI, Macfarlane GJ, et al. Genetic variation in the hypotha-lamic-pituitary-adrenal stress axis influences susceptibility to musculoskeletal pain: results from the EPIFUND study. Ann Rheum Dis 31 Aug 2009. [Online].
121. Korszun A, Young EA, Engleberg NC, et al. Follicular phase hypothalamic-pituitary-gonadal axis function in women with fibromyalgia and chronic fatigue syndrome. J Rheumatol 2000;27:1526–30.
122. Akkus S, Delibas N, Tamer MN. Do sex hormones play a role in fibromyalgia? Rheumatology 2000;39:1161–3.
123. Gur A, Cevik R, Sarac AJ, et al. Hypothalamic-pituitary-gonadal axis and cortisol in young women with primary fibromyalgia: the potential roles of depression, fatigue, and sleep disturbance in the occurrence of hypocortisolism. Ann Rheum Dis 2004;63:1504–6.
124. Okifuji A, Turk DC. Sex hormones and pain in regularly menstruating women with fibromyalgia syndrome. J Pain 2006;7:851–9.
125. Vamvakopoulos NC, Chrousos GP. Evidence of direct estrogenic regulation of human corticotropin-releasing hormone gene expression. Potential implications for the sexual dimorphism of the stress response and immune/inflammatory reaction. J Clin Invest 1993;92:1896–902.
126. Tsigos C, Chrousos GP. Hypothalamic-pituitary-adrenal axis, neuroendocrine factors and stress. J Psychosom Res 2002;53:865–71.
127. Waxman J, Zatzkis SM. Fibromyalgia and menopause. Examination of the rela-tionship. Postgrad Med 1986;80:165–7, 170–1.
128. Dessein PH, Shipton EA, Stanwix AE. Neuroendocrine deficiency-mediated development and persistence of pain in fibromyalgia: a promising paradigm? Pain 2000;86:213–5.
129. Lautenbacher S, Rollman GB. Possible deficiencies of pain modulation in fibro-myalgia. Clin J Pain 1997;13:189–96.
130. Bennett RM. Emerging concepts in the neurobiology of chronic pain: evidence of abnormal sensory processing in fibromyalgia. Mayo Clin Proc 1999;74: 385–98.
131. Staud R. Evidence of involvement of central neural mechanisms in generating fibromyalgia pain. Curr Rheumatol Rep 2002;4:299–305.
132. Baranauskas G, Nistri A. Sensitization of pain pathways in the spinal cord: cellular mechanisms. Prog Neurobiol 1998;54:349–65.
133. Woolf CJ. Pain: moving from symptom control toward mechanism-specific pharmacologic management. Ann Intern Med 2004;140:441–51.
134. Latremoliere A, Woolf CJ. Central sensitization: a generator of pain hypersensi-tivity by central neural plasticity. J Pain 2009;10:895–926.
135. Buskila D, Neumann L. Musculoskeletal injury as a trigger for fibromyalgia/posttraumatic fibromyalgia. Curr Rheumatol Rep 2000;2:104–8.

136. Wallace DJ, Linker-Israeli M, Hallegua D, et al. Cytokines play an aetiopathogenetic role in fibromyalgia: a hypothesis and pilot study. Rheumatology 2001;40:743–9.

137. Watkins LR, Maier SF. Immune regulation of central nervous system functions: from sickness responses to pathological pain. J Intern Med 2005;257:139–55.

138. Vaeroy H, Helle R, Fokrre O, et al. Elevated CSF levels of substance P and high incidence of Raynaud phenomenon in patients with fibromyalgia: new features for diagnosis. Pain 1988;32:21–6.

139. Russell IJ, Orr MD, Littman B, et al. Elevated cerebrospinal fluid levels of substance P in patients with fibromyalgia syndrome. Arthritis Rheum 1994;37:1593–601.

140. Watkins LR, Wiertelak EP, Furness LE, et al. Illness-induced hyperalgesia is mediated by spinal neuropeptides and excitatory amino acids. Brain Res 1994;664:17–24.

141. Schwarz MJ, Spath M, Muller-Bardorff H, et al. Relationship of substance P, 5-hydroxyindole acetic acid and tryptophan in serum of fibromyalgia patients. Neurosci Lett 1999;259:196–8.

142. Sarchielli P, Mancini ML, Floridi A, et al. Increased levels of neurotrophins are not specific for chronic migraine: evidence from primary fibromyalgia syndrome. J Pain 2007;8:737–45.

143. Harris RE, Sundgren PC, Pang Y, et al. Dynamic levels of glutamate within the insula are associated with improvements in multiple pain domains in fibromyalgia. Arthritis Rheum 2008;58:903–7.

144. de Souza JB, Potvin S, Goffaux P, et al. The deficit of pain inhibition in fibromyalgia is more pronounced in patients with comorbid depressive symptoms. Clin J Pain 2009;25:123–7.

145. Russell IJ, Vaeroy H, Javors M, et al. Cerebrospinal fluid biogenic amine metabolites in fibromyalgia/fibrositis syndrome and rheumatoid arthritis. Arthritis Rheum 1992;35:550–6.

146. Russell IJ, Michalek JE, Vipraio GA, et al. Platelet 3H-imipramine uptake receptor density and serum serotonin levels in patients with fibromyalgia/fibrositis syndrome. J Rheumatol 1992;19:104–9.

147. Yunus MB, Dailey JW, Aldag JC, et al. Plasma tryptophan and other amino acids in primary fibromyalgia: a controlled study. J Rheumatol 1992;19:90–4.

148. Basbaum AI, Fields HL. Endogenous pain control systems: brainstem pathways and endorphin circuitry. Annu Rev Neurosci 1984;7:309–38.

149. Clark FM, Proudfit HK. The projections of noradrenergic neurons in the A5 catecholamine cell groups to the spinal cord in the rat: anatomical evidence that A5 neurons modulate nociception. Brain Res 1993;616:200–13.

150. Kageyama K, Tozawa F, Horiba N, et al. Serotonin stimulates corticotropin-releasing factor gene expression in the hypothalamic paraventricular nucleus of conscious rats. Neurosci Lett 1998;243:17–20.

151. Moldofsky H, Scarisbrick P. Induction of neurasthenic musculoskeletal pain syndrome by selective sleep stage deprivation. Psychosom Med 1975;38:35–44.

152. Moldofsky H, Scarisbrick P, England R, et al. Musculoskeletal symptoms and non-REM sleep disturbance in patients with "fibrositis syndrome" and healthy subjects. Psychosom Med 1975;37:341–51.

153. Nishizawa S, Benkelfat C, Young SN, et al. Differences between males and females in rates of serotonin synthesis in human brain. Proc Natl Acad Sci U S A 1997;94:5308–13.

154. Gracely RH, Petzke F, Wolf JM, et al. Functional magnetic resonance imaging evidence of augmented pain processing in fibromyalgia. Arthritis Rheum 2002;46:1333–43.

155. Bradley LA, McKendree-Smith NL, Alarcon GS, et al. Is fibromyalgia a neurologic disease? Curr Pain Headache Rep 2002;6:106–14.
156. Fishbain D. Evidence-based data on pain relief with antidepressants. Ann Med 2000;32:305–16.
157. Arnold LM. Duloxetine and other antidepressants in the treatment of patients with fibromyalgia. Pain Med 2007;8(Suppl 2):S63–74.
158. Lawson K. Tricyclic antidepressants and fibromyalgia: what is the mechanism of action? Expert Opin Investig Drugs 2002;11:1437–45.
159. Arnold LM, Keck PE Jr, Welge JA. Antidepressant treatment of fibromyalgia. A meta-analysis and review. Psychosomatics 2000;41:104–13.
160. Tofferi JK, Jackson JL, O'Malley PG. Treatment of fibromyalgia with cyclobenzaprine: a meta-analysis. Arthritis Rheum 2004;51:9–13.
161. Goldenberg DL, Burckhardt C, Crofford L. Management of fibromyalgia syndrome. JAMA 2004;292:2388–95.
162. Beliles K, Stoudemire A. Psychopharmacologic treatment of depression in the medically ill. Psychosomatics 1998;39:S2–19.
163. Nørregaard J, Volkmann H, Danneskiold-Samsø B. A randomized controlled trial of citalopram in the treatment of fibromyalgia. Pain 1995;61:445–9.
164. Anderberg UM, Marteinsdottir I, von Knorring L. Citalopram in patients with fibromyalgia – a randomized, double-blind, placebo-controlled study. Eur J Pain 2000;4:27–35.
165. Wolfe F, Cathey MA, Hawley DJ. A double-blind placebo controlled trial of fluoxetine in fibromyalgia. Scand J Rheumatol 1994;23:255–9.
166. Goldenberg D, Mayskiy M, Mossey C, et al. A randomized, double-blind cross-over trial of fluoxetine and amitriptyline in the treatment of fibromyalgia. Arthritis Rheum 1996;39:1852–9.
167. Arnold LM, Hess EV, Hudson JI, et al. A randomized, placebo-controlled, double-blind, flexible-dose study of fluoxetine in the treatment of women with fibromyalgia. Am J Med 2002;112:191–7.
168. Patkar AA, Masand PS, Krulewicz S, et al. A randomized, controlled trial of controlled release paroxetine in fibromyalgia. Am J Med 2007;120:448–54.
169. Millan MJ. Descending control of pain. Prog Neurobiol 2002;66:355–474.
170. Fishbain DA, Cutler R, Rosomoff HL, et al. Evidence-based data from animal and human experimental studies on pain relief with antidepressants: a structured review. Pain Med 2000;1:310–6.
171. Harvey AT, Rudolph RL, Preskorn SH. Evidence of the dual mechanisms of action of venlafaxine. Arch Gen Psychiatry 2000;57:503–9.
172. Zijlstra TR, Barendregt PJ, van de Laar MAF. Venlafaxine in fibromyalgia: results of a randomized, placebo-controlled, double-blind trial. 66th Annual Meeting of the American College of Rheumatology, New Orleans, LA, October 24–29, 2002.
173. Bymaster FP, Dreshfield-Ahmad LJ, Threlkeld PG, et al. Comparative affinity of duloxetine for serotonin and norepinephrine transporters in vitro and in vivo, human serotonin receptor subtypes, and other neuronal receptors. Neuropsychopharmacology 2001;25:871–80.
174. Eli Lilly and Company, Cymbalta (duloxetine), package insert. Indianapolis (IN), June 2008.
175. Arnold LM, Lu Y, Crofford LJ, et al. A double-blind, multicenter trial comparing duloxetine to placebo in the treatment of fibromyalgia patients with or without major depressive disorder. Arthritis Rheum 2004;50: 2974–84.

176. Arnold LM, Rosen A, Pritchett YL, et al. A randomized, double-blind, placebo-controlled trial of duloxetine in the treatment of women with fibromyalgia with or without major depressive disorder. Pain 2005;119:5–15.

177. Russell IJ, Mease PJ, Smith TR, et al. Efficacy and safety of duloxetine for treatment of fibromyalgia in patients with or without major depressive disorder: results from a 6-month, randomized, double-blind, placebo-controlled, fixed-dose trial. Pain 2008;136:432–44.

178. Gahimer J, Wernicke J, Yalcin I, et al. A retrospective pooled analysis of duloxetine safety in 23,983 subjects. Curr Med Res Opin 2007;23:175–84.

179. Greist J, McNamara RK, Mallinckrodt CH, et al. Incidence and duration of antidepressant-induced nausea: duloxetine compared with paroxetine and fluoxetine. Clin Ther 2004;26:1446–55.

180. Wernicke JF, Lledo A, Raskin J, et al. An evaluation of the cardiovascular safety profile of duloxetine: findings from 42 placebo-controlled studies. Drug Saf 2007;30:437–55.

181. Forest Pharmaceuticals, Inc. Savella (milnacipran), package insert. June 2009.

182. Gendreau RM, Thorn MD, Gendreau JF, et al. Efficacy of milnacipran in patients with fibromyalgia. J Rheumatol 2005;32:1975–85.

183. Clauw DJ, Mease P, Palmer RH, et al. Milnacipran for the treatment of fibromyalgia in adults: a 15-week, multicenter, randomized, double-blind, placebo-controlled, multiple-dose clinical trial. Clin Ther 2008;30:1988–2004.

184. Mease PJ, Clauw DJ, Gendreau M, et al. The efficacy and safety of milnacipran for treatment of fibromyalgia. A randomized, double-blind, placebo-controlled trial. J Rheumatol 2009;36:398–409.

185. Dooley DJ, Taylor CP, Donevan S, et al. Ca^{2+} channel $\alpha_2\delta$ ligands: novel modulators of neurotransmission. Trends Pharmacol Sci 2007;28:75–82.

186. Field MJ, Cox PJ, Stott E, et al. Identification of the alpha2-delta-1 subunit of voltage-dependent calcium channels as a molecular target for pain mediating the analgesic actions of pregabalin. Proc Natl Acad Sci U S A 2006;103:17537–42.

187. Taylor CJ, Angelotti T, Fauman E. Pharmacology and mechanism of action of pregabalin: the calcium channel α_2–δ (alpha$_2$-delta) subunit as a target for antiepileptic drug discovery. Epilepsy Res 2007;73:137–50.

188. Pfizer Inc, Lyrica (pregabalin), package insert. New York; June 2007.

189. Crofford LJ, Rowbotham MC, Mease PJ, et al. Pregabalin for the treatment of fibromyalgia syndrome. Results of a randomized, double-blind, placebo-controlled trial. Arthritis Rheum 2005;52:1264–73.

190. Mease PJ, Russell IJ, Arnold LM, et al. A randomized, double-blind, placebo-controlled, phase III trial of pregabalin in the treatment of patients with fibromyalgia. J Rheumatol 2008;35:502–14.

191. Arnold LM, Russell IJ, Diri EW, et al. A 14-week, randomized, double-blinded, placebo-controlled monotherapy trial of pregabalin in patients with fibromyalgia. J Pain 2008;9:792–805.

192. Crofford LJ, Mease PJ, Simpson SL, et al. Fibromyalgia relapse evaluation and efficacy for durability of meaningful relief (FREEDOM): a 6-month, double-blind, placebo-controlled trial with pregabalin. Pain 2008;136:419–31.

193. Pfizer Inc, Neurontin (gabapentin), package insert. New York; January 2007.

194. Arnold LM, Goldenberg DL, Stanford SB, et al. Gabapentin in the treatment of fibromyalgia. A randomized, double-blind, placebo-controlled, multicenter trial. Arthritis Rheum 2007;56:1336–44.

195. Rossy LA, Buckelew SP, Dorr N, et al. A meta-analysis of fibromyalgia treatment interventions. Ann Behav Med 1999;21:180–91.

196. Goldenberg DL, Felson DT, Dinerman H. A randomized, controlled trial of amitriptyline and naproxen in the treatment of patients with fibromyalgia. Arthritis Rheum 1986;29:1371–7.
197. Fossaluzza V, De Vita S. Combined therapy with cyclobenzaprine and ibuprofen in primary fibromyalgia syndrome. Int J Clin Pharmacol Res 1992;12:99–102.
198. Clark S, Tindall E, Bennett RM. A double blind crossover trial of prednisone versus placebo in the treatment of fibrositis. J Rheumatol 1985;12:980–3.
199. Bennett RM, Kamin M, Karim R, et al. Tramadol and acetaminophen combination tablets in the treatment of fibromyalgia pain: a double-blind, randomized, placebo-controlled study. Am J Med 2003;114:537–45.
200. Senay EC, Adams EH, Geller A, et al. Physical dependence on Ultram® (tramadol hydrochloride): both opioid-like and atypical withdrawal symptoms occur. Drug Alcohol Depend 2003;69:233–41.
201. Kemple KL, Smith G, Wong-Ngan J. Opioid therapy in fibromyalgia – a four year prospective evaluation of therapy selection, efficacy, and predictors of outcome. Arthritis Rheum 2003;48:S88.
202. Wolfe F, Anderson J, Harkness D, et al. A prospective, longitudinal, multicenter study of service utilization and costs in fibromyalgia. Arthritis Rheum 1997;40:1560–70.
203. Bennett RM, Jones J, Turk DC, et al. An internet survey of 2,596 people with fibromyalgia. BMC Musculoskelet Disord 2007;8:27.
204. Chu LF, Clark DJ, Angst MS. Opioid tolerance and hyperalgesia in chronic pain patients after one month of oral morphine therapy: a preliminary prospective study. J Pain 2006;7:43–8.
205. King T, Gardell LR, Wang R, et al. Role of NK-1 neurotransmission in opioid-induced hyperalgesia. Pain 2005;116:276–88.
206. Drewes AM, Andreasen A, Jennum P, et al. Zopiclone in the treatment of sleep abnormalities in fibromyalgia. Scand J Rheumatol 1991;20:288–93.
207. Gronblad M, Nykanen J, Konttinen Y, et al. Effect of zopiclone on sleep quality, morning stiffness, widespread tenderness and pain and general discomfort in primary fibromyalgia patients. A double-blind randomized trial. Clin Rheumatol 1993;12:186–91.
208. Moldofsky H, Lue FA, Mously C, et al. The effect of zolpidem in patients with fibromyalgia: a dose ranging, double blind, placebo controlled, modified crossover study. J Rheumatol 1996;23:529–33.
209. Russell IJ, Fletcher EM, Michalek JE, et al. Treatment of primary fibrositis/fibromyalgia syndrome with ibuprofen and alprazolam. A double-blind, placebo-controlled study. Arthritis Rheum 1991;34:552–60.
210. Quijada-Carrera J, Valenzuela-Castano A, Povedano-Gomez J, et al. Comparison of tenoxicam and bromazepan in the treatment of fibromyalgia: a randomized, double-blind, placebo-controlled trial. Pain 1996;65:221–5.
211. Russell IJ, Perkins AT, Michalek JE. Sodium oxybate relieves pain and improves function in fibromyalgia syndrome: a randomized, double-blind, placebo-controlled, multicenter clinical trial. Arthritis Rheum 2009;60:299–309.
212. Nicholson KL, Balster RL. GHB: a new and novel drug of abuse. Drug Alcohol Depend 2001;63:1–22.
213. Griffiths RR, Johnson MW. Relative abuse liability of hypnotic drugs: a conceptual framework and algorithm for differentiating among compounds. J Clin Psychiatry 2005;66(Suppl 9):31–41.
214. Busch AJ, Barber KA, Overend TJ, et al. Exercise for treating fibromyalgia syndrome. Cochrane Database Syst Rev 2007;(4):CD003786.

215. Arnold LM. Biology and therapy of fibromyalgia. New therapies in fibromyalgia. Arthritis Res Ther 2006;8:212.
216. Clark SR, Jones KD, Burckhardt CS, et al. Exercise for patients with fibromyalgia: risks versus benefits. Curr Rheumatol Rep 2001;3:135–46.
217. Williams DA, Cary MA, Groner KH, et al. Improving physical functional status in patients with fibromyalgia: a brief cognitive behavioral intervention. J Rheumatol 2002;29:1280–6.
218. Thieme K, Turk DC, Flor H. Responder criteria for operant and cognitive-behavioral treatment of fibromyalgia syndrome. Arthritis Rheum 2007;57:830–6.
219. Oliver K, Cronan TA, Walen HR, et al. Effects of social support and education on health care costs for patients with fibromyalgia. J Rheumatol 2001;28:2711–9.
220. King SJ, Wessel J, Bhambhani Y, et al. The effects of exercise and education, individually or combined, in women with fibromyalgia. J Rheumatol 2002;29:2620–7.
221. Rooks DS, Gautam S, Romeling M, et al. Group exercise, education, and combination self-management in women with fibromyalgia: a randomized trial. Arch Intern Med 2007;167:2192–200.
222. Holdcraft LC, Assefi N, Buchwald D. Complementary and alternative medicine in fibromyalgia and related syndromes. Best Pract Res Clin Rheumatol 2003; 17:667–83.
223. Mayhew E, Ernst E. Acupuncture for fibromyalgia–a systematic review of randomized clinical trials. Rheumatology (Oxford) 2007;46:801–4.

Women at a Dangerous Intersection: Diagnosis and Treatment of Depression and Related Disorders in Patients with Breast Cancer

Tal Weinberger, MD[a,b], Anique Forrester, MD[c],
Dimitri Markov, MD[b,d], Keira Chism, MD[b,e,*],
Elisabeth J.S. Kunkel, MD[a,b]

KEYWORDS

- Breast cancer • Depression • Pharmacotherapy
- Psychotherapy • Insomnia

In the popular culture of illness and treatment, breast cancer holds a strange sort of popularity. From the proliferation of pink-ribboned events, to Race for the Cure, to wig-removing protests on the hit TV show Sex and the City, the light of our collective attention seems to shine on women with breast cancer. A variety of psychiatric disorders have also entered popular consciousness, with ideas about diagnosis and treatment of individuals with obsessive compulsive disorder and substance-use problems on reality TV, nightly advertisements for antidepressants, and the revealing tales of celebrity mental illness. Despite all this attention, evidence-based options for diagnosis and treatment of psychiatric disorders in women with breast cancer remain scarce and inconclusive. Yet there is a growing body of evidence that depression, anxiety, and insomnia, when they occur concomitantly with breast cancer, are

[a] Consultation-Liaison Psychiatry, Thomas Jefferson University, 1020 Sansom Street, Suite 1652, PA 19107, USA
[b] Department of Psychiatry and Human Behavior, Thomas Jefferson University, 1020 Sansom Street, Suite 1652, Philadelphia, PA 19107, USA
[c] Department of Psychiatry and Human Behavior, Thomas Jefferson University, 833 Chestnut Street, 2nd Floor, Philadelphia, PA 19107, USA
[d] Department of Medicine, Thomas Jefferson University, 1020 Sansom Street, Suite 1652, Philadelphia, PA 19107, USA
[e] Consultation-Liaison Psychiatry, Methodist Hospital, Philadelphia, PA, USA
* Corresponding author. Department of Psychiatry and Human Behavior, Thomas Jefferson University, 1020 Sansom Street, Suite 1652, Philadelphia, PA 19107.
E-mail address: keira.chism@jefferson.edu

Psychiatr Clin N Am 33 (2010) 409–422
doi:10.1016/j.psc.2010.01.005
0193-953X/10/$ – see front matter © 2010 Elsevier Inc. All rights reserved.

recognizable and treatable. Evidence for the effect of these treatments on mortality, although logical, remains inferential.

DIAGNOSIS OF DEPRESSION IN PATIENTS WITH BREAST CANCER

In the United States, the lifetime risk of developing breast cancer in women is 12%. The incidence of newly diagnosed cases projected for 2009 is approximately 192,370.[1] One of the primary concerns faced by medical practitioners and their patients is the psychosocial stigma associated with a diagnosis of breast cancer and the distress that many patients and their families face after being confronted with this serious illness. A dilemma for many is how to distinguish so-called normal distress from a more serious set of symptoms that may indicate the presence of depression and hence, the need for psychiatric intervention.

One of the first forays into this problem came from Roth and colleagues[2] with the development of the Distress Thermometer, a simple screening tool that correlated a specific set of problems to the level of distress experienced by patients diagnosed with prostate cancer.[3] The advantage of this tool was that a cut-off point could be defined which indicated that, above a certain level of distress, patients required referral for further evaluation of their symptoms and possibly for psychiatric treatment. In a later study by Hegel and colleagues,[4] 41% of patients with a diagnosis of breast cancer were found to have distress; only 11% of the patients with distress were diagnosed with major depression.[5] The goal for behavioral health care providers is to develop specific ways of identifying clinically significant levels of distress in patients with cancer, and once identified, how to determine whether these symptoms indicate a need for further evaluation of an underlying depression.

The importance of this evaluation lies in the clear evidence that emotional distress and underlying depression can affect health outcomes in women diagnosed with breast cancer. One of the major areas of investigation is health-related quality of life. With major medical advancements leading to earlier detection and treatment, many women are living longer with breast cancer. Now research focuses on how coping with this illness affects survival rates and quality of life. In a systematic review by Montazeri[6] comparing all the major instruments that measure disease-specific quality of life, all proved to be valid and reliable in measuring how quality of life can affect patient outcomes. Some of the breast cancer specific measures include the European Organization for Research and Treatment of Cancer Breast Cancer Quality of Life Questionnaire (EORTC QLQ-BR 23), the Functional Assessment of Chronic Illness Therapy-Breast (FCIT-B), Breast Cancer Chemotherapy Questionnaire (BCQ), and the Satisfaction with Life Domains Scale for Breast Cancer (SLDS-BC). The major areas of psychological distress for women diagnosed with breast cancer relate to fear of death, body image concerns, dealing physically and emotionally with the side effects of treatment, and integration of new medical demands in the context of women's prior image of self and family. Another major focus of research has been the correlation between coping skills and medical outcomes. In 2007, Kenne Sarenmalm and colleagues[7] discussed the relationship between coping ability and quality of life. They found that, patients with less ability to cope reported more severe physical symptoms, experienced more distress, and felt worse about their prognosis. Each of these contributed to a decreased quality of life.

The goal in the treatment of breast cancer is to manage progression of the disease; most patients desire a cancer-free outcome. In pursuit of these goals, many patients engage in multiple treatment modalities including surgery, chemotherapy, and radiation, each of which can have devastating physical, emotional, and spiritual effects, on patients and their families. According to Rowland,[8] the most important time to identify patients who may be at higher risk for depression is during the first year after the diagnosis of breast cancer. Many clinicians believe that it is critical to initiate treatment of depression during this year, when many of the most aggressive therapies are implemented.

Distress clearly affects quality of life. Symptoms such as pain, fatigue, insomnia, and anxiety elicited in quality of life screenings are also symptoms that may indicate an underlying depression. The prevalence of depression in patients with breast cancer is estimated at about 10% to 25%, but there is no definitive meta-analysis of the depression prevalence data. One of the most consistent findings is that the rate of diagnosis of depression in breast cancer is third, after the prevalence of depression in pancreatic and oropharyngeal cancers.[9,10] The high rate of depression in patients with breast cancer highlights why it is important to identify it and then to provide appropriate resources and treatment. Maguire and colleagues[11] examined patients with breast cancer after undergoing mastectomy and found that treating clinicians and health care professionals failed to identify patients with depression. They also learned that affected patients tended not to disclose psychological symptoms. Whether this failure to disclose was caused by shame, psychiatric stigma, or lack of confidence in the treatment team member's ability to assist them effectively, was unclear.

The main issue for treating physicians and psychiatrists is the accurate diagnosis of depression in patients with breast cancer. According to Aapro,[12] there is a general misconception that patients with cancer have higher rates of depression than patients with other medical conditions. The incidence of depression in patients with breast cancer is similar to the incidence of depression in other medical illnesses, yet, earlier indications of distress and more clinician sensitivity to the effects of depression on emotional well-being and medical outcome has led to better identification of depression in this population.[13] Recognition of depression in patients with breast cancer now occurs at higher rates than in other populations of medically ill patients.

The diagnosis of major depression by DSM-IV criteria includes physical symptoms that may be indistinguishable from the symptoms that occur with the cancer itself or from the side effects of treatments and medications. Insomnia, loss of appetite, poor energy, and impaired concentration act as confounding factors in the assessment of individual patients for depression. One proposed solution to this quandary is the elimination of somatic symptoms from measures of depression in patients with cancer in favor of an emphasis on psychological symptoms of distress. These symptoms include suicidality, guilt, helplessness, and hopelessness.[14] Hopwood and colleagues,[15] and later Ibbotson and colleagues,[16] examined this approach when they compared the Hospital Anxiety and Depression Scale (HADS), which was designed for general physical illness, with the Rotterdam Symptom Checklist (RSCL), which looks specifically at cancer. Both of these measures had high positive predictive values for accurately identifying symptoms of depression and anxiety in patients with advanced cancer. Several factors can predispose patients with cancer to a higher risk of depression: previous history of psychiatric illness; strong family history of psychiatric illness and specifically mood disorders; poor social support; and higher self-reported levels of distress related to the cancer diagnosis and issues surrounding treatment.

Whether or not physical symptoms are included in diagnostic measures to help practitioners recognize patients who may be at higher risk for depression, the goal of identification is to provide appropriate interventions that may help to improve quality of life and decrease morbidity for these patients. Clinicians must improve their screening of patients who experience psychological distress, especially within the first year after diagnosis. It is crucial to establish adequate communication and provide emotional tools to the patient who then may feel more comfortable disclosing distressing symptoms. For example, work by Moorey and colleagues[17] and Greer and Moorey[18] indicates that adjuvant psychological therapy (APT), a therapy focused on implementing elements of cognitive behavioral therapy (CBT) and brief psychotherapy targeted specifically to patients with cancer, may be helpful in this early stage to help foster a more realistic outlook on prognosis and have a positive effect on quality of life. More time and research should be devoted to ways in which patient who have breast cancer can benefit from early intercession from practitioners who can then provide resources designated specifically to address depression. There is a clear benefit to pursuing psychiatric intervention, including medications and therapy, to treat underlying depression in addition to improving patient morbidity and mortality with medical treatment of breast cancer.

SLEEP PROBLEMS IN PATIENTS WITH BREAST CANCER

Insomnia as a symptom encompasses difficulty with initiating or maintaining sleep, early morning awakenings, or poor quality of sleep. In addition, reporting a symptom of insomnia carries an expectation of daytime impairment. Classification schemes for insomnia as a specific diagnosis or disorder have been included in the Diagnostic and Statistical Manual of Mental Disorders (DSM-IV).[19]

Patients with cancer commonly report sleep-related problems, such as insomnia, daytime sleepiness, and fatigue.[20] Patients with breast cancer frequently report dissatisfaction with their sleep and complain of symptoms of insomnia.[21] They experience frequent awakenings when undergoing radiation therapy or chemotherapy,[22] and their insomnia may persist for many years after cancer therapy. Up to 44% of patients with breast cancer reported symptoms of insomnia 2 to 6 years after their diagnosis,[23,24] which indirectly implies that symptoms of insomnia may persist for years, even after successful management of breast cancer. Koopman and colleagues[25] reported that up to 63% of patients with metastatic breast cancer complained of insomnia symptoms. In a study by Savard and colleagues,[26] 51% of women with breast cancer who were treated with radiation therapy reported symptoms of insomnia, and 19% of these patients met the criteria for insomnia disorder, which was chronic in most patients. Poor sleep in patients with cancer was shown to predict decreased quality of life.[20,27] Patients with breast cancer have restless sleep (higher levels of nighttime activity were shown in studies that used actigraphy) as well as lower levels of daytime activity, a pattern of disruption of sleep-wake cycle, which also suggests a disruption of other circadian rhythms.

Even before starting chemotherapy, patients with breast cancer may display altered circadian rhythms.[28–30] Patients who have cancer frequently report severe daytime fatigue before, during, and often many years after, chemotherapy. Causes and contributing factors to this cancer-related fatigue (CRF) include anemia, effects of chemotherapy, radiation therapy, and inflammation. Sleep of poor quality has not been viewed as a factor in CRF, however Stepanski and Burgess suggest that daytime sleepiness and poor sleep quality need to be considered to understand all causes of CRF.[20]

Historically, insomnia in patients with cancer was viewed as a secondary condition, believed to be caused by, or associated with, pain, anxiety, depression, chemotherapy, or some other aspect of cancer; thus, treatment of the underlying causes would alleviate the insomnia. Current thinking suggests that the insomnia that accompanies any medical or psychiatric illness is a comorbid disorder. For example, a patient may develop insomnia at the time of diagnosis with cancer, but the insomnia may persist for many years after successful therapy for cancer, and at that point, insomnia will require independent management.[20,26]

Savard and colleagues[31] showed the effectiveness of CBT in the treatment of insomnia in patients with nonmetastatic breast cancer. Treated patients reported significant improvement in subjective sleep parameters and decreased use of hypnotic medications. CBT may be a reasonable intervention for patients with breast cancer who have a comorbid insomnia.

Several psychotherapeutic approaches are effective for treatment of insomnia. Studies show that psychotherapeutic approaches are no less effective than pharmacotherapy in the management of insomnia.[32] What is collectively called CBT for insomnia actually encompasses a combination of different psychotherapeutic approaches **Box 1**.[33]

Psychotherapy is effective for both primary and comorbid insomnia. There is no evidence that allows us to predict which specific type of psychotherapy should be prescribed for a given patient. Therefore, best practice is implementation of a combination of the therapeutic approaches mentioned earlier.

MEDICATIONS FOR MOOD AND ANXIETY DISORDERS IN PATIENTS WHO HAVE BREAST CANCER

Mood and anxiety disorders have been shown to affect multiple parameters in patients with cancer, including quality of life, perception of pain, and compliance with oncological treatment. Some studies evaluating the effects of antidepressant treatment in patients who have cancer have not differentiated between different types of cancer. In a study of 73 women with cancer meeting criteria for major depressive disorder, the antidepressant mianserin (a compound similar to mirtazapine) was found to be more effective than placebo in reducing the severity and duration of depression.[34] In a double-blind placebo-controlled trial comparing fluoxetine with desipramine in women with advanced cancer, both medications were effective in treating mood and anxiety symptoms, and fluoxetine was found to have a nonsignificant advantage in several quality-of-life measures.[35] Fluoxetine was found to be superior to placebo in improving depressive symptoms and quality of life in patients with advanced solid tumors. Greater improvements were shown in patients with more severe symptoms at baseline. No differences in survival were found between the treatment and placebo groups.[36]

Many other studies have examined the benefits of antidepressant medication in patients with a diagnosis of breast cancer, excluding other malignancies. Reasons to evaluate this population independently of patients with other malignancies include the unique effect of this illness and its cancer treatments on body image, as well as the potential effect of hormonal therapy and chemotherapy on mood. Breast cancer

---

Box 1
Effective therapies encompassed by CBT in the treatment of insomnia

Sleep hygiene education

Sleep restriction therapy

Cognitive therapy

Stimulus-control therapy

Relaxation therapy

Paradoxic intention

affects women almost exclusively, and as women have twice the baseline rate of depression as men,[37] this might result in a higher rate of depression in patients with breast cancer compared with patients with other cancers.

Unfortunately, the patient populations and the methodologies of the different studies tend to be heterogeneous. Some studies evaluate only women who meet criteria for major depressive disorder, some only include women with adjustment disorders, and some include all women with depressive symptoms, regardless of diagnosis. In terms of breast cancer diagnosis, some studies include only women with advanced metastatic disease, whereas others include women with early-stage disease, and still others include all women with breast cancer, regardless of stage. Some studies measure only improvement in symptoms, whereas others track the percentage of women achieving remission (likely a more clinically relevant measure).[38] Furthermore, some only measure improvement in mood symptoms, whereas others also include measures of quality of life.

Few studies measure the effect of symptomatic improvement on compliance with oncological treatment or survival. Antidepressants have already been established as an effective treatment of depression in the general population, and they are likely to be equally effective for depression in this specific subpopulation. Therefore, an important reason to study the effect of antidepressants in this population should be to assess the effect of psychiatric treatment of mood symptoms on oncological outcomes, including compliance with treatment and survival.

In a multicenter double-blind study, women with breast cancer were randomized to either paroxetine (20–40 mg/d) or amitriptyline (75–150 mg/d). Although women with breast cancer at any stage without cerebral metastases were included, all subjects did meet criteria for major depression. Paroxetine and amitriptyline improved depressive symptomatology at the end point, with no statistically significant differences between the 2 groups. The magnitude of improvement for both groups corresponded to a change from moderately to mildly ill on the Clinical Global Improvement severity of illness scale. There was also a demonstrated improvement in the quality of life of patients in both treatment groups.[39] No measure of the number of patients achieving remission was used. There was no placebo control. There was no measure of effect of treatment or treatment response on compliance with oncologic treatment or medical outcome.

In a small (n = 20), open-label, 8-week study, patients with a DSM-IV diagnosis of major depressive disorder and breast cancer at any stage were treated with reboxetine, a norepinephrine reuptake inhibitor. Depressive symptoms decreased significantly, and the study showed significant changes in measures of coping strategies. Specifically, measures of hopelessness and anxious preoccupation with illness improved significantly. The investigators cite evidence that these are significant dysfunctional cognitive patterns in patients with cancer. One then could speculate that improvement in these coping strategies might be associated with more adaptive illness behavior and perhaps even improved illness outcome. However, the effect on compliance with treatment or survival was not assessed in this study. There was no control group, making it difficult to assess whether improvements in coping strategies were associated more with the medication or with the support that comes with being part of a clinical trial.[40]

In another small study, 18 women with breast cancer at any stage were randomized to receive either trazodone or clorazepate (a long-acting benzodiazepine). All women met criteria for an adjustment disorder. Measures of quality of life as well as depression and anxiety improved more with trazodone than clorazepate. These differences did not achieve statistical significance, possibly because of the small sample size. Again, effects on compliance with treatment or survival were not assessed.[41]

In the only placebo-controlled study assessing efficacy of antidepressant treatment in patients with breast cancer (other than studies of patients with breast cancer on hormone therapy or chemotherapy, which are examined separately), 35 women who met criteria for major depressive disorder with breast cancer at any stage were randomized to paroxetine, desipramine, or placebo for 6 months. Different psychiatric symptoms improved in each of the 3 groups during the study, similar to the 3 studies described earlier (which were conducted without a placebo control group). However, in this study there was no significant difference between the 2 treatment groups and the placebo group in the rates of response or remission. The investigators hypothesize that this may have been a result of the small sample size or the heterogeneity of the patient population, which consisted of women in different stages of breast cancer.[42] This study clearly underscored the need for further placebo-controlled studies.

THE EFFECT OF HORMONAL THERAPY OR CHEMOTHERAPY ON MOOD

Breast cancer treatments potentially confer additional psychiatric risk, above the baseline risk of depression in a patient with breast cancer. Increased levels of depression are found in perimenopausal patients, and in women taking antiestrogen treatments, such as tamoxifen, raloxifen, and letrozole; the antiestrogens may induce a menopausal state and may potentially contribute to increased levels of depression.[43] Patients undergoing chemotherapy also report higher rates of depression.[44] Hormonal shifts related to either chemical or surgical menopause may affect mood.[44] Abrupt termination of menses is associated with depression.[45]

Estrogen has been associated with increased serotonergic and noradrenergic activity and may therefore have antidepressant properties. The antiestrogen properties of tamoxifen may counteract the antidepressant effects of estrogen and could produce depressive symptoms.[45] In one study, symptoms of acute estrogen deficiency correlated with the severity of psychiatric symptoms reported by 44% of 222 patients with breast cancer.[24]

Studies have investigated whether tamoxifen causes treatment-emergent depression, with conflicting results. In one trial, an oncologist evaluated patients receiving tamoxifen and patients not receiving tamoxifen for symptoms of depression. Of the patients receiving tamoxifen, 15% became depressed, as opposed to 3% of the patients not on tamoxifen, which represented a significant difference between the 2 groups. In the depressed group receiving tamoxifen, onset of symptoms was temporally related to initiation of tamoxifen. The oncologist assessing the patients was not blinded to which patients were receiving tamoxifen, which could have potentially affected his evaluation.[46] In another study, dysphoria and insomnia were almost ubiquitous in women whose breast cancer treatment induced estrogen insufficiency.[47]

A large retrospective trial examined the administrative database of a large insurance company. The records of patients with breast cancer receiving tamoxifen and not receiving tamoxifen were examined for a diagnosis of major depressive disorder or a prescription for an antidepressant. There was no significant difference in recorded diagnosis of major depression or in treatment of depression between the tamoxifen and no-tamoxifen groups.[48] However, as it is well known that depression is under diagnosed in patients with cancer, this may not have been a reliable method of assessing the incidence of depression in these patients. In addition, the group not treated with tamoxifen was more likely to have been treated with chemotherapy, which is an independent risk factor for depression. This may have inflated the depression risk in the patients not receiving tamoxifen.

Tamoxifen may cause subtle psychiatric symptoms that do not meet the criteria for a full major depressive episode.[45] These symptoms may then escape detection by rating scales used to measure depression in clinical trials. Further research needs to be done to clarify this phenomenon.

MEDICATION TREATMENT OF PSYCHIATRIC SYMPTOMS IN PATIENTS ON HORMONAL THERAPY OR CHEMOTHERAPY

Several studies have examined the effect of antidepressant treatment on patients undergoing chemotherapy or hormonal therapy. Outcome measures include depressive symptoms, quality of life, and compliance with oncological treatment. Many different antidepressants have been studied and found to be effective.

One hundred and ninety-three patients with early-stage breast cancer, who were receiving either hormonal therapy, chemotherapy, or both, were randomized to fluoxetine or placebo. Patients with mild, transient depressive symptoms were included, and patients were excluded if they met criteria for major depressive disorder. Fluoxetine use was associated with a higher rate of completion of all forms of adjuvant treatment, a higher quality of life, and a decrease in depressive symptoms. Patients with higher baseline scores of depressive symptoms were more likely to benefit from fluoxetine treatment.[43]

In a small case series of patients with gynecological (uterine, ovarian, or cervical) or breast cancer undergoing treatment with chemotherapy, radiation, or tamoxifen, mirtazapine was found to improve symptoms of nausea, anxiety, depression, and insomnia.[44] In another trial, patients with cancer (stages of illness not specified) undergoing chemotherapy were randomized to either paroxetine or placebo. Paroxetine was found to significantly reduce depression but not fatigue.[49]

In a small, open-label, single-arm study of patients with breast cancer who had completed a course of chemotherapy and who were receiving adjunctive hormonal therapy, buproprion was found to decrease depressive symptoms and improve sexual function, but had no significant effect on quality of life measures. None of these patients met criteria for depression at baseline.[50] In a placebo-controlled trial of patients with early-stage breast cancer taking tamoxifen, sertraline was found to have no significant effect on hot flash frequency. A nonsignificant trend toward improvement in depressive symptoms and quality of life was found in the sertraline group.[51]

Another potential issue in concurrent treatment with antidepressants and tamoxifen is the potential for drug-drug interactions. Tamoxifen is essentially a prodrug, and is converted to its more potent metabolite, endoxifen, by the cytochrome p450 enzyme CYP2D6. Therefore, medications that are inhibitors of CYP2D6 could potentially decrease the potency of tamoxifen and adversely affect breast cancer outcomes. Women treated with tamoxifen were found to have low serum concentrations of endoxifen when concurrently treated with the strong 2D6 inhibitors, such as fluoxetine or paroxetine, and intermediate concentrations of endoxifen when concurrently treated with weak 2D6 inhibitors, such as sertraline and citalopram. Venlafaxine, which does not inhibit CYP2D6, had little effect on endoxifen concentrations.[52]

PSYCHOLOGICAL INTERVENTIONS

In a landmark study by Spiegel and colleagues,[53] patients with metastatic breast cancer were randomized to either supportive-expressive group therapy (SEGT) or to a control group, which received only routine oncological treatment. In the treatment group, patients were encouraged to express their feelings about their illness and its effect on their lives, to be appropriately assertive with medical providers, and to discuss physical problems. The group learned hypnosis techniques for pain management, and also focused on finding personal meaning in illness. The mean survival time for the treatment group (37.6 months) was found to be significantly longer than the survival time for the control group (18.9 months). Many unsuccessful attempts were made to replicate these results. In a larger multicenter trial, women with metastatic breast cancer were randomized to SEGT or to a control group. Women assigned to the therapy group reported significantly less sadness, anxiety, anger, and confusion than women in the control group, and had significantly less worsening of pain than women in the control group. Women who were more distressed and who experienced more pain at baseline benefited more from the treatment group than women who experienced less pain and distress. However, SEGT did not prolong survival in this study.[54] In another study, SEGT improved quality of life in women with metastatic breast cancer, helped treat depression, and prevented new onset of depressive symptoms. Again, survival time was not affected by the intervention.[55]

In another study of SEGT in patients with metastatic breast cancer (survival time was not assessed), group therapy was found to significantly decrease trauma symptoms, with the women with the highest baseline level of symptoms demonstrating the most benefit. The overall reduction in trauma symptoms was found to be mediated by a large decrease in avoidance symptoms. The reduction of avoidance symptoms in the SEGT treatment arm was hypothesized to be a result of the features of SEGT common to effective trauma therapies, including exposure to the feared stimulus and a focus on coping with life threat.[56]

Researchers also examined the effectiveness of CBT. In a randomized controlled trial with patients with any form of cancer (not exclusively breast cancer), patients were randomized to a CBT group or a control group. Some techniques used by the group leaders included identifying negative automatic thoughts and challenging them, using role playing to cope with anticipated stressful events, encouraging activities that fostered a sense of accomplishment and pleasure, identifying personal strengths and encouraging open communication, and teaching progressive muscle relaxation to manage severe anxiety. The treatment group demonstrated improvement over the control group for several parameters, including anxiety, depression, and distress.[57]

In another trial where women with metastatic breast cancer were randomized to individual cognitive therapy (CT) or wait-list control, the women in the CT group had significantly fewer depressive symptoms than the control group. Psychological intervention and improvement in mood and anxiety symptoms did not have a significant effect on parameters of immunological function.[58] In a group therapy called cognitive-existential group therapy, women with early-stage breast cancer assigned to the treatment group had reduced anxiety and improved family functioning compared with matched controls. This therapy modality combined education, cognitive reappraisal, and promotion of enhanced coping with existentially oriented and supportive-expressive strategies.[59]

Other psychosocial treatment modalities have also been studied in patients with breast cancer. In a randomized controlled trial with women experiencing their first breast cancer recurrence, a peer-delivered telephone intervention did not improve measures of depression or psychosocial distress.[60] Another study did demonstrate benefit from 2 brief interventions: a brief series of nutritional sessions and a brief series of educational sessions. These brief interventions reduced depressive symptoms and enhanced physical functioning.[61] Individuals with more negative social interactions, who were more pessimistic in outlook, and who had fewer intrapersonal resources, achieved greater incremental benefit from the nutrition intervention.[62] In a small randomized clinical trial, an exercise intervention did not decrease depressive symptoms in women with breast cancer receiving hormonal therapy.[63] This study may have been confounded by small sample size and low levels of preintervention depressive symptoms in the treatment and control groups.

In a meta-analysis of psychosocial interventions for patients with cancer (not exclusively breast cancer), different treatment modalities were separated into categories, including cognitive behavioral interventions, informational and educational treatments, nonbehavioral psychotherapy, social support by nonprofessionals, and unusual treatments that combined different treatment approaches. No significant differences in efficacy were noted between the different treatment approaches. There was no clear difference between patients with early illness with good prognosis and patients with advanced metastatic disease in terms of their level of benefit from psychotherapy. There was no difference between studies that only recruited subjects with clear psychiatric symptoms and those that included all patients with cancer regardless of level of distress.[64] The diversity of treatment modalities, the broad range of outcomes studied (effects on pain, treatment side effects, psychological distress, and quality of life), and the small sample size for each category may have affected their results.[65]

In another meta-analysis of patients with cancer and depression, and a second meta-analysis of patients with cancer and anxiety, studies of psychotherapeutic interventions that target psychiatrically symptomatic patients with cancer were found to produce more robust results than those that include all patients with cancer regardless of distress level. In general, effect sizes tended to be higher in studies of psychotherapeutic treatment of anxiety than in studies of depression. Group therapy was found to be at least as effective, if not more effective, than individual therapy.[65]

As with medication trials, investigations of psychotherapeutic treatment of patients with breast cancer tend to be done on a diverse population, with diverse study methodologies, and diverse outcomes measured. However, a few general conclusions can be drawn. First, many different psychotherapy modalities seem to be effective in reducing psychiatric symptoms in patients with breast cancer. Group therapies seem to be at least as effective as individual therapies. As group therapy is significantly less expensive than individual therapy, this seems to be the wisest method of allocating scarce resources.[65] Another consistent, but somewhat unexpected finding that repeats itself throughout multiple studies is that patients with early illness and late metastatic disease seem to benefit equally from psychotherapeutic interventions. Some investigators suggest that cognitive behavioral techniques may be more effective in early illness, and supportive-expressive techniques may be more helpful in women with more advanced disease and poorer prognosis.[59] This theory has yet to be definitively confirmed or refuted.

Some relevant issues to be addressed in further research are:

1. Does psychotherapy modality matter and what are the essential components of an effective psychotherapeutic treatment of depression? More comparisons between different psychotherapy modalities, such as CBT and supportive-expressive therapy, should be conducted to confirm or refute the tentative conclusion in Meyer and Mark's[64] meta-analysis that all modalities are equally effective.
2. Are psychotherapeutic interventions best targeted at all patients with cancer, with the goal of preventing psychiatric morbidity, or should they be used only in patients with psychiatric symptoms? One study[55] demonstrated clear benefit in preventing new psychiatric symptoms in asymptomatic patients with a psychotherapeutic intervention. However, in a meta-analysis, the effect size of the psychotherapeutic

interventions targeting patients with psychiatric symptoms was greater than the effect size of those interventions targeting all patients with cancer.[65] One fairly consistent result throughout multiple studies is that patients with more severe symptoms benefit from an intervention more than those with milder symptoms. This would seem to favor targeting more symptomatic patients.

3. Does psychotherapy have an effect on course of illness? Survival has been looked at in multiple studies, but the initial results of Spiegel and colleagues[53] showing longer survival times in patients undergoing SEGT have not been replicated. Survival could also could be evaluated more closely in studies of other psychotherapy modalities. Other parameters to evaluate could include measures of immunological function and compliance with oncological treatment, cancer recurrence rates, and/or other cancer outcome measures.

SUMMARY

The advances in diagnostic and treatment modalities in breast cancer have led to prolonged survival of people with this disease. Many health practitioners now conceptualize cancer as a chronic illness, akin to diabetes or hypertension. With prolonged survival comes the recognition that quality of life is an important indicator of treatment success, and management of comorbidities is a crucial component of maintaining remission. Depression, anxiety, and insomnia, whether syndromal or symptomatic, affect a variety of quality of life indicators, and depression has been shown to lead to significant mortality. Identification of depression, anxiety, and insomnia in patients with breast cancer is a vital aspect of managing the illness. Several instruments, as well as clinicians' awareness, contribute to the trend of earlier and more frequent identification of depression in women with breast cancer. Good treatments exist for depression, anxiety, and insomnia in the context of breast cancer. Treatment may be pharmacologic or psychotherapeutic, or both. Science cannot yet show the best treatment for individual patients, nor can it prove that treatment of depression in women with breast cancer affects cancer-free outcomes. It is hoped that in the race toward the cure, our understanding of the interaction between mind and body will lead to depression-free breast cancer survival.

REFERENCES

1. American Cancer Society. What are the key statistics for breast cancer? (2009, May 13). Available at: www.cancer.org. Accessed July 1, 2009.
2. Roth A, Kornblith AB, Batel-Copel L, et al. Rapid screening for psychologic distress in men with prostate carcinoma; a pilot study. Cancer 1998;82:1904–8.
3. Kash KM, Mago R, Duffany S, et al. Psycho-oncology: review and update. Curr Psychiatry Rep 2006;8:246–52.
4. Hegel MT, Moore CP, Collins ED, et al. Distress, psychiatric syndromes and impairment of function in women with newly diagnosed breast cancer. Cancer 2006;107:2924–31.
5. Fann J, Thomas-Rich AM, Katon WJ, et al. Major depression after breast cancer: a review of epidemiology and treatment. Gen Hosp Psychiatry 2008;30:112–26.
6. Montazeri A. Health-related quality of life in breast cancer patients: A bibliographic review of literature from 1974 to 2007. J Exp Clin Cancer Res 2008;27:32.
7. Kenne Sarenmalm E, Ohlén J, Jonsson T, et al. Coping with recurrent breast cancer: predictors of distressing symptoms and health-related quality of life. J Pain Symptom Manage 2007;34:24–39.

8. Rowland J. Anxiety and the blues after breast cancer: how common are they? CNS Spectrums 1999;40–54.

9. Massie M. Prevalence of depression in patients with cancer. J Natl Cancer Inst Monogr 2004;32:57–71.

10. McDaniel JM. Depression in patients with cancer. Diagnosis, biology, and treatment. Arch Gen Psychiatry 1995;52:89–99.

11. Maguire GP, Lee EG, Bevington DJ, et al. Psychiatric problems in the first year after mastectomy. BMJ 1978;19:963–5.

12. Aapro MC. Depression in breast cancer patients: the need for treatment. Ann Oncol 1999;10:627–36.

13. Massie MJ, Holland JC. Depression and the cancer patient. J Clin Psychiatry 1990;(Suppl 51):12–7 [discussion: 18–9].

14. Mermelstein HT, Lesko L. Depression in patients with cancer. Psychooncology 1992;17:199–215.

15. Hopwood P, Howell A, Maguire P. Screening for psychiatric morbidity in patients with advanced breast cancer. Validation of two self-report questionnaires. Br J Cancer 1991;64:353–6.

16. Ibbotson T, Maguire P, Selby P, et al. Screening for anxiety and depression in cancer patients: the effects of disease and treatment. Eur J Cancer 1994;30A: 37–40.

17. Moorey S, Greer S, Bliss J, et al. A comparison of adjuvant psychological therapy and supportive counseling in patients with cancer. Psychooncology 1998;7: 218–28.

18. Greer S, Moorey S. Psychological therapy for patients with cancer: a new approach. New York: Oxford: Heinemann Medical Books; 1989.

19. American Psychiatric Association. Diagnostic and statistical manual of mental disorders. 4th edition. Washington, DC: American Psychiatric Association; 1994.

20. Stepanski EJ, Burgess HJ. Sleep and cancer. Sleep Med Clin 2007;2:67–75.

21. Knobf MT. Physical and psychological distress associated with adjuvant chemotherapy in women with breast cancer. J Clin Oncol 1986;4(5):678–84.

22. Berger AM, Farr L. The influence of daytime inactivity and nighttime restlessness on cancer-related fatigue. Oncol Nurs Forum 1999;26(10):1663–71.

23. Kurtz ME, Kurtz JC, Given CW, et al. Loss of physical functioning among patients with cancer: a longitudinal view. Cancer Pract 1993;1(4):275–81.

24. Couzi RJ, Helzlsouer KJ, Fetting JH. Prevalence of menopausal symptoms among women with a history of breast cancer and attitudes toward estrogen replacement therapy. J Clin Oncol 1995;13(11):2737–44.

25. Koopman C, Bita N. Sleep disturbance in women with metastatic breast cancer. Breast J 2002;8(6):362–70.

26. Savard J, Sebastien S, Blanchet J. Prevalence, clinical characteristics, and risk factors for insomnia in the context of breast cancer. Sleep 2001;24(5):583–90.

27. Fortner BV, Stepanski EJ, Wang SC, et al. Sleep and quality of life in breast cancer patients. J Pain Symptom Manage 2002;24:471–80.

28. Ancoli-Israel S, Liu L, Marler M, et al. Fatigue, sleep, and circadian rhythms prior to chemotherapy for breast cancer. Support Care Cancer 2006;14:201–9.

29. Berger AM, Farr LA, Kunh BR, et al. Values of sleep/wake, activity/rest, circadian rhythms, and fatigue prior to adjuvant breast cancer therapy. J Pain Symptom Manage 2007;33:398–409.

30. Savard J, Liu L, Natarajan L, et al. Breast cancer patients have progressively impaired sleep-wake activity rhythms during chemotherapy. Sleep 2009;32(9): 1155–60.

31. Savard J, Sebastien S, Ivers H, et al. Randomized study on the efficacy of cognitive-behavioral therapy for insomnia secondary to breast cancer, part I: Sleep and psychological effects. J Clin Oncol 2005;23(25):6083–96.
32. Yang C-M, Spielman AJ, Glovinsky PB. Nonpharmacologic strategies in the management of insomnia. Psychiatr Clin North Am 2006;29:895–921.
33. Morgenthaler T, Kramer M, Alessi C, et al. Practice parameters for the psychological and behavioral treatment of insomnia: an update. An American Academy of Sleep Medicine report. Sleep 2006;29(11):1415–9.
34. Costa D, Mogos I, Toma T. Efficacy and safety of mianserin in the treatment of depression on women with cancer. Acta Psychiatr Scand 2007;72(Suppl 320):85–92.
35. Holland JC, Romano SJ, Heiligenstein JH, et al. A controlled trial of fluoxetine and desipramine in depressed women with advanced cancer. Psychooncology 1998; 7(4):291–300.
36. Fisch MJ, Loehrer PJ, Kristeller J, et al. Fluoxetine versus placebo in advanced cancer outpatients: a double-blinded trial of the Hoosier Oncology Group. J Clin Oncol 2003;21(10):1937–43.
37. Rihmer Z, Angst J. Mood disorders: epidemiology. In: Sadock BJ, Sadock VA, editors. Kaplan & Sadock's comprehensive textbook of psychiatry. 8th edition. Philadelphia: Lippincott, Williams & Wilkins; 2005. p. 1575–82.
38. Keller MB. Past, present, and future directions for defining optimal treatment outcome in depression: remission and beyond. JAMA 2003;289(29):3152–60.
39. Pezzela G, Moslinger-Gehmayr R, Contu A. Treatment of depression in patients with breast cancer: a comparison between paroxetine and amitriptyline. Breast Cancer Res Treat 2001;70:1–10.
40. Grassi LG, Biancosino B, Marmai L, et al. Effect of reboxetine on major depressive disorder in breast cancer patients: an open label study. J Clin Psychiatry 2004;65:515–20.
41. Razavi D, Kormoss N, Collard A, et al. Comparative study of the efficacy and safety of trazodone versus clorazepate in the treatment of adjustment disorders in cancer patients: a pilot study. J Int Med Res 1999;27(6):264–72.
42. Musselman DL, Somerset WI, Guo Y, et al. A double-blind, multicenter, parallel-group study of paroxetine, desipramine, or placebo in breast cancer patients (stages I, II, III, and IV) with major depression. J Clin Psychiatry 2006;67:288–96.
43. Navari RM, Brenner MC, Wilson MN. Treatment of depressive symptoms in patients with early stage breast cancer undergoing adjuvant therapy. Breast Cancer Res Treat 2008;112:197–201.
44. Thompson DS. Mirtazapine for the treatment of depression and nausea in breast and gynecological oncology. Psychosomatics 2000;41(4):356–9.
45. Thompson DS, Spanier CA, Vogel VG. The relationship between tamoxifen, estrogen, and depressive symptoms. Breast J 1999;5(6):375–82.
46. Cathcart CK, Jones SE, Pumroy CS, et al. Clinical recognition and management of depression in node negative breast cancer patients treated with tamoxifen. Breast Cancer Res Treat 1993;27:277–81.
47. Duffy LS, Greenberg DB, Younger J, et al. Iatrogenic acute estrogen deficiency and psychiatric syndromes in breast cancer patients. Psychosomatics 1999; 40(4):304–8.
48. Lee KC, Ray GT, Hunkeler EM, et al. Tamoxifen treatment and new-onset depression in breast cancer patients. Psychosomatics 2007;48:205–10.
49. Roscoe JA, Morrow GR, Hickok JT, et al. Effect of paroxetine hydrochloride (Paxil) on fatigue and depression in breast cancer patients receiving chemotherapy. Breast Cancer Res Treat 2005;89:243–9.

50. Mathias C, Cardeal Mendez CM, Ponde de Sena E, et al. An open-label, fixed-dose study of buproprion effect on sexual function scores in women treated for breast cancer. Ann Oncol 2006;17:1792–6.
51. Kimmick GG, Lovato J, McQuellon R, et al. Randomized, double-blind, placebo-controlled, crossover study of sertraline (Zoloft) for the treatment of hot flashes in women with early stage breast cancer taking tamoxifen. Breast J 2006;12(2): 114–22.
52. Henry NL, Stearns V, Flockhart DA, et al. Drug interactions and pharmacogenomics in the treatment of breast cancer and depression. Am J Psychiatry 2008; 165(10):1251–5.
53. Spiegel D, Bloom JR, Kraemer HC, et al. Effect of psychosocial treatment on survival of patients with metastatic breast cancer. Lancet 1989;2:888–91.
54. Goodwin PJ, Leszcz M, Ennis M, et al. The effect of group psychosocial support on survival in metastatic breast cancer. N Engl J Med 2001;345(24): 1719–26.
55. Kissane DW, Grabsch B, Clarke DM, et al. Supportive-expressive group therapy for women with metastatic breast cancer: survival and psychosocial outcome from a randomized controlled trial. Psychooncology 2007;16:277–86.
56. Classen C, Butler LD, Koopman C, et al. Supportive-expressive group therapy and distress in patients with metastatic breast cancer. Arch Gen Psychiatry 2001;58:494–501.
57. Greer S, Moorey S, Baruch JDR, et al. Adjuvant psychological therapy for patients with cancer: a prospective randomized trial. BMJ 1992;304(14):675–80.
58. Savard J, Simard S, Giguere I, et al. Randomized clinical trial on cognitive therapy for depression in women with metastatic breast cancer: psychological and immunological effects. Palliat Support Care 2006;4(3):219–37.
59. Kissane DW, Bloch S, Smith GS, et al. Cognitive-existential group psychotherapy for women with primary breast cancer: a randomised controlled trial. Psychooncology 2003;12:532–46.
60. Cook Gotay C, Moinpour CM, Unger JM, et al. Impact of a peer-delivered telephone intervention for women experiencing a breast cancer recurrence. J Clin Oncol 2007;25(15):2093–9.
61. Scheier MF, Helgeson VS, Schultz R, et al. Interventions to enhance physical and psychological functioning among younger women who are ending nonhormonal adjuvant treatment for early-stage breast cancer. J Clin Oncol 2005;23(19): 4298–311.
62. Scheier MF, Helgeson VS, Schultz R, et al. Moderators of interventions designed to enhance physical and psychological functioning among younger women with early-stage breast cancer. J Clin Oncol 2007;25(36):5710–4.
63. Payne JP, Held J, Thorpe J, et al. Effect of exercise on biomarkers, fatigue, sleep disturbances, and depressive symptoms in older women with breast cancer receiving hormonal therapy. Oncol Nurs Forum 2008;35(4):635–42.
64. Meyer TJ, Mark MM. Effects of psychosocial interventions with adult cancer patients: a meta-analysis of randomized experiments. Health Psychol 1995; 14(2):101–8.
65. Sheard T, Maguire P. The effect of psychological interventions on anxiety and depression in cancer patients: results of two meta-analyses. Br J Cancer 1999; 80(11):1770–80.

Obesity in Women

Leila Azarbad, PhD[a],*, Linda Gonder-Frederick, PhD[b]

KEYWORDS
- Obesity • Overweight • Weight gain
- Women • Women's health

The prevalence of obesity in women has reached epidemic proportions in the United States. According to the National Health and Nutrition Examination Survey (NHANES), approximately 62% of American women greater than 20 years of age are overweight.[1] One out of every 3 women is obese, and approximately 6.9% of women meet criteria for extreme obesity.[1] Projected estimates suggest that if current trends continue, 42.5% of American adult women will be obese in 2010, 50.3% will be obese by 2020, and 58% will be obese by 2030.[2] Obesity carries tremendous adverse medical consequences for men and women. In women, obesity is associated with increased risk of hypertension,[3,4] metabolic syndrome,[5] insulin resistance,[6] dyslipidemia,[4] systemic inflammation,[7] cardiovascular disease,[5] sleep apnea,[8] polycystic ovarian syndrome,[9] stroke,[10] and mortality.[11] Obesity has also been linked to increased incidence of various female cancers, including endometrial and postmenopausal breast cancer, as well as colon and kidney cancers.[5] Data from the Nurses' Health study suggests that weight gain alone accounts for 16% of postmenopausal breast cancer.[12]

Although the chronic medical sequelae associated with obesity affect both sexes, obesity seems to be associated with greater perceived physical impairments among women.[13,14] Compared with normal-weight individuals, women who are overweight and mildly obese report poorer perceived physical health, whereas only men who are moderately obese report poorer perceived health. These differences were independent of actual medical comorbidities.[13] The heightened disease burden that is experienced by obese women may be influenced in part by weight-related stigma, discrimination, and body image disturbances, all of which have been shown to be more pronounced among women than men.[15,16]

The economic consequences of obesity are also placing an increased burden at the individual, health care system, and societal levels. In 2000, direct medical costs of

a Department of Behavioral Sciences, Rush University Medical Center, 1653 West Congress Parkway, Chicago, IL 60612, USA
b Department of Psychiatry and Neurobehavioral Sciences, University of Virginia Health System, Box 800223, Charlottesville, VA 22908, USA
* Corresponding author.
E-mail address: Leila_Azarbad@rush.edu

Psychiatr Clin N Am 33 (2010) 423–440
doi:10.1016/j.psc.2010.01.003
0193-953X/10/$ – see front matter © 2010 Elsevier Inc. All rights reserved.

obesity were estimated at $61 billion, and indirect costs, such as absenteeism, lowered productivity, and morbidity were estimated at $56 billion.[2] Among women aged 45 to 54 years, lifetime cost of obesity rises with increased body mass index (BMI, calculated as weight in kilograms divided by the square of height in meters).[2] Lifetime obesity costs for individuals who are normal weight, overweight, class 1 obese, and class II obese are estimated at $18,800, $23,200, $28,700, and $35,300, respectively.[17]

This article reviews the major biological, hormonal, environmental, and behavioral processes that contribute to the increased prevalence of obesity in women, presenting risk factors for obesity that are unique to women. The negative social and psychological effects of obesity for women are explored, including the effect of obesity on mental health. The problem of obesity for women with psychiatric disorders is reviewed, and the relationship between psychotropic medications and weight gain is discussed. Treatment options for women are presented in a stepped care model, focusing on identifying appropriate interventions for different groups of obese women.

DEFINITION AND ASSESSMENT OF OBESITY

Obesity is most commonly assessed by the BMI, first proposed by the World Health Organization and later adopted by the National Institutes of Health.[18] A BMI of 25.0 to 29.9 defines overweight, 30.0 to 34.9 defines class I obesity, 35.0 to 39.9 defines class II obesity, and 40.0 and greater defines class III (extreme) obesity.[18] Overweight, obesity, and extreme obesity generally correspond to body weights 20%, 40%, and 100% more than healthy weights, respectively.[19] Although BMI is the most common measure of obesity, distribution of adipose tissue is more directly related to medical comorbidities than total adipose tissue or BMI.[20] Specifically, central (abdominal) obesity, which promotes visceral adipose tissue, is more strongly linked to cardiovascular disease, type II diabetes, metabolic syndrome, and hypertension than BMI or gluteal/femoral adiposity.[5] Women with a waist-hip circumference ratio more than 35 have been shown to be at increased risk for all of the diseases listed.[5]

Men and women differ with respect to the distribution and total amount of adipose tissue. Regardless of cultural background or dietary habits, women have a higher percentage of body fat than men.[21] However, women tend to accumulate fat in the gluteal/femoral regions (gynoid or female-pattern obesity), whereas men tend to accumulate fat in the central/abdominal region (android or male-pattern obesity).[20] Because of these differences, obese men tend to be at greater risk for development of medical comorbidities than obese women.[22]

GENETIC AND HORMONAL INFLUENCES ON OBESITY
Genetic Transmission of Obesity

It is widely established that obesity is to some extent an inherited disease, with genetic factors accounting for 25% to 40% of the variance in body weight.[23] Among first-degree relatives (parents, siblings, offspring, and dizygotic twins), moderate correlations (0.20–0.30) have been found for obesity.[21] Correlations are higher in adult monozygotic twins (0.60–0.70), regardless of whether they are raised together or apart.[21] In a twin study of obesity in 1242 monozygotic and 828 dizygotic twin pairs, the monozygotic within-pair correlation (0.82) was significantly greater than dizygotic within-pair correlation (0.48).[24] Further support for the role of genetic factors in obesity transmission is evident in studies of overfeeding in humans, which have illustrated that certain individuals possess greater genetic propensity for weight gain when exposed to similar conditions of positive energy balance.[25,26] An early study exposed 12 mono-zygotic twin pairs to a sedentary lifestyle and a 1000 kcal/d caloric surplus for 6 days per week for 100 days and found 3 times more variation in weight gain and fat mass between pairs than within pairs.[25] More recent research suggests that a rare genetic variant in the visfatin gene may protect against obesity,[27] although further research is needed.

Endocrine Influences on Obesity

The hormone insulin is secreted by the pancreas and is responsible for changing glucose to energy, making insulin central to metabolic control.[28] Increased BMI and the presence of visceral and hepatic adiposity have been associated with higher levels of fasting insulin and reduced insulin sensitivity.[28] Women have higher levels of adiposity, less lean mass, and less visceral and hepatic adipose tissue than men, which may contribute to the observed increase in insulin sensitivity in women.[28] Insulin resistance is fundamental to the development of type 2 diabetes and has been associated with body composition and sex hormones.[28] Currently, approximately 8.1 million American women have diabetes, with 90% to 95% having type 2 diabetes.[29] Women are at particularly high risk for development of type 2 diabetes, given the increasing life span of women and the increase in ethnic minority populations in the United States.[29]

Ghrelin is a hormone produced in the gastric mucosa of the stomach and pancreas and is responsible for stimulating appetite.[30] Ghrelin levels are increased during fasting, increase before meals, and decrease after food consumption. Ghrelin levels and their effects on body weight are present in utero or from birth, and chronic ghrelin administration increases body weight in laboratory animals and humans.[31] Circulating ghrelin levels have been shown to increase in individuals with anorexia or bulimia nervosa[32,33] and individuals who lose weight via low-calorie diets.[34] Conversely, circulating ghrelin decreases in obese persons relative to their normal-weight counterparts.[31] Ghrelin also increases appetite and food intake to a greater extent in obese relative to lean individuals, suggesting that ghrelin blockage may promote weight loss in obese individuals.[35]

In contrast to ghrelin and other gastrointestinal hormones linked to appetite stimulation, the hormone leptin is associated with appetite inhibition.[30] Leptin is produced in the white adipose tissue and reflects levels of subcutaneous adipose tissue and recent food intake, with higher levels of circulating leptin indicating greater adiposity.[30] Obese individuals have higher levels of leptin than normal-weight counterparts,[20] and prepubescent females have higher leptin levels than men, even after controlling for differences in body composition.[22] However, the precise influence of leptin on weight gain remains unclear. Although there is no relationship between leptin and future weight gain in normal-weight individuals, increased leptin levels are associated with increased weight gain in overweight individuals[36,37] and decreased weight gain in obese individuals.[38,39] Among leptin-deficient individuals, leptin replacement therapy decreases hunger ratings and self-reported liking of food images, and increases postprandial satiety.[40]

Numerous other hormones and hormonal interactions can affect appetite, satiety, and food intake but are beyond the scope of this review. These hormones include resistin, pancreatic polypeptide-fold peptides, proglucagon products, peptide YY, oxyntomodulin, glucagonlike peptide (GLP-1, GLP-2), and cholecystokinin. Hivert and colleagues[30] have published a comprehensive review of endocrinological mechanisms involved in metabolism, appetite, and satiety.

REPRODUCTIVE TRANSITIONS AND OBESITY
Pregnancy and Weight Gain

The hormonal transitions associated with pregnancy and menopause present a unique risk factor for obesity in women. In May 2009, the Institute of Medicine[41] issued a new set of guidelines on weight gain during pregnancy, which recommended specific ranges of weight gain based on BMI categories. The recommended pregnancy weight gain for normal weight, overweight, and obese women is 11.4 to 15.9 kg (25–35 lb), 6.8 to 11.4 kg (15–25 lb), and 5 to 9 kg (11–20 lb), respectively. These new guidelines were in response to significant increases in gestational weight gain, with more than 43% of pregnant women gaining more weight than recommended.[42] Rates of overweight and obesity at conception have also steadily increased, with 45% of women starting pregnancy as overweight or obese, reflecting a near twofold increase since 1983.[42]

Pregnancy also increases the risk of future weight gain.[43,44] Gunderson[43] found that under- or normal-weight women who exceeded the recommended guidelines for pregnancy weight gain were at 3 times greater risk for becoming overweight post partum. Longitudinal data show that the weight gain and increased central adiposity that occur following a first pregnancy persist long-term, independent of age, demographic, and behavioral factors.[45] A longitudinal study showed that 1 birth increased the risk of overweight/obesity in a 10-year period relative to no births.[46] Consistent positive associations exist between gestational weight and postpartum weight, with gestational weight accounting for an estimated 20% to 35% of long-term changes in maternal body weight.[43,47] At 1 year post partum, approximately 13% to 20% of women experience substantial weight retention (eg, maintaining at least 5 kg more than their preconception weight).[43] In women who are obese, weight gain during pregnancy seems to be more variable, with greater or lesser weight gain relative to their normal-weight counterparts.[48] Pregnancy also changes body fat distribution, with overweight and obese women showing greater increases in central obesity following pregnancy.[49]

Obesity greatly increases the risk for reproductive problems in women and obstetric complications in the mother and infant. A review of risks associated with maternal obesity[44] concluded that maternal obesity increases the risk for infertility, miscarriage, thromboembolic complications, hypertensive complications, stillbirth, preterm delivery, cesarean section, birth defects, fetal overgrowth, and gestational diabetes. Further, fetuses of obese mothers have greater body fat and insulin resistance than those of lean mothers, suggesting that maternal obesity poses metabolic risk to fetuses in utero.[50]

Menopause and Weight Gain

Perimenopause leads to increases in body weight and changes in weight distribution.[51,52] The median age for natural menopause among white women is 51 years and is much earlier for surgically induced menopause, generally before age 45 years.[53] Consistent with weight gain that accompanies the perimenopausal period, women reach their peak weight in their 40s, 50s, and 60s.[1] Women gain approximately 0.45 kg (1 lb) per year during perimenopause, resulting in a 4.5- to 6.8-kg (10–15-lb) weight gain from age 45 to 55 years.[52,54] In early postmenopausal women, increased total body fat and weight gains of 5 kg in a 36-month period have been observed.[52] Menopause is also accompanied by a transition to central obesity, which increases the risk for cardiovascular disease and diabetes in postmenopausal women.[55] Perimenopausal weight gain is directly related to decreases in estrogen,[22] which have direct effects on visceral fat, appetitive hormonal signals, and cardiovascular functioning.

Decreases in estrogen have been linked to a redistribution of fat from a gynoid to an android pattern,[52,54] as well as greater resistance to leptin[56] and insulin.[54] Reduced estrogen also produces abnormal plasma lipids, increased blood pressure, increased sympathetic tone, endothelial dysfunction, and vascular inflammation, which, combined with increased central adiposity and leptin/insulin resistance, increase the risk of obesity and cardiovascular disease in postmenopausal women.[54]

Hormone replacement therapy (HRT) reduces menopause-related increases and redistribution of body weight.[51,52,57] A randomized, controlled trial examining the effects of combined estrogen-progestogen therapy on postmenopausal women found that hormone therapy did not affect total body fat mass or total lean body mass but prevented increases in abdominal fat.[57] Early postmenopausal women taking HRT for 36 months prevented increase in body fat or fat on the trunk or arms and had lower increases in total body fat than the control group.[51] Data from randomized trials and reappraisal of the data from the Women's Health Initiative indicate that HRT improves insulin sensitivity[54] and may reduce cardiovascular disease risk if initiated within several years of menopause onset.[54,58,59] Further review of the outcome of the Women's Health Initiative is given by Prentice and colleagues.[59]

BEHAVIORAL AND ENVIRONMENTAL CONTRIBUTORS TO OBESITY

Although biological factors may increase the likelihood that an individual will be obese, lifestyle influences such as dietary intake and lack of sufficient physical activity play a crucial role in the emergence and maintenance of excess weight. Horgen and Brownell[60] suggest that the modern toxic environment, consisting of convenient, high-fat foods, increasing portion sizes in restaurants and fast-food chains, and television advertising aimed at encouraging children to purchase processed and calorie-dense foods, has significantly contributed to the obesity epidemic in the United States. Further compounding this toxic food environment are increases in technological advances, such as video games, the Internet, and elevators and escalators, which promote sedentary lifestyles.[61] In addition, the lower cost of high-fat/carbohydrate and fast food may further promote weight gain among women and families of lower socioeconomic status.[62] Physical inactivity, another primary contributor to obesity, is more common among women than men.[63] More than 25% of American women do not engage in any form of physical activity, and more than 60% do not engage in the recommended amount (30 minutes moderate-intensity activity 6 or more days per week or 20 minutes vigorous-intensity physical activity 4 or more days per week.).[63] Factors likely contributing to decreased physical activity in women include limited time or energy for exercise as a result of multiple social, occupational, and caregiving roles, as well as financial limitations/poverty.

Sleep and Obesity

A growing body of evidence shows a relationship between reduced sleep and weight gain. Short sleep duration has consistently been found to correlate with BMI[64,65] and a variety of adverse health outcomes, including diabetes,[66] heart disease,[67] and obesity,[64,68] even after controlling for family history of weight problems, physical activity, and demographic variables.[64] For each additional hour of nightly sleep, risk of obesity decreases 24%.[65] Given the increase in social and occupational demands in the last several decades, women increasingly report sleep debt and daytime sleepiness. Data from the 1998 National Sleep Foundation (NSF) Women and Sleep poll found that an average woman aged 30 to 60 years sleeps only 6 hours and 41 minutes during the work week, less than the recommended 7 to 9 hours.[69] In the 2002 NSF

Sleep in America poll, women reported a higher frequency of insomnia than men (63% vs 54%), as well as a greater prevalence of daytime sleepiness.[70]

Several studies have found a U-shaped relationship between sleep duration and BMI, with minimum BMI typically occurring around 7 hours of sleep.[71–73] In a longitudinal study of more than 68,000 middle-aged women, Patel and colleagues[68] found that women sleeping 5 or fewer hours showed weight increases an average of 1.14 kg higher in 16 years relative to women who slept 7 or more hours. Although the exact mechanisms underlying this association are not known, 2 epidemiological studies have shown that sleep deprivation decreases leptin and increases ghrelin levels,[73,74] which may contribute to the increased hunger and caloric intake often observed in sleep-deprived individuals.[75] Sleep-deprived individuals also tend to prefer carbohydrate and high-fat foods[76,77] and may exhibit limited daytime physical activity and movement,[68,78] which further promote weight gain.

Psychological Stress and Obesity

There is increasing evidence that psychological stress plays a role in the development and maintenance of obesity.[79] Nearly half of Americans express concern about the amount of stress in their lives and report unhealthy coping strategies, such as overeating and smoking.[80] Under stressful situations, animals and humans tend to prefer high-fat, high-calorie foods,[81,82] and women report more frequent stress eating than men.[81]

Individual differences in stress sensitivity and the hypothalamic-pituitary-adrenal (HPA) axis affect stress-induced eating behavior in women.[83,84] Women showing higher cortisol reactivity in response to stress consume more calories and prefer more sweet, high-fat foods than women showing lower reactivity.[84,85] Because excessive cortisol also stimulates accumulation of abdominal adiposity, chronic stress can significantly increase the risk for central obesity, metabolic syndrome, and a host of other medical problems.[82] In addition to promoting a preference for palatable foods and increased caloric intake, stress may also reduce time for physical activity and other health-promoting behaviors. The association between stress and weight gain seems to affect not only adults but also children, who have a significantly higher obesity risk cross-sectionally and longitudinally when there is psychological stress in the family.[86] Thus, individuals who experience chronic psychological stress from a young age may be particularly vulnerable to the development of obesity in later life.

EFFECT OF OBESITY ON QUALITY OF LIFE AND PSYCHOLOGICAL STATUS
Social and Occupational Functioning

Obesity is associated with significant social, occupational, and economic burdens for women. Obese women tend to be lower in socioeconomic status and make less money than their nonobese counterparts.[87] Although some of the occupational and economic burden is secondary to obesity-related physical disability and comorbidity, negative attitudes and attributions toward overweight people also play a significant role. Numerous studies have documented that obese individuals experience greater social stigma and discrimination worldwide than lean individuals.[88] Negative affect toward obese individuals can be observed in children as young as 3 years old, who rate larger body shapes more negatively than normal-weight or thin figures.[89] Negative attitudes toward obese individuals also exist among health care professionals, including those specializing in obesity treatment.[90] There is even an antifat bias among obese individuals themselves, who show greater negative implicit attitudes toward others who are overweight.[91]

In addition to social stigma, obese people report greater levels of institutional and daily interpersonal discrimination. In 1 study, individuals with class 1 and II obesity were 40% and 50% more likely to report experiencing major discrimination than normal-weight individuals.[88] Likelihood of discrimination seems to increase as BMI increases, with rates as high as 84% for individuals with class III obesity.[88] Reported workplace discrimination occurs at all stages of employment, including selection, compensation, promotion, discipline, and termination,[92] with 1 study finding that weight accounted for 35% of the variance in hiring decisions.[93] Workplace discrimination can even occur toward individuals who are in mere proximity to obese persons. Male job applicants were rated more poorly when accompanied by an obese woman instead of a normal-weight woman.[15] Women seem to be more prone to obesity-related stigma and discrimination than men,[92–94] presumably secondary to increased societal pressure on women to strive for beauty and thinness. Although research shows a reluctance to hire obese applicants of both genders, this bias is stronger against women than men.[92,93]

Obesity and Psychological Status in the General Population

Early studies of psychopathology in the obese population focused on the search for unifying characteristics that would describe the obese personality, but no consistent personality profiles were found.[95] These studies also yielded mixed results with respect to psychological differences between obese and nonobese individuals,[96] with some reporting greater psychopathology and distress among obese individuals and others reporting less psychopathology and distress. However, many of these early studies had significant methodological limitations, including use of small convenience samples, variable criteria to define overweight/obesity, limited objective psychological assessment, and failure to examine gender differences or include control groups.[16]

More recently, large population studies have addressed these methodological problems, investigating the relationship between obesity and mental health using nationally representative samples of more than 32,000 [97,98] and more than 40,000 individuals.[99] All studies concluded that excess weight has greater adverse psychological consequences for women than for men. Istvan and colleagues[97] found a positive, although weak, correlation between BMI and depressive symptoms as measured by the Center for Epidemiologic Studies Depression scale,[100] with smoking status moderating this relationship. Women in the highest BMI quintile (BMI ≥ 28.96) who had ever smoked reported greater depression than women of similar smoking status at lower BMI quintiles. Women with the highest BMIs were 38% more likely to report clinically significant symptoms of depression compared with those with lower BMIs. No relationship was found between BMI and depression among men or among women who had never smoked. Carpenter and colleagues[99] found evidence for slightly increased risk of depression, suicidal ideation, and suicide attempts among obese women. Relative to normal-weight women, obese women were 37% more likely to have experienced a depressive episode in the last year, 20% more likely to report suicidal ideation, and 23% more likely to have made a suicide attempt. Among men, obesity was associated with reduced risk of depression and suicide attempts, whereas being underweight was associated with increased risk of depression, suicidal ideation, and suicide attempt. When extended to population data, this finding means that if 10% of normal-weight women experienced depression in the last year,[101] then approximately 13.7% of obese women would experience depression during that period. In 2003, Onyike and colleagues[98] conducted a third population study that updated the study by Istvan and colleagues[97] and analyzed data from NHANES-III.

Results were similar to earlier studies, with increased risk of depression among obese women but not among men. Taken together, these population studies indicate that there is an increased risk for depression in the obese, but this occurs far more frequently in obese women than men. Although this increased risk is certainly important, research does not support early beliefs that excess weight typically leads to significant psychological disturbances. The results of these population studies show that most obese individuals are not clinically depressed.

Obesity and Psychological Functioning in Clinical Populations

In contrast to results of population studies, research in clinical settings has consistently found that obese individuals seeking weight loss treatment exhibit more psychopathology than the general population.[102,103] A review of literature from the 1960s and 1970s[104] found at least 10 studies showing higher increases on depression, hypochondriasis, and impulsivity scales in obese individuals presenting for treatment. However, these studies were limited by the absence of control groups. An early controlled study[103] found that obese treatment seekers showed greater psychopathology and distress than obese non-treatment seekers and normal-weight controls. A subsequent meta-analysis found a moderate effect size (mean D = 0.52) for differences in rates of depression between obese persons seeking treatment and those in the general population.[96]

A later study compared psychological status and eating-related parameters across 3 demographically matched groups: obese individuals seeking treatment in a hospital-based weight reduction program, obese individuals not seeking treatment, and normal-weight individuals.[102] Obese treatment seekers had higher levels of psychopathology on the Borderline Symptom Inventory (BSI) and the Binge Scale than nontreatment seekers and higher levels of overall psychological distress than normal-weight controls. Although significantly higher, mean scores on the BSI for obese treatment seekers did not reach criteria for diagnosis of borderline personality disorder. Similar BSI results have been found in previous comparisons of obese treatment seekers and nontreatment seekers.[105]

Obesity and Psychological Distress: Temporal Associations and Risk Factors

Although the research described earlier shows an association between mental health problems and obesity in some subgroups, it does not address the question of causality: does obesity lead to depression and other psychiatric problems, or do depression and psychiatric problems lead to obesity? A review of the literature on temporal sequencing of obesity and psychopathology has concluded that depression seems to precede obesity in adolescence but follows obesity onset in later adulthood.[95] Based on these findings, these investigators recommended that obese individuals who present for weight loss treatment with comorbid depression receive treatment of their mood disturbance before initiating any weight program or intervention.[95] Clinical experience concurs with this recommendation because the low mood, anhedonia, lowered motivation, and negative and distorted thinking that accompany depression often interfere with individuals' abilities to comply with weight loss treatment, further setting them up for treatment failure and lowered self-esteem.

Given the heterogeneity in mental health status in the obese, it is important to identify factors that increase risk of psychological distress in this population. Three primary risk factors have been identified: gender, extreme obesity, and binge eating disorder (BED).[95] The research reporting that being female and obese is associated with a greater risk of depression than being male and obese was discussed earlier.[97–99] In addition to being female, extremely obese individuals (BMI $\geq$40) are at greater risk for psychological distress than those who are moderately obese.[106,107] This finding may be secondary to increased medical comorbidities and impairments in health-related quality of life, and the possibility of increased weight-related stigma and discrimination in extreme obesity. BED has also consistently emerged as a risk factor for greater psychopathology in obesity, independent of treatment-seeking status.[16,108,109] BED is more prevalent among obese individuals than in the general population[110,111] and among overweight women than men.[110] Compared with obese nonbinge eaters, obese binge eaters exhibit higher levels of depression and borderline personality disorder, lower levels of self-esteem, and greater prevalence of any other axis I disorder, including substance abuse or dependence.[112–115]

PSYCHIATRIC DISORDERS, PSYCHOTROPIC MEDICATIONS, AND OBESITY

Obesity is more prevalent in individuals with bipolar disorder[116,117] and schizophrenia[118,119] than in the general population. In individuals with bipolar disorder, obesity is associated with more frequent manic and depressive episodes, as well as greater percentage of recurrence and shorter time to recurrence of depressive episodes.[117] Of individuals with schizophrenia, 42% have a BMI of 27 or higher, compared with 27% of the general population, a discrepancy that is largely attributed to the high prevalence of obesity among young women with schizophrenia.[118] Antipsychotic medications used to treat schizophrenia, bipolar disorder, and other psychotic disorders are commonly associated with clinically significant weight gain, with weight gain highest in patients treated with olanzapine (2.3 kg/mo), clozapine (1.7 kg/mo), and quetiapine (1.8 kg/mo).[120] In 2004, the US Food and Drug Administration (FDA) issued a warning that all atypical antipsychotics have the propensity to induce weight gain. Subsequently, a consensus statement[121] developed by several medical associations recommended frequent assessment of weight (at 4, 8, and 12 weeks) in patients taking antipsychotic medications and switching to another medication if a weight gain of more than 5% occurs.

Among antidepressants, the largest class of prescribed medication among women, tricyclic antidepressants (TCAs) and monoamine oxidase inhibitors are most commonly associated with weight gain.[122] A review of 5 studies[123] found that weight gain in patients taking TCAs varied from −0.4 kg to 4.12 kg per month of therapy, depending on the drug, dose, and duration of treatment. Newer antidepressant agents, such as selective serotonin reuptake inhibitors (SSRIs), have been shown to produce weight loss in the short-term but weight gain in the long-term.[124] Of the SSRIs, paroxetine is most prone to promoting weight gain and results in greater weight gain compared with fluoxetine and sertaline, with patients receiving paroxetine for more than 1 year having an average weight gain of 11 kg.[125] Case studies of patients using fluoxetine report a mean weight gain of 9 kg.[126] Mood stabilizers, such as lithium, also lead to weight gain with long-term use, ranging from 5 kg in a 1- to 2-year period to between 4.5 and 15.6 kg in a 2-year period.[127] Little is known about the effects of anxiolytic agents on weight gain.[122]

With all psychotropic medications, the decision to consider switching medications should be made with careful consideration of clinical response and changes in BMI. Clinicians should also respond to women's concerns about psychotropic-induced weight gain by either suggesting weight loss treatment or considering alternate treatment options when clinically appropriate.

OBESITY TREATMENT

Decisions about type of obesity treatment should be based on BMI, health risks, history of weight loss efforts, and psychological/behavioral readiness for weight loss.[128,129] A stepped care decision-making process has been outlined for interventions that range from low-intensity, low-cost approaches (self-directed diet and exercise when BMI is <27, and self-help, commercial, or behavioral programs when BMI is between 27 and 29) to aggressive and expensive interventions (pharmacotherapy, low-calorie diets for BMI 30–39, and bariatric surgery for BMI ≥40).[130] Low-cost weight loss interventions, such as self-help, commercial programs, or behavioral weight loss programs are often the first line of intervention attempted by obese individuals, particularly women. Weight Watchers International is the world's largest commercial program, with approximately 600,000 active members in North America,[131] most of whom are women. There is evidence that Weight Watchers produces significant weight loss,[132,133] with greater weight loss 1 year after treatment (5.0 kg) than a self-help program.[133]

Hospital-based or medical clinic-based behavioral weight loss programs are another popular weight loss treatment among women. The average participant is a middle-aged woman weighing approximately 90 kg.[134] Behavioral programs typically consist of weekly meetings for several months and emphasize caloric restriction, physical activity, self-monitoring, enhancing stimulus control, problem solving, and relapse prevention.[134] A review of the major behavioral weight loss trials from 1996 to 1999 indicated that average weight loss is 9.6 kg in 21 weeks.[135] Although behavioral programs can produce initial weight loss, they typically fail to produce weight loss maintenance.[136] Most patients regain more than one-third of their initial weight loss in the first year of follow-up, resulting in an average weight loss of 5.2 kg at 40-week follow-up.[134]

Physical activity is another cornerstone of many behavioral programs. Despite the documented benefits of physical activity programs on weight loss in women, physical activity alone results in less weight loss than caloric restriction. Meta-analysis has indicated that 21 weeks of aerobic activity produces a 2.9-kg weight loss, whereas 15 weeks of caloric restriction produces an 11-kg weight loss.[137] Physical activity as a sole method for weight loss is particularly difficult in obese individuals, whose mobility is often limited. Although physical activity alone has not been shown to produce substantial weight loss, it is the most consistent predictor of weight loss maintenance.[134] Data from the National Weight Control Registry, a group of 1047 men and women who have lost 13.6 kg or more (>30 lb) and maintained the loss for at least 1 year, indicate that successful weight loss maintainers exercised daily for an average of 1 hour or more.[138]

Pharmacotherapy, in conjunction with behavioral therapy, is recommended for individuals with BMI 30 or greater or 27 to 30 with 1 or more obesity-related medical comorbidities.[139] Among individuals with a BMI of 30 or greater, women report using weight loss medications at a much higher rate than men (10% vs 3%).[140] Currently, 2 weight loss medications are approved by the FDA for long-term use: orlistat and sibutramine. Orlistat is a minimally absorbable agent that inhibits pancreatic and gastric lipases and blocks gastrointestinal uptake of roughly 30% of ingested fat.[135] Sibutramine inhibits reuptake of serotonin and norepinephrine, resulting in appetite suppression.[135] Orlistat and sibutramine result in losses of 7% to 10% of initial weight 4 to 6 months after treatment onset, then weight loss slows and stops.[141–143] Maintained weight losses of 7% to 8% of initial weight are reported beyond 1 year in patients who continue with drug treatment, although weight regain is common once medication is discontinued.[144] Lifestyle trials and pharmacotherapy interventions seem to consistently produce an approximate 3.2-kg weight loss that is sustained for 2 years and associated with improvements in blood pressure, diabetes, and cardiovascular risk factors.[135]

Bariatric surgery, the most invasive type of weight loss treatment, is recommended for individuals with BMI 40 or greater or BMI 35 or greater with serious comorbid disease who have failed to lose and maintain weight loss via nonsurgical means.[145] Prevalence of women of reproductive age[18–45] who undergo bariatric surgery has increased dramatically, accounting for nearly 49% of all patients from 1998 to 2005.[146] Bariatric surgery can produce substantial weight reduction, with an average loss of two-thirds of excess weight within 1 to 2 years,[147] depending on the type of surgery and the patient's ability to implement lifestyle changes. Weight loss surgery corrects type 2 diabetes in most patients and hypertension in two-thirds to three-quarters of patients.[147] Substantial improvements in obstructive sleep apnea, cardiac function, lipid profile, joint pain, and a variety of other medical problems are also observed.[147]

SUMMARY

Obesity carries a unique disease burden on women and is influenced by a variety of biological, environmental, and cultural factors. Reproductive hormonal changes observed in pregnancy and menopause increase the risk for obesity in women. Lifestyle factors, such as lack of physical activity, chronic sleep debt, and psychological stress, are common among women and also contribute to the development and maintenance of excess weight. Most obese individuals in the general population are psychologically healthy. However, compared with obese men, obese women experience greater weight-related stigma and discrimination and are at greater risk for development of depression. Rates of obesity are higher among individuals with bipolar disorder and schizophrenia, particularly among young women, and can be further exacerbated by use of psychotropic medications that are associated with clinically significant weight gain. Obesity treatment of women should take into consideration degree of obesity, health risks, past weight loss attempts, and individual differences in motivation and readiness for treatment.

ACKNOWLEDGMENTS

The authors would like to thank Megan Greear for her invaluable editorial assistance in the preparation of this manuscript.

REFERENCES

1. Ogden CL, Carroll MD, Curtin LR, et al. Prevalence of overweight and obesity in the United States, 1999–2004. JAMA 2006;295(13):1549–55.
2. Gavard JA. Health care costs of obesity in women. Obstet Gynecol Clin North Am 2009;36:213–26.
3. Pi-Sunyer FX. Medical hazards of obesity. Ann Intern Med 1993;119:655.
4. Plaisted CS, Istfan NW. Metabolic abnormalities of obesity. In: Blackburn GL, Kanders BS, editors. Obesity pathophysiology, psychology, and treatment. Boston: Chapman & Hall; 1994. p. 80.
5. Hu FB. Overweight and obesity in women: health risks and consequences. J Womens Health 2003;12:163–72.

6. Carey DG, Jenkins AB, Campbell LV, et al. Abdominal fat and insulin resistance in normal and overweight women: direct measures reveal a strong relationship in subjects at both low and high risk of NIDDM. Diabetes Care 1996;45:633.

7. Visser M, Bouter LM, McQuillan GM, et al. Elevated C-reactive protein levels in overweight and obese adults. JAMA 1999;282:2131.

8. Guilleminault CM, Quera-Salva MA, Partinen M, et al. Women and the obstructive sleep apnea syndrome. Chest 1988;93:104–9.

9. Gambineri A, Pelusi C, Vicennati V, et al. Obesity and the polycystic ovary syndrome. Int J Obes Relat Metab Disord 2002;26:883.

10. Rexrode KM, Hennekens CH, Willett WC, et al. A prospective study of body mass index, weight change, and risk of stroke in women. JAMA 1997;277:1539.

11. Manson JE, Willett WC, Stampfer MJ, et al. Body weight and mortality among women. N Engl J Med 1995;333:667.

12. Huang Z, Hankinson SE, Colditz GA, et al. Dual effects of weight and weight gain on breast cancer risk. JAMA 1997;278:1407.

13. Mond J, Baune BT. Overweight, medical comorbidity, and health-related quality of life in a community sample of women and men. Obesity 2009;17(8):1627–34.

14. Larsson U, Karlsson J, Sullivan M. Impact of overweight and obesity on health-related quality of life–a Swedish population study. Int J Obes 2002;26:47–424.

15. Hebl MR, Mannix LM. The weight of obesity in evaluating others: a mere proximity effect. Pers Soc Psychol Bull 2003;29:28–38.

16. Wadden TA, Womble LG, Stunkard AJ, et al. Psychosocial consequences of obesity and weight loss. In: Wadden TA, Stunkard AJ, editors. Handbook of obesity treatment. New York: Guilford Press; 2002. p. 144–72.

17. Thompson D, Edelsberg J, Coditz G, et al. Lifetime health and economic consequences of obesity. Arch Intern Med 1999;159:2177–83.

18. NHLBI Obesity Education Initiative Expert Panel on the Identification, Evaluation, and Treatment of Overweight and Obesity in Adults. Practical guide: identification, evaluation, and treatment of overweight and obesity in adults. Washington, DC: National Institutes of Health; 2000.

19. Foster GD, Kendall PC. The realistic treatment of obesity: changing the scales of success. Clin Psychol Rev 1994;14:701–36.

20. Mayes JS, Watson GH. Direct effects of sex steroid hormones on adipose tissue and obesity. Obes Rev 2004;5:197–216.

21. Price RA. Genetics and common obesities: background, current status, strategies, and future prospects. In: Wadden TA, Stunkard AJ, editors. Handbook of obesity treatment. New York: Guilford Press; 2002. p. 73–94.

22. Shi H, Clegg DJ. Sex differences in the regulation of body weight. Physiol Behav 2009;97:199–204.

23. Bouchard C. Genetic influences on body weight and shape. In: Brownell KD, Fairburn CG, editors. Eating disorders and obesity: a comprehensive handbook. New York: Guilford Press; 1995. p. 21–6.

24. Watson NF, Goldberg J, Arguelles L, et al. Genetic and environmental influences on insomnia, daytime sleepiness, and obesity in twins. Sleep 2006;29:645–9.

25. Bouchard C, Tremblay A, Despres JP, et al. The response to long-term overfeeding in identical twins. N Engl J Med 1980;322:1477–82.

26. Bouchard C. Current understanding of the etiology of obesity: genetic and nongenetic factors. Am J Clin Nutr 1991;53:1561S–5S.

27. Blakemore AIF, Meyre D, Delplanque J, et al. A rare variant in the visfatin gene (NAMPT/PBEF1) is associated with protection from obesity. Obesity 2009;17:1549–53.

28. Geer EB, Shen W. Gender differences in insulin resistance, body composition, and energy balance. Gend Med 2009;6:60–75.
29. American Diabetes Association. Available at: http://www.diabetes.org/type-1-diabetes/women-diabetes.jsp. Accessed September 15, 2009.
30. Hivert MF, Langlois MF, Carpentier AC. The entero-insular axis and adipose tissue-related factors in the prediction of weight gain in humans. Int J Obes 2007;31:731–42.
31. Cummings DE. Ghrelin and the short- and long-term regulation of appetite and body weight. Physiol Behav 2006;89:71–84.
32. Nedvidkova J, Krykorkova I, Bartak V, et al. Loss of meal-induced decrease in plasma ghrelin levels in patients with anorexia nervosa. J Clin Endocrinol Metab 2003;88:678–82.
33. Kojima S, Nakahara T, Nagai N, et al. Altered ghrelin and peptide YY responses to meals in bulimia nervosa. Clin Endocrinol (Oxf) 2005;62:74–8.
34. Cummings ED, Weigle DS, Frayo RS, et al. Plasma ghrelin levels after diet-induced weight loss or gastric bypass surgery. N Engl J Med 2002;346:1623–30.
35. Druce MR, Wren AM, Park AJ, et al. Ghrelin increases food intake in obese as well as lean subjects. Int J Obes (Lond) 2005;29:1130–6.
36. Lissner L, Karlsson C, Lindroos AK, et al. Birth weight, adulthood BMI, and subsequent weight gain in relation to leptin levels in Swedish women. Obes Res 1999;7:150–4.
37. van Rossum CT, Hoebee B, van Baak MA, et al. Genetic variation in the leptin receptor gene, leptin, and weight gain in young adult Dutch adults. Obes Res 2003;377–86.
38. Ravussin E, Pratley RE, Maffei M, et al. Relatively low plasma leptin concentrations precede weight gain in Pima Indians. Nat Med 1997;3:238–40.
39. Lindroos AK, Lossner I, Carlsson B, et al. Familial predisposition for obesity may modify the predictive value of serum leptin concentrations for long-term weight change in obese women. Am J Clin Nutr 1998;67:1119–23.
40. Farooqi IS, Bullmore E, Keogh J, et al. Leptin regulates striatal regions and human eating behavior. Science 2007;317:1355.
41. Institute of Medicine. Weight gain during pregnancy: reexamining the guidelines. Washington, DC: National Academy of Sciences; 2009.
42. Centers for Disease Control & Prevention. Pediatric and pregnancy nutrition surveillance system. Available at: http://www.cdc.gov/pednss/pnss_tables/tables_health_indicators.htm. Accessed September 17, 2009.
43. Gunderson E. Childbearing and obesity in women: weight before, during, and after pregnancy. Obstet Gynecol Clin North Am 2009;36:317–32.
44. Yogev Y, Catalano PM. Pregnancy and obesity. Obstet Gyn Clin N Am 2009;36:285–300.
45. Smith DE, Lewis CE, Carveny JL, et al. Longitudinal changes in adiposity associated with pregnancy: the CARDIA Study. Coronary Artery Risk Development in Young Adults Study. JAMA 1994;271:1747–51.
46. Williamson DF, Madans J, Parnuk E, et al. A prospective study of childbearing and 10-year weight gain in US white women 25 to 45 years of age. Int J Obes Relat Metab Disord 1994;18:561–9.
47. Gunderson EP, Abrams B, Selvin S. The relative importance of gestational gain and maternal characteristics associated with the risk of becoming overweight after pregnancy. Int J Obes Relat Metab Disord 2000;24:1660–8.

48. Wells CS, Schwalberg R, Noonan G, et al. Factors influencing inadequate and excessive weight gain in pregnancy: Colorado, 2000–2002. Matern Child Health J 2006;10:55–62.

49. Soltani H, Fraser RB. A longitudinal study of maternal anthropometric changes in normal weight, overweight, and obese women during pregnancy and post-partum. Br J Nutr 2000;84:95–101.

50. Catalano PM, Farrell K, Thomas A, et al. Perinatal risk factors for childhood obesity and metabolic dysregulation. Am J Clin Nutr 2009.

51. Gambacciani M, Ciaponi M, Cappagli B, et al. Prospective evaluation of body weight and body fat distribution in early postmenopausal women with and without hormonal replacement therapy. Maturitas 2001;39:125–32.

52. Gambacciani M, Ciaponi M, Cappagli B, et al. Climacteric modifications in body weight and fat distribution. Climacteric 1999;2:37–44.

53. Crawford SL, Casey VA, Avis NE, et al. A longitudinal study of weight and the menopause transition: results from the Massachusetts Women's Health Study. Menopause 2000;7(2):96–104.

54. Rosano GMC, Vitale C, Marazzi G, et al. Menopause and cardiovascular disease: the evidence. Climacteric 2007;10:19–24.

55. Ryan AS, Nicklas BJ, Berman DM. Hormone replacement therapy, insulin sensitivity, and abdominal obesity in postmenopausal women. Diabetes Care 2002;25:127–33.

56. Shi H, Seeley RJ, Clegg DJ. Sexual differences in the control of energy homeostasis. Front Neuroendocrinol 2009;30:396–404.

57. Haarbo J, Marslew U, Gotfredsen A, et al. Postmenopausal hormone replacement therapy prevents central distribution of body fat after menopause. Metabolism 1991;40:1323–6.

58. Phillips LS, Langer RD. Postmenopausal hormone therapy: critical reappraisal and a unified hypothesis. Fertil Steril 2005;83:558–66.

59. Prentice RL, Langer R, Stefanick ML, et al. Combined postmenopausal hormone therapy and cardiovascular disease: toward resolving the discrepancy between observational studies and the Women's Health Initiative clinical trial. Am J Epidemiol 2005;162:404–14.

60. Horgen KB, Brownell KD. Policy change as a means for reducing the prevalence and impact of alcoholism, smoking, and obesity. In: Miller WR, Heather N, editors. Treating addictive behaviors. 2nd edition. New York: Plenum; 1998. p. 105–18.

61. Horgen KB, Brownell KD. Confronting the toxic environment: environmental and public health actions in a world crisis. In: Wadden TA, Stunkard AJ, editors. Handbook of obesity treatment. New York: Guilford Press; 2002. p. 95–106.

62. Drewnowski A, Darmon N, Briend A. Replacing fats and sweets with vegetables and fruits–a question of cost. Am J Public Health 2004;94:1555–9.

63. Centers for Disease Control. Physical activity and health: report of the surgeon general. Atlanta (GA): U.S. Department of Health and Human Services, CDC; 1996.

64. Hasler G, Buysse DJ, Klaghofer R, et al. The association between short sleep duration and obesity in young adults: a 13-year prospective study. Sleep 2004;27(4):661–6.

65. Vioque J, Torres A, Quiles J. Time spent watching television, sleep duration and obesity in adults living in Valencia, Spain. Int J Obes Relat Metab Disord 2000; 24:1683–8.

66. Ayas NT, White DP, Al-Delaimy WK, et al. A prospective study of self-reported sleep duration and incident diabetes in women. Diabetes Care 2003;26:380–4.
67. Ayas NT, White DP, Manson JE, et al. A prospective study of sleep duration and coronary heart disease in women. Arch Intern Med 2003;163:205–9.
68. Patel SR, Malhotra A, White DP, et al. Association between reduced sleep and weight gain in women. Am J Epidemiol 2006;164:947–54.
69. National Sleep Foundation. 1998 "Sleep in America" poll. Washington, DC: National Sleep Foundation; 1998.
70. National Sleep Foundation. 2002 "Sleep in America" poll. Washington, DC: National Sleep Foundation; 2002.
71. Kripke DF, Garfinkel L, Wingard DL, et al. Mortality associated with sleep duration and insomnia. Arch Gen Psychiatry 2002;59:131–6.
72. Gottlieb DJ, Redline S, Nieto FJ, et al. Association of usual sleep duration with hypertension: the Sleep Heart Health Study. Sleep 2006;29:1009–14.
73. Taheri S, Lin L, Austin D, et al. Short sleep duration is associated with reduced leptin, elevated ghrelin, and increased body mass index. PLoS Med 2004;1:e62.
74. Chaput JP, Despres JP, Bouchard C, et al. Short sleep is associated with reduced leptin levels and increased adiposity: results from the Quebec Family Study. Obesity 2007;15:253–61.
75. Patel SR, Hu FB. Short sleep duration and weight gain: a systematic review. Obesity 2008;16:643–53.
76. Dinges DF, Chugh DK. Physiologic correlates of sleep deprivation. In: Kinney JM, Tucker HN, editors. Physiology, stress and malnutrition: functional correlates, nutritional intervention. New York: Lippincott-Raven; 1997. p. 1–27.
77. Spiegel K, Tasali E, Penev P, et al. Brief communication: sleep curtailment in healthy young men is associated with decreased leptin levels, elevated ghrelin levels, and increased hunger and appetite. Ann Intern Med 2004;141:846–50.
78. Patel SR, Malhotra A, Gottlieb DJ, et al. Correlates of long sleep duration. Sleep 2006;29:881–9.
79. Tamashiro KLK, Hegeman MA, Sakai RR, et al. Chronic stress in a changing dietary environment. Physiol Behav 2006;89:536–42.
80. Stambor Z. Stressed out nation. Monitor on Psychology 2006;37:28.
81. Zellner DA, Loaiza S, Gonzalez Z, et al. Food selection changes under stress. Physiol Behav 2006;87:789–93.
82. Adam TC, Epel ES. Stress, eating and the reward system. Physiol Behav 2007;91:449–58.
83. Teegarden SL, Bale TL. Effects of stress on dietary preference and intake are dependent on access and stress sensitivity. Physiol Behav 2008;93:713–23.
84. Epel E, Lapidus R, McEwen B, et al. Stress may add bite to appetite in women: a laboratory study of stress-induced cortisol and eating behavior. Psychoneuroendocrinology 2001;26(1):37–49.
85. Newman E, O'Connor DB, Conner M. Daily hassles and eating behaviour: the role of cortisol reactivity status. Psychoneuroendocrinology 2007;32:125–32.
86. Koch F, Sepa A, Ludvigsson J. Psychological stress and obesity. J Pediatr 2008;153(6):839–44.
87. Sargent JD, Blanchflower DG. Obesity and stature in adolescence and earning in young adulthood. Arch Pediatr Adolesc Med 1994;148:681–7.
88. Carr D, Friedman MA. Is obesity stigmatizing? Body weight, perceived discrimination, and psychological well-being in the United States. J Health Soc Behav 2005;46(3):244–59.

89. Cramer P, Steinwert T. Thin is good, fat is bad: how early does it begin? J Appl Dev Psychol 1998;19:429–51.
90. Schwartz MB, Chambliss HO, Brownell KD, et al. Weight bias among health professionals specializing in obesity. Obes Res 2003;11:1033–9.
91. Wang SS, Brownell KD, Wadden TA. The influence of the stigma of obesity on overweight individuals. Int J Obes (Lond) 2004;28:1333–7.
92. Roehling MV. Weight-based discrimination in employment: psychological and legal aspects. Pers Psychol 1999;52:969–1017.
93. Pingitore R, Dugoni BL, Tindale RS, et al. Bias against overweight job applicants in a simulated employment interview. J Appl Psychol 1994;79:900–17.
94. Hebl MR, Heatherton TF. The stigma of obesity in women: the difference is black and white. Pers Soc Psychol Bull 1998;24:417–26.
95. Fabricatore AN, Wadden TA. Psychological aspects of obesity. Clin Dermatol 2004;22:332–7.
96. Friedman MA, Brownell KD. Psychological correlates of obesity: moving to the next research generation. Psychol Bull 1995;117:3–20.
97. Istvan J, Zavela K, Weidner G. Body weight and psychological distress in NHANES I. Int J Obes 1992;16:999–1003.
98. Onyike CU, Crum RM, Lee HB, et al. Is obesity associated with major depression? Results from the Third National Health and Nutrition Examination Survey. Am J Epidemiol 2003;158(12):1139–47.
99. Carpenter KM, Hasin DS, Allison DB, et al. Relationships between obesity and DSM-IV major depressive disorder, suicide ideation, and suicide attempts: results from a general population study. Am J Public Health 2000;90:251–7.
100. Radloff S. The CES-D scale: a self-report depression scale for research in the general population. Appl Psychol Meas 1977;1:385–401.
101. Kessler RC, McGonagle KA, Zhao S, et al. Lifetime and 12-month prevalence of DSM-III-R psychiatric disorders in the United States. Arch Gen Psychiatry 1994;51:8–19.
102. Fitzgibbon ML, Stolley MR, Kirschenbaum DS. Obese people who seek treatment have different characteristics than those who do not seek treatment. Health Psychol 1993;12:342–5.
103. Prather RC, Williamson DA. Psychopathology associated with bulimia, binge eating, and obesity. Int J Eat Disord 1988;7:177–84.
104. Wadden TA, Stunkard AJ. Social and psychological consequences of obesity. Ann Intern Med 1985;103:1062–7.
105. Fitzgibbon ML, Kirschenbaum DS. Distressed binge eaters as a distinct subgroup among obese individuals. Addict Behav 1991;16:441–51.
106. Zavela K, Weidner G. Body weight and psychological distress in NHANES. Int J Obes (Lond) 1992;16:999–1003.
107. Wadden TA, Sarwer DB, Womble LG, et al. Psychosocial aspects of obesity and obesity surgery. Surg Clin North Am 2001;81:1001–24.
108. Telch CF, Stice E. Psychiatric comorbidity in women with binge eating disorder: prevalence rates from a non-treatment seeking sample. J Consult Clin Psychol 1998;66:768–76.
109. French SA, Jeffery RW, Sherwood NE, et al. Prevalence and correlates of binge eating in a nonclinical sample of women enrolled in a weight gain prevention program. Int J Obes (Lond) 1999;23:555–85.
110. Spitzer RL, Devlin M, Walsh BT, et al. Binge-eating disorder: its further validation in a multisite study. Int J Eat Disord 1993;13:137–50.

111. Bruce B, Agras WS. Binge eating in females: a population-based investigation. Int J Eat Disord 1992;12:365–73.
112. Yanovski SZ, Nelson JE, Dubbert BK, et al. Association of binge eating disorder and psychiatric comorbidity in obese subjects. Am J Psychiatry 1993;150: 1472–9.
113. Specker S, de Zwaan M, Raymond N, et al. Psychopathology in subgroups of obese women with and without binge eating disorder. Compr Psychiatry 1994; 35:185–90.
114. Telch CF, Agras WS. Obesity, binge eating and psychopathology: are they related? Int J Eat Disord 1994;15:53–61.
115. Mussell MP, Mitchell JE, de Zwaan M, et al. Clinical characteristics associated with binge eating in obese females: a descriptive study. Int J Obes 1996;20: 324–31.
116. Fagiolini A, Frank E, Houck PR, et al. Prevalence of obesity and weight change during treatment in patients with bipolar 1 disorder. J Clin Psychiatry 2002;63: 528–33.
117. Fagiolini A, Kupfer DJ, Houck PR, et al. Obesity as a correlate of outcome in patients with bipolar 1 disorder. Am J Psychiatry 2003;160:112–7.
118. Allison DB, Fontaine KR, Heo M, et al. The distribution of body mass index among individuals with and without schizophrenia. J Clin Psychiatry 1999;60: 215–20.
119. Homel P, Casey D, Allison DB. Changes in body mass index for individuals with and without schizophrenia, 1987–1996. Schizophr Res 2002;55:277–84.
120. Wetterling T. Body weight gain with atypical antipsychotics. A comparative review. Drug Saf 2001;24:59–73.
121. Diabetes Care. Consensus development conference on antipsychotic drugs and obesity and diabetes 2004;27(2):596–601.
122. Masand PS. Weight gain associated with psychotropic drugs. Expert Opin Pharmacother 2000;1(3):377–89.
123. Garland EJ, Remick RA, Zis AP. Weight gain associated with antidepressants and lithium. J Clin Psychopharmacol 1988;8:323–30.
124. Schwartz TL, Nihalani N, Jindal S, et al. Psychiatric medication induced obesity: a review. Obes Rev 2004;5:115–21.
125. Fava M, Judge R, Hoog SL, et al. Fluoxetine versus sertraline and paroxetine in major depressive disorder: changes in weight with long term treatment. J Clin Psychiatry 2000;61:863–7.
126. Sussman N, Ginsberg D. Rethinking side effects of the selective serotonin reuptake inhibitors: sexual dysfunction and weight gain. Psychiatr Ann 1988;28:89–97.
127. Chen Y, Silverstone T. Lithium and weight gain. Int Clin Psychopharmacol 1990; 5(3):217–25.
128. Wadden TA, Osei S. The treatment of obesity: an overview. In: Wadden TA, Stunkard AJ, editors. Handbook of obesity treatment. New York: Guilford Press; 2002. p. 229–48.
129. Wadden TA, Phelan S. Behavioral assessment of the obese patient. The treatment of obesity: an overview. In: Wadden TA, Stunkard AJ, editors. Handbook of obesity treatment. New York: Guilford Press; 2002. p. 186–228.
130. Wadden TA, Brownell KD, Foster GD. Responding to the global epidemic. J Consult Clin Psychol 2002;70(3).
131. Womble LG, Wang SS, Wadden TA. Commercial and self-help weight loss programs. In: Wadden TA, Stunkard AJ, editors. Hand book of obesity treatment. New York: Guilford Press; 2002. p. 395–415.

132. Lowe MR, Miller-Kovach K, Frye N, et al. An initial evaluation of a commercial weight loss program: short-term effects on weight, eating behavior, and mood. Obes Res 1999;7:51–9.
133. Heshka S, Anderson JW, Atkinson RL, et al. Self-help weight loss versus a structured commercial program after 1 year: a randomized controlled study [addendum]. FASEB J 2000;14:37.
134. Wing R. Behavioral weight control. In: Wadden TA, Stunkard AJ, editors. Handbook of obesity treatment. New York: Guilford Press; 2002. p. 301–16.
135. Powell LH, Calvin JE, Calvin JE. Effective obesity treatments. Am Psychol 2007; 62:234–46.
136. Perri MG, Corsica JA. Improving the maintenance of weight lost in behavioral treatment of obesity. In: Wadden TA, Stunkard AJ, editors. Handbook of obesity treatment. New York: Guilford Press; 2002. p. 357–82.
137. Miller WC, Koceja DM, Hamilton EJ. A meta-analysis of the past 25 years of weight loss research using diet, exercise or diet plus exercise intervention. Int J Obes (Lond) 1997;21:941–7.
138. McGuire MT, Wing RR, Klem ML, et al. Long-term maintenance of weight loss: do people who lose weight through various weight loss methods use different behaviors to maintain their weight? Int J Obes (Lond) 1998;22:572–7.
139. NHLBI Obesity Education Initiative Expert Panel on the Identification, Evaluation, and Treatment of Overweight and Obesity in Adults. Executive summary of the clinical guidelines on the identification, evaluation, and treatment of overweight and obesity in adults. Arch Intern Med 1998;158:1855–67.
140. Yanovski SZ, Yanovski JA. Drug therapy. N Engl J Med 2002;346(8):591–602.
141. Sjostrom L, Rissanen A, Anderson TE, et al. Randomized placebo-controlled trial of orlistat for weight loss and prevention of weight regain in obese patients. Lancet 1998;352:167.
142. Jones SP, Smith IG, Kelly F, et al. Long-term weight loss with sibutramine. Int J Obes 1995;19(Suppl 2):41.
143. Davidson MH, Hauptman J, DiGirolamo M, et al. Weight control and risk factor reduction in obese subjects treated for 2 years with orlistat: a randomized control trial. JAMA 1999;281:235–42.
144. Bray GA. Drug treatment of obesity. In: Wadden TA, Stunkard AJ, editors. Handbook of obesity treatment. New York: Guilford Press; 2002. p. 317–38.
145. National Institutes of Health, National Heart, Lung, and Blood Institute and National Institute of Diabetes and Digestive and Kidney Diseases. Clinical guidelines on the identification, evaluation, and treatment of overweight and obesity in adults. Bethesda (MD): NIH; 1998.
146. Maggard MA, Yermilov LZ. Pregnancy and fertility following bariatric surgery: a systematic review. JAMA 2008;19:2286–96.
147. Latifi R, Kellum JM, De Maria EJ, et al. Surgical treatment of obesity. In: Wadden TA, Stunkard AJ, editors. Handbook of obesity treatment. New York: Guilford Press; 2002. p. 339–56.

Complementary and Alternative Medicine for the Treatment of Depressive Disorders in Women

Kristina M. Deligiannidis, MD[a,b,c,*], Marlene P. Freeman, MD[d]

KEYWORDS

- Complementary/alternative treatment • S-Adenosylmethionine
- Omega-3 fatty acids • St John's wort • Acupuncture
- Depression • Women

Complementary and alternative medicine (CAM) therapies are commonly practiced in the United States and are used more frequently among women than men. This article reviews several CAM treatments for depressive disorders in women, with a focus on major depressive disorder (MDD) across the reproductive life cycle. An emphasis on CAM treatments for MDD was selected because of the large evidence base compared with other psychiatric disorders. The CAM treatments selected for review are those with high clinical importance resulting from available data and prevalence of use. In

This work was supported by the University of Massachusetts Medical School Department of Psychiatry and the University of Massachusetts Medical School Center for Psychopharmacologic Research and Treatment.

Disclosures: Dr Kristina M. Deligiannidis has received grant/research support from the Worcester Foundation for Biomedical Research and Forest Research Institute. In the past 12 months, Dr Marlene P. Freeman has received research support from the US Federal Drug Administration, Forest, Lilly and Glaxo SmithKline. She has received honoraria for consulting and continuing medical education programs from PamLab, and an honorarium for medical editing from DSM Nutritionals.

[a] Depression Specialty Clinic, UMass Memorial Medical Center, University of Massachusetts Medical School, Worcester, MA 01605, USA

[b] Women's Mental Health Specialty Clinic, UMass Memorial Medical Center, University of Massachusetts Medical School, Worcester, MA 01605, USA

[c] Center for Psychopharmacologic Research and Treatment, University of Massachusetts Medical School, 361 Plantation Street, Worcester, MA 01605, USA

[d] Perinatal and Reproductive Psychiatry Program, Massachusetts General Hospital, Harvard Medical School, 185 Cambridge Street, 2nd Floor, Boston, MA 02114, USA

* Corresponding author. Center for Psychopharmacologic Research and Treatment, University of Massachusetts Medical School, 361 Plantation Street, Worcester, MA 01605.

E-mail address: kristina.deligiannidis@umassmemorial.org

women, omega-3 fatty acids, exercise, and folate are interventions that may be attractive to incorporate with standard treatments for MDD, because of low risk, benefits for general health, and evidence suggesting an adjunctive role in the treatment of MDD. S-Adenosylmethionine (SAMe) and bright light therapy may be reasonable therapeutic options for some individuals, as there is evidence to support monotherapy in MDD. St John's wort (*Hypericum perforatum*) has the most consistent evidence of efficacy in mild to moderate depression, but carries a risk of potential drug-drug interactions. As with standard antidepressants, SAMe, bright light therapy, and St John's wort have been associated with emergent hypomania or mania after treatment initiation, and this may be especially important in women who have bipolar disorder. Further studies are necessary before acupuncture can be recommended in the treatment of MDD. In general, although some treatments seem promising, well-powered rigorous studies are necessary to elucidate the role of CAM in the treatment of psychiatric disorders in women.

MOOD DISORDERS ACROSS THE REPRODUCTIVE LIFE CYCLE: MENSTRUAL CYCLE, ANTEPARTUM AND POSTPARTUM PERIODS, AND THE MENOPAUSAL TRANSITION
Menstrual Cycle

Women commonly experience mood, behavioral, and somatic symptoms in the luteal phase of the menstrual cycle. Symptoms can vary in intensity and duration, and may include depressed mood or dysphoria, anxiety, irritability, loss of energy, change in appetite or sleep, breast tenderness, or bloating. For most women, premenstrual syndrome (PMS) symptom severity is mild and functioning is not impaired. However, about 4.6% to 6.4% of women have more severe signs and symptoms accompanied by impaired social, occupational, or personal functioning and meet diagnostic criteria for premenstrual dysphoric disorder (PMDD).[1–3] Subthreshold PMDD has been reported in 18.6% to 20.7% of women.[4,5] The earliest PMS studies in CAM, including several with omega-3 fatty acids, bright light, and exercise, predate the new term PMDD, such that it is necessary to extrapolate findings from the older literature. Despite lack of rigorous clinical data, women often use CAM treatments, including vitamin and mineral supplements, exercise, and diet changes rather than standard antidepressants or oral contraceptives.[6] Thus, the rigorous investigation of CAM therapies in the treatment of severe PMS and PMDD is warranted.

Antepartum and Postpartum Periods

Women have greater 1-year and lifetime prevalence rates of MDD compared with men.[7,8] Hormonal fluctuations associated with reproductive events are believed to contribute to the higher prevalence of depression observed in women.[9,10] Estimates of prevalence for minor and major depression in the periods during pregnancy and the postpartum period vary widely, from 14% to 25%, depending on the different diagnostic criteria, time points, and specifics regarding the population studied, and overall study design.[9,11–18] Antenatal depression is associated with an increased risk of underutilization of prenatal care,[19] increased somatic symptoms and physician visits during pregnancy,[20,21] obstetric complications,[22] preterm birth,[23,24] negative childbirth experience,[20] and postpartum depression (PPD).[25]

Annually in the United States, it is estimated that 1 in 8 women develop depression after birth.[11,26–28] Untreated PPD is associated with consequences for the infant that include prolonged infant crying, infant colic,[29] insecure attachment between mother and child,[30] increased infant cortisol levels,[31] decreased general intelligence quotient and language skills,[32] and abnormal infant socioemotional development.[33,34]

For decades, the safety and efficacy of antidepressant treatment during pregnancy and lactation were not adequately studied. Only recently were treatment guidelines published by representatives from the American Psychiatric Association and the American College of Obstetrics and Gynecology regarding treatment algorithms for antenatal management of depression.[35] Women may be particularly motivated to seek treatment other than standard medications during pregnancy or while breast-feeding. Therefore, although CAM therapies have been less rigorously studied than standard antidepressants, many women may seek CAM treatments because they may believe they are a safer alternative to prescribed antidepressant treatment.

Menopausal Transition

The perimenopause refers to the transition characterized by hormonal fluctuation and changes in menstrual patterns, and this lasts typically for several years before meno-pause.[36] Women have higher prevalence rates of MDD during the perimenopausal transition compared with rates found in premenopausal women.[37] Recently, in 2 large prospective epidemiological studies, investigators reported an increased risk of new onset of MDD during the perimenopause.[38,39] Although estrogen may have antide-pressant effects,[40,41] many women seek nonhormonal interventions for mood and somatic symptoms associated with the menopausal transition. Since the results of the Women's Health Initiative were published in 2002, the use of replacement hormones has become less common as the risks and benefits are reevaluated.[42] Associated with the decrease in prescriptions for hormonal therapies for perimeno-pausal symptoms was a corresponding increase in antidepressant prescriptions for perimenopausal women.[43,44] Antidepressants, particularly those with mechanisms of action on serotonergic neurotransmission, and other psychotropic medications are frequently used to treat the mood, insomnia, and vasomotor symptoms in meno-pausal and perimenopausal women.[45] Because the use of hormonal therapies has become more controversial, CAM therapies may be attractive to women for the poten-tial treatment of mood and vasomotor symptoms.

WHAT IS CAM? DEFINITIONS, BELIEFS AND CHALLENGES

CAM refers to treatments that are not considered standard or established practices in Western medicine. Complementary approaches specifically refer to those that are consistent with the Western biomedical concepts, whereas the term alternative applies to those more philosophically separate from traditional Western medical prac-tices. The term integrative medicine is perhaps a more constructive term, as it refers to an approach to medical care that incorporates standard Western medicine and CAM. As defined by the National Institutes of Health's National Center for Complementary and Alternative Medicine (NCCAM), CAM is "a group of diverse medical and health care systems, practices, and products that are not presently considered to be part of conventional medicine" (NCCAM, 2002). Because the NCCAM definition refers to what CAM treatments are not, rather than what they are, it is essentially impossible for the scientific community to make broad conclusions about CAM therapies.

Differing beliefs about CAM can create challenges for patients and clinicians alike. Some individuals perceive CAM treatments as safer because they are deemed natural, even when evidence is lacking or suggests otherwise. Clinicians might not prescribe CAM if they lack education about these treatments or perceive these treatments as ineffective.[46] Clinicians may in addition find it difficult to translate research findings into evidence-based practice because of the limited evidence base for some CAM treatments.

A limited evidence base may arise from several specific methodological challenges inherent to research in CAM. For example, few CAM treatments have been adequately studied in treatment trials with validated diagnoses as inclusion criteria and with validated assessment tools used to measure outcomes. The randomized controlled trial (RCT), considered essential for determination of efficacy, is sometimes extremely challenging when adequate control conditions are difficult to design. For example, control conditions are challenging to create in exercise and acupuncture interventions. When studies are not controlled, the high rate of placebo response in MDD makes trial results difficult to interpret. In addition, some alternative medical practices are enmeshed in a broader cultural context and belief system that makes them difficult to evaluate in controlled trials. These challenges must be overcome so that clinicians and patients may discuss the risks and benefits of CAM treatment so that safety and efficacy are optimized for each individualized treatment plan.

PREVALENCE OF USE

CAM treatments are commonly used. In the past couple of decades, CAM use has incrementally increased. Currently 40% of adult Americans use at least 1 CAM treatment annually.[47–49] In general, women use CAM treatments more frequently than men and are more likely to have disorders such as MDD and anxiety disorders for which CAM treatments are commonly sought.[50–54] In addition, when women use CAM therapies for psychiatric indications, they may do so in the context of reproductive life events (eg, menstrual cycle, pregnancy, lactation, and menopausal transition). Therefore, particular study is warranted regarding the safety and efficacy of commonly used CAM treatments among women of all ages. Despite the growing prevalence of CAM use, psychiatry generally lacks adequately powered, well-designed studies of CAM treatments in which diagnoses are verified at study entry and outcomes are clearly defined and assessed before and after treatment.

DEPRESSIVE DISORDERS AND SPECIFIC CAM TREATMENTS OF FOCUS

Because CAM therapies include a large number of diverse modalities that have varying amounts of study, the authors have selected treatments to review based on prevalence of use and the availability of randomized, placebo-controlled data. This review focuses on specific CAM treatments and considerations for their use in women, with selected treatments, including SAMe, omega-3 fatty acids, St John's wort, bright light therapy, acupuncture, and exercise. Although not an exhaustive review of all CAM treatments, the use of these treatments is widespread, and it is compelling to know about these to inform clinical practice.

SAMe

SAMe is a naturally occurring molecule in the body. It is produced from the amino acid L-methionine through the 1-carbon cycle, a metabolic pathway that requires adequate concentrations of folate and vitamin B_{12}.[55,56] SAMe is involved in the methylation of entities with important biological roles in psychiatric disorders, including neurotransmitters, phospholipids, and cellular receptors and channels.[55]

A systematic review has found that SAMe, studied in doses of 200 to 1600 mg per day, is efficacious in the treatment of MDD.[57] In addition, Mischoulon and Fava's 2002 review[55] of placebo-controlled RCTs found SAMe significantly more efficacious than placebo in 6 of 8 studies, and equivalent to placebo in 2 others. When compared with tricyclic antidepressants (TCAs), SAMe was at least equivalent in efficacy to TCAs in most RCTs and performed better than imipramine in 1. Two meta-analyses have similarly found that SAMe seems superior to placebo and equivalent to TCAs, although adequate studies comparing it with newer antidepressants are lacking.[58–60]

Studies to evaluate the efficacy of SAMe have generally been of short duration (6 weeks or shorter), but meet rigorous standards for evidence for efficacy as monotherapy in MDD.[61] Fewer studies have evaluated SAMe as an augmentation strategy in MDD. Alpert and colleagues[62] assessed SAMe (maximum daily dose of 1600 mg) in a 6-week open trial as an adjunctive treatment in partial and nonresponders to selective serotonin reuptake inhibitors (SSRIs) or venlafaxine (N = 30). The response and remission rates were 50% and 43%, respectively, using the Hamilton Depression Rating Scale (HAM-D).

SAMe has been reported to be generally well tolerated, with infrequently reported side effects that include mild gastrointestinal symptoms, sweating, dizziness, irritability, and anxiety. In the treatment of bipolar depression, however, mania has been reported.[55,56,63,64]

SAMe in the treatment of antepartum and postpartum depression

No data are available regarding the efficacy of SAMe in antepartum depression. Although not specifically studied for MDD during pregnancy, SAMe had been used in treatment studies in pregnant women with liver disease. As it may have a protective role in liver function and the treatment of liver diseases, SAMe has been assessed as a treatment of cholestasis in pregnancy. In a review by the Agency for Healthcare Research and Quality,[57] 8 trials were identified in which SAMe was assessed for cholestasis in pregnancy. Five systematically assessed tolerability and side effects, with no evidence of adverse events or side effects for mothers or for their infants.

In a placebo-controlled study of women with postpartum depressive symptoms, Cerutti and colleagues[65] observed significant decreases in depressive symptoms with SAMe compared with the placebo group. A quick onset of response was noted after 10 days of treatment, with significantly greater improvement in the SAMe group compared with the placebo group. One limitation of this study was that investigators did not report the validation of the diagnosis of MDD.

Considerations in breastfeeding

There have not been systematic studies that address the safety of SAMe in the context of breastfeeding. There have been no reports of side effects or adverse events when breastfeeding mothers have been treated with SAMe. SAMe given in large doses to nursing rats has not been shown to cause neonatal adverse effects.[66]

SAMe in the treatment of depressive disorders during the menopausal transition

Salmaggi and colleagues[67] randomized 80 women with MDD or dysthymia who were within 6 and 36 months of natural or surgical menopause to SAMe or placebo after a 1-week single-blind placebo lead-in. Participants received either SAMe (1600 mg) or placebo daily for 30 days. There was a significantly greater improvement in depressive symptoms with SAMe by day 10 compared with placebo. SAMe was well tolerated, with side effects noted as minimal and transient.

Folate

Folate is necessary for homocysteine and 5-methyltetrahydrofolate (5-MTHF) formation, also known as methylfolate. Methylfolate is the immediate precursor of SAMe. An adequate supply of vitamin B_{12} is required to convert methionine from 5-MTHF.[68] Some patients with depression may be folate deficient, and experience impaired methylation and monoamine neurotransmitter metabolism.[69] The C677T polymorphism of the methylenetetrahydrofolate reductase gene is associated with

MDD and with poor conversion of folate into 5-methylfolate.[70,71] For those patients who do not efficiently metabolize folate, methylfolate is available and may be an important option. Low folate blood levels have been associated with a poorer response to treatment with antidepressants in MDD[68,72] and higher folate levels at baseline seem associated with a better response.[73] Current data are inadequate to suggest the efficacy of folate or methylfolate as a monotherapy for MDD.

Folate has been studied in a placebo-controlled trial as an adjunctive treatment to fluoxetine, with significantly greater improvement in the folate group, a difference most pronounced in women.[74] 94% of women who received fluoxetine with the addition of folate (500 μg per day) were treatment responders, compared with 61% of those who received fluoxetine and placebo. Those who received folate were less likely to experience side effects.

Folate in the treatment of antepartum and postpartum depression

There have been no studies published on the efficacy of folate monotherapy or augmentation therapy for antepartum or postpartum depression. One epidemiological study of 865 women who completed nutritional questionnaires during pregnancy and who recorded an Edinburgh Postnatal Depression Score (EPDS) between 2 and 9 months post partum did not report that higher folate intake during pregnancy resulted in lower rates of PPD.[75] However, folate in doses typical in multivitamins and prenatal vitamins is considered low risk, and known to protect against birth defects in early pregnancy. For the prevention of birth defects, 0.4 to 1 mg per day is recommended for women of reproductive age. High rates of unplanned pregnancy make folate supplementation important in women of reproductive age, regardless of plans to conceive. Considering the modest evidence that supports folate as an augmentation strategy and the attractive risk/benefit profile, folate can be represented as a reasonable adjunctive strategy for MDD that carries little risk and may decrease birth defects in the case of pregnancies.

Folate in the treatment of depressive disorders during the menopausal transition

No studies to date have evaluated the efficacy and tolerability of folate monotherapy or augmentation therapy in the treatment of MDD during the menopausal transition.

Omega-3 Fatty Acids

According to a recent national epidemiological survey of CAM use in the United States, omega-3 fatty acids are among the most commonly used CAM treatments.[47] Omega-3 fatty acids have received the most rigorous study to date in RCTs for the adjunctive treatment of MDD. Few controlled monotherapy studies have been completed. The preponderance of the current evidence suggests a role for omega-3 fatty acids as an adjunctive treatment of MDD[76,77] rather than monotherapy,[78,79] and some data support use in bipolar depression.[80] In general, the evidence base is limited by underpowered studies and inconsistent findings. The well-established health benefits of omega-3 fatty acids make them an important consideration from a public health standpoint. For example, the American Heart Association has issued specific recommendations for intake of omega-3 fatty acids based on the cardiovascular benefits of adequate consumption and supplementation.[81]

Omega-3 fatty acids are nutritional compounds with well-established benefits for human health and particular benefits for fetal and infant development.[81–83] Eicosapentaenoic acid (EPA) and docosahexaenoic acid (DHA) are 2 crucial omega-3 fatty acids found in fish. Meta-analyses of RCTs report a statistically significant antidepressant benefit of omega-3 fatty acids in mood disorders overall, but there has been noted heterogeneity in study designs and results, and they are best studied as an augmentation treatment.[80,84] In 2006, the Omega-3 Fatty Acids Subcommittee, assembled by the Committee on Research on Psychiatric Treatments of the American Psychiatric Association, recommended that patients with a mood disorder should consume 1 g EPA + DHA daily. Current evidence may support the use of 1 to 9 g supplement of EPA + DHA daily for patients with mood disorders, although use of greater than 3 g daily should be monitored by a physician.[85]

Omega-3 fatty acids in the treatment of premenstrual mood exacerbation and PMDD

The literature is sparse concerning the use of omega-3 fatty acids in PMS or PMDD. An early epidemiological study found that lower dietary intake of essential polyunsaturated omega-3 fatty acids was associated with menstrual pain.[86] A subsequent study found that 1080 mg EPA + 720 mg DHA + 1.5 mg vitamin E taken daily for 2 months resulted in a marked reduction in menstrual symptoms from baseline in adolescents with dysmenorrhea, including mood symptoms.[87] Three of 4 RCTs found no benefit of 3 to 6 g evening primrose oil, which contains the omega-6 fatty acid γ-linolenic acid,[88–91] in the reduction of menstrual symptoms versus placebo. One study found a small additional benefit of 3 g of omega-6 fatty acid taken for 4 menstrual cycles in reducing menstrual and depressive symptoms compared with that observed with placebo, but that study did not confirm PMS diagnoses and was not double-blinded.[88] Overall, there is insufficient evidence to support the efficacy of omega-3 or omega-6 fatty acid treatment of PMS or PMDD.

Omega-3 fatty acids in the treatment of antepartum and postpartum depression

Maternal omega-3 fatty acid intake has well-documented obstetrical and infant outcome benefits.[83,92,93] In rats, maternal brain DHA levels decrease when omega-3 fatty acid intake is deficient during pregnancy.[94] Despite increased demand for omega-3 fatty acids during pregnancy, dietary intake by pregnant and postpartum women in the United States has been noted as deficient, with dietary intake during pregnancy even more diminished after issuances from the US Food and Drug Administration of mercury advisories regarding fish intake during pregnancy.[95,96]

In a cross-national epidemiological study, Hibbeln[97] reported that per capita seafood intake was significantly inversely associated with depressive symptoms in postpartum women. In addition, in a large cohort study, Golding and colleagues[98] recently reported that higher levels of omega-3 fatty acid consumption during pregnancy are associated with lower rates of depressive symptoms during pregnancy and throughout the postpartum year. The association remained after adjustment for socioeconomic and demographic variables.

However, Browne and colleagues[99] did not find an association between prenatal fish consumption and PPD in a group that was not at risk for PPD. It is possible that the inclusion of subjects who eat white and oily fish in the fish-eating group of that study lessened the ability to detect a between-group difference because white fish contain significantly less omega-3 fatty acids than oily fish. Similarly, Miyake and colleagues[100] did not detect an inverse relationship between fish intake and later risk of PPD, although these investigators noted that their study population had a high overall intake of oily fish and that the protective effect of omega-3 fatty acids may be demonstrable only in populations with low oily fish intake.

Recently, in a large Danish prospective cohort study of more than 54,000 women, subjects who self-reported the lowest fish intake during pregnancy were at increased risk of being treated for depression with an antidepressant up to 1 year post partum.[101] Although lowest omega-3 fatty acid consumption was associated with higher rates of treatment with an antidepressant, the investigators found that fish intake was strongly associated with sociodemographic characteristics. Therefore, in studies of fish consumption and risk of depression, it is important to assess covariates that may influence omega-3 fatty acid intake.

A small case-controlled study reported that women with lower third-trimester omega-3 fatty acid levels were approximately 6 times more likely to suffer from antenatal depression than those with higher levels.[102] Women at greater risk for depression had lower omega-3 polyunsaturated fatty acid levels, including DHA but not EPA.

Our group conducted an open-label study of omega-3 fatty acids in depression during pregnancy, and a randomized dose-finding study of omega-3 fatty acids in postpartum women.[85,103] Both provided promising preliminary data regarding feasibility, tolerability, and efficacy. However, 3 small randomized placebo-controlled trials have been conducted in which investigators assessed omega-3 fatty acids versus placebo for perinatal depression, and these have produced inconsistent findings. In 2, investigators did not detect a difference between omega-3 fatty acids and placebo.[104,105] However, Su and colleagues[106] reported a significant benefit of omega-3 fatty acids compared with placebo in antenatal depression. The RCTs conducted to date have several limitations. All included small numbers of subjects and were of short duration (up to 8 weeks). In the 2 studies that failed to find a difference between placebo, omega-3 fatty acid and placebo groups improved significantly from study entry, suggesting that other factors related to study participation were associated with improvement.[104,105] Dose may be especially important for further study, as the positive 2008 study by Su and colleagues used the highest dose. Omega-3 fatty acid supplements have been well tolerated by perinatal women[107] and seem free of significant levels of mercury or other contaminants.[108]

Omega-3 fatty acids in the treatment of depressive disorders during the menopausal transition

Although CAM treatments are often sought for hot flashes and other perimenopausal symptoms, few have evidence of benefit from RCTs. For example, Newton and colleagues[109] did not find an advantage of black cohosh (*Cimicifuga racemosa*), a multibotanical plus black cohosh, or a multibotanical with soy over placebo for the treatment of hot flashes. However, in a recent 8-week placebo-controlled RCT, omega-3 fatty acids were found efficacious in the treatment of hot flashes in women 40 to 55 years old who were experiencing psychological distress.[110] Women received 1200 mg per day of omega-3 fatty acids (1050 mg EPA and 150 mg DHA per day). Both groups experienced improved quality of life scores throughout the study.

Bright Light Therapy

Bright light therapy was first assessed as a treatment of seasonal MDD, and has subsequently been shown to be effective for nonseasonal unipolar depression.[111–115] Hypomania has been reported as an adverse event in the treatment of seasonal affective disorder, and switches to mixed state have been associated with light therapy used in patients with bipolar disorder.[115–117] Chronobiological interventions have been investigated in women at times of reproductive hormonal flux because estrogen and progesterone modulate circadian rhythmicity. Gonadal hormones affect the phase and amplitude of the circadian system: perturbation of this rhythmicity has been implicated in the development of mood disorders in women, and interventions such as bright light therapy have beneficial treatment effects in MDD.[118]

Bright light therapy in the treatment of premenstrual mood exacerbation and PMDD

A few studies support the efficacy of bright white light therapy during the symptomatic luteal phase of the menstrual cycle in women with PMDD. Women who received 1 week's treatment of either morning bright light (42%), evening bright light (21%), or evening dim light (26%) had a 50% or greater reduction in HAM-D ratings to a value less than 8.[119] Irritability and physical symptoms were significantly reduced after each of the light treatments compared with baseline. In a separate study, women treated with half an hour of evening light box therapy had fewer depression and premenstrual tension scores compared with women who received placebo (red light).[120]

Bright light therapy in the treatment of antepartum and postpartum depression

Two small studies that assessed bright light therapy in antepartum depression suggest potential efficacy. In a small open pilot trial, pregnant women received 60 minutes of bright light therapy in the morning.[121] Of 16 participants who received at least 3 weeks of bright light therapy, depression scores improved by a mean of 49%, and among the 7 subjects who completed at least 5 weeks, scores improved by 59%. Two patients reported treatment-related nausea but no other significant side effects were reported. In a small double-blind study, pregnant women (N = 10) were randomized to bright light therapy or a dim light placebo condition for 10 weeks.[122] One participant who received bright light therapy experienced the onset of hypomania. Bright light therapy produced a significantly greater antidepressant response rate than placebo, with significant differences after 5 weeks. In a small study of women with PPD (N = 15), participants were assigned randomly to bright light or a placebo dim light condition.[123] Both groups experienced significant improvement from baseline, without differences in response. Larger, controlled studies are needed to better evaluate the efficacy of bright light therapy in antepartum MDD and PPD, and patients should be monitored carefully for emergent symptoms of mania when bright light therapy is initiated.

Bright light therapy in the treatment of depressive disorders during the menopausal transition

No studies have specifically evaluated the efficacy and tolerability of bright light therapy in the treatment of MDD during the menopausal transition.

Exercise

Exercise is well known for its contribution to optimal health. Studies specifically looking at the effect of exercise on mood generally agree that regular exercise is associated with mood-enhancing and antidepressant effects. Several trials reported that aerobic exercise has antidepressant effects,[124,125] and epidemiological data suggest that regular exercise is associated with decreased risk of depressive symptoms.[126,127] Treatment research is difficult with exercise, as adequate study control conditions and maintenance to treatment assignment pose challenges in study design. Dose and adherence to exercise protocols are important considerations of study.[128]

Exercise in the treatment of premenstrual mood exacerbation and PMDD

Two small nonrandomized controlled studies and 2 small randomized studies have evaluated the effects of exercise on PMS signs and symptoms; all reported positive findings. Decreases in breast tenderness and fluid retention,[129–131] personal stress, anxiety,[130] depression,[130,131] muscle stiffness, cramps, anxiety, tension, and restlessness[132] have been associated with either conditioning or aerobic exercise interventions.

Exercise in the treatment of antepartum and postpartum depression

Regular exercise is recommended for most pregnant women. According to recommendations from the American College of Obstetricians and Gynecologists, pregnant women without medical contraindications should engage in 30 minutes of moderate intensity exercise most days.[133]

Studies in pregnancy have mainly focused on women without depression rather than those with validated mood disorders. In 1 prospective study of pregnant women without MDD, those who engaged in regular exercise reported significantly fewer depressive symptoms in the first and second trimesters than those who did not exercise, a difference not observed later in the third trimester.[134] In a Taiwanese study of 80 women at 6 weeks post partum with EPDS scores of 10 or greater (considered at risk for PPD), women were randomized to 3 exercise sessions weekly or treatment as usual.[135] Women assigned to the exercise arm had significantly more improvement on their EPDS scores at 5 months post partum than controls.

St John's Wort

Hypericum perforatum, commonly referred to as St John's wort or goat weed, has been used for its medicinal properties since the times of ancient Greece. Over the past decade there has been increasing interest in its study as a treatment of MDD, and a considerable evidence base has developed backing its efficacy in the treatment of minor depression and mild to moderate MDD. Evidence has been less consistent for moderate to severe MDD. Its study is of particular interest in the study of depressive disorders given several of its bioactive substances, including hypericin, hyperforin, and flavinoids,[136] have affinity for neurotransmitter systems important to the pathophysiology and pharmacotherapy for MDD. In vitro receptor assays indicate that individual bioactive components of St John's wort have activity at γ-aminobutyric acid A (GABA$_A$), GABA$_B$, N-methyl-D-aspartic acid (NMDA), μ-, κ- and δ-opioid and 5-hydroxytryptamine (5-HT$_6$ and 5-HT$_7$) receptors.[137–140]

Two large meta-analyses in 2004 and 2005 compared the efficacy of St John's wort versus placebo or standard antidepressants in the treatment of depressive symptoms or MDD.[141,142] Results from the individual studies were mixed with a more robust effect seen in patients with mild to moderate depressive symptoms. St John's wort, at daily dosage 300 to 1200 mg, had a significant advantage compared with placebo in these smaller studies, but in larger placebo-controlled studies in which patients met criteria for MDD, the effect size was smaller. St John's wort had similar efficacy to TCAs or SSRI antidepressants, and better efficacy than the standard antidepressant in a subgroup of patients with MDD of mild to moderate severity.[142] There is less of a consensus that St John's wort is efficacious in severe MDD.

The phase I metabolism and adenosine triphosphate (ATP)-binding cassette (ABC) membrane transport of St John's wort have been studied in regards to drug metabolism and drug-herb interactions. St John's wort, which contains high concentrations of the bioactive component hyperforin, induces the cytochrome P450 system (CYP3A4) and inhibits ABCB1, a membrane-bound transporter that facilitates transport across the intestinal lumen and the blood-brain barrier.[143,144] St John's wort may interact with medications such as SSRIs, oral contraceptives, and hormone replacement,[145,146] resulting in a diminished level of the 3A4 substrate. Reduced levels of oral contraceptives could result in ovulation; unplanned pregnancies have been reported, as a result of suspected drug-herb interactions.[147]

St John's wort in the treatment of antepartum and postpartum depression

Few studies have evaluated the safety of St John's wort during pregnancy, and no RCTs have been published that have evaluated the efficacy or safety of St John's wort for antepartum or postpartum depression. There are no data on animal or human placental transfer of the bioactive components of St John's wort. There is a limited body of animal data, most of which has reported a lack of adverse effects on the progress of gestation during organogenesis,[148–152] although a small number of animal studies have raised concerns regarding exposure to the key St John's wort metabolites hypericum and hypercin.[149,153,154] Limited data in 54 human pregnancies indicated no increased risk of major malformations or prematurity rate for infants born to women taking St John's wort during pregnancy and matched controls.[155]

Considerations in breastfeeding

St John's wort is excreted into breast milk at undetectable to low levels, comparable with other antidepressants, and its bioactive components are either undetectable or at the limit of quantification in infant plasma.[156,157] In 1 small prospective observational cohort study of nursing women (N = 33) treated with hypericum, increased rates of adverse events including colic, drowsiness, and lethargy were reported in breastfed newborns compared with infants of matched depressed and nondepressed controls.[96] None of the reported events required medical intervention.[158] Between groups, there was no difference in either maternal reports of decreased milk volume or infant weight as recorded by medical records over the first year.

St John's wort in the treatment of depressive disorders during the menopausal transition

No studies have evaluated St John's wort as a monotherapy for depression occurring during the menopausal transition; however, a couple of studies have evaluated the efficacy of a combination of St John's wort and other phytotherapies for menopausal and psychological complaints. In a double-blind RCT of late-perimenopausal and postmenopausal women, the combination of St John's wort and chaste tree/berry (*Vitex agnus-castus*) therapy was found no more effective in the management of hot flashes and other menopausal symptoms than placebo.[159] However, a double-blind RCT of a fixed combination of St John's wort and black cohosh was found superior to placebo in reducing menopausal and depressive symptoms as measured by the Menopause Rating Scale (MRS) and the HAM-D. Active treatment effects were seen at 8 (34.8% reduction in MRS score, 30% reduction in HAM-D score) and 16 (50% reduction in MRS score, 41.8% reduction in HAM-D score) week study time points.[160] The combined herbal treatment was well tolerated.

Acupuncture

According to traditional Chinese medicine, the body is seen as a balance of 2 forces: yin and yang; maintenance of this balance is associated with health and imbalance is associated with a blockage of vital energy (qi). Acupuncture stimulates anatomical points on the body, often with thin metallic needles (manual acupuncture), which serves to restore qi flow that has been blocked by trauma. Controlled trials evaluating acupuncture as a treatment of MDD have been mixed.[161–164] A recent meta-analysis of 8 RCTs evaluated the efficacy of manual, electro-, or laser acupuncture versus sham treatment in patients with MDD or depressive neurosis.[165] Acupuncture was found to significantly reduce HAM-D or Beck Depression Inventory scores but there was no significant effect of acupuncture on either the response or remission rate.

Assessment of the evidence base for acupuncture is challenging for clinicians practicing primarily Western medicine, as many studies are published in Asian languages, diagnostic and symptom assessments may not be standardized across studies, and acupuncture techniques may vary across studies.[166] In addition, establishing an effective placebo for acupuncture research is challenging. Three types of placebo have been traditionally used: nonspecific acupuncture, sham acupuncture, and placebo needles.[167]

Acupuncture in the treatment of antepartum and postpartum depression

There are few data on the safety or efficacy of acupuncture during pregnancy or in the postpartum period. Some acupuncture points have been reported to enhance cervical ripening at term and advance labor and delivery.[168–170]

In 1 small RTC, 61 pregnant women with MDD were randomized to receive 8 weeks of treatment with either active acupuncture, active control acupuncture, or massage.[171] Response rates were higher for active acupuncture (69%) compared with the control acupuncture (47%) or massage groups (32%), and responders to the acute treatment during pregnancy had lower depression scores in the postpartum period than nonresponders. Tolerability of the different treatment modalities was not reported.

Acupuncture in the treatment of depressive disorders during the menopausal transition

Several RCTs, and a couple of systematic reviews, have investigated whether acupuncture therapy reduces vasomotor symptoms associated with natural menopause, with divergent results. The recent Cho and Whang systematic review[172] evaluated 11 RCTs of varying methodological quality, 6 of which compared active with sham or placebo acupuncture. Only 1 of those 6 RCTs reported a significant reduction in vasomotor symptoms between active and placebo groups. In several trials active and placebo or sham acupuncture reduced vasomotor symptoms, without significant between-group differences.

The effectiveness of acupuncture plus self-care versus self-care alone on hot flashes was studied in postmenopausal women in an RCT conducted in Norway.[173] Women who received 10 acupuncture treatment sessions plus education on self-care experienced a statistically significant reduction in mean hot flash frequency (5.8 per 24 hours) compared with women receiving only education on self-care (3.7 per 24 hours). Women who received the combined therapy also had significant improvements in somatic and sleep symptoms as measured by the Women's Health Questionnaire. There was no sham or placebo acupuncture control group in this study.

A few RCTs that used nonspecific, sham, or placebo acupuncture as a control reported reduction of menopausal vasomotor symptoms between active and control groups,[174–177] but other studies have not been able to show a significant difference between active and placebo or sham acupuncture.[178,179] In addition, some studies that reported a positive benefit of acupuncture treatment of vasomotor symptoms did not include a placebo or sham control.[173] Currently there is not enough evidence to support recommendation of acupuncture in the treatment of vasomotor symptoms related to natural menopause.

SUMMARY

As many patients will not experience remission from psychiatric disorders with standard treatments, and CAM use is growing in prevalence, it is important to consider the potential role of CAM treatments when use is supported by an evidence base of efficacy and safety. Pursuing CAM treatments in lieu of standard evaluation and treatments carries the risk of delaying other possibly efficacious treatment. The popularity of many CAM treatments necessitates that health care providers actively and respectfully inquire about CAM use and understand their risks and benefits.

However, with appropriate consideration of benefit and harm evidence, some of the better-studied CAM treatments can expand the list of treatment options available to patients. Almost 40% of the adult US population currently uses some form of CAM treatment, with anxiety, depression, and insomnia among the top 10 health conditions for which CAM is most frequently used.[180,181] Given the acceptability of CAM, inclusion of evidence-based CAM therapies in clinical practice may help to engage some individuals who may be wary of standard treatments. In addition, CAM therapies may increase treatment strategies for patients who have not remitted with standard treatments or have had difficulty tolerating them.

Further study is necessary to delineate the role of specific CAM therapies in PMS, PMDD, antepartum and postpartum depression, lactation, and the menopausal transition. Further well-designed, adequately powered studies are warranted to assess CAM therapies not only in MDD, which has the largest evidence base, but also in anxiety and psychotic disorders, which have received much less investigation. Future research should evaluate these treatments with large enough sample sizes in men and women to discern any gender-based differences in efficacy or tolerability, as has been shown for synthetic antidepressants.

REFERENCES

1. Cohen LS, Soares CN, Otto MW, et al. Prevalence and predictors of premenstrual dysphoric disorder (PMDD) in older premenopausal women. The Harvard Study of Moods and Cycles. J Affect Disord 2002;70(2): 125–32.
2. Rivera-Tovar AD, Frank E. Late luteal phase dysphoric disorder in young women. Am J Psychiatry 1990;147(12):1634–6.
3. Sternfeld B, Swindle R, Chawla A, et al. Severity of premenstrual symptoms in a health maintenance organization population. Obstet Gynecol 2002;99(6): 1014–24.
4. Steiner M, Macdougall M, Brown E. The premenstrual symptoms screening tool (PSST) for clinicians. Arch Womens Ment Health 2003;6(3):203–9.
5. Wittchen HU, Becker E, Lieb R, et al. Prevalence, incidence and stability of premenstrual dysphoric disorder in the community. Psychol Med 2002;32(1): 119–32.
6. Kraemer GR, Kraemer RR. Premenstrual syndrome: diagnosis and treatment experiences. J Womens Health 1998;7(7):893–907.
7. Regier DA, Boyd JH, Burke JD Jr, et al. One-month prevalence of mental disorders in the United States. Based on five epidemiologic catchment area sites. Arch Gen Psychiatry 1988;45(11):977–86.
8. Blazer DG, Kessler RC, McGonagle KA, et al. The prevalence and distribution of major depression in a national community sample: the National Comorbidity Survey. Am J Psychiatry 1994;151(7):979–86.
9. Llewellyn AM, Stowe ZN, Nemeroff CB. Depression during pregnancy and the puerperium. J Clin Psychiatry 1997;58(Suppl 15):26–32.
10. Warner R, Appleby L, Whitton A, et al. Demographic and obstetric risk factors for postnatal psychiatric morbidity. Br J Psychiatry 1996;168(5): 607–11.
11. Cox JL, Murray D, Chapman G. A controlled study of the onset, duration and prevalence of postnatal depression. Br J Psychiatry 1993;163:27–31.

12. O'Hara MW, Gorman LL, Wright EJ. Description and evaluation of the Iowa Depression Awareness, Recognition, and Treatment Program. Am J Psychiatry 1996;153(5):645–9.

13. Bennett HA, Einarson A, Taddio A, et al. Prevalence of depression during pregnancy: systematic review. Obstet Gynecol 2004;103(4):698–709.

14. Dietz PM, Williams SB, Callaghan WM, et al. Clinically identified maternal depression before, during, and after pregnancies ending in live births. Am J Psychiatry 2007;164(10):1515–20.

15. Reck C, Stehle E, Reinig K, et al. Maternity blues as a predictor of DSM-IV depression and anxiety disorders in the first three months postpartum. J Affect Disord 2009;113(1–2):77–87.

16. Vesga-Lopez O, Blanco C, Keyes K, et al. Psychiatric disorders in pregnant and postpartum women in the United States. Arch Gen Psychiatry 2008;65(7): 805–15.

17. Forman DN, Videbech P, Hedegaard M, et al. Postpartum depression: identification of women at risk. BJOG 2000;107(10):1210–7.

18. Gaynes BN, Gavin N, Meltzer-Brody S, et al. Perinatal depression: prevalence, screening accuracy, and screening outcomes. Evid Rep Technol Assess (Summ) 2005;119:1–8.

19. Marcus SM. Depression during pregnancy: rates, risks and consequences– Motherisk Update 2008. Can J Clin Pharmacol 2009;16(1):e15–22.

20. Andersson L, Sundstrom-Poromaa I, Bixo M, et al. Point prevalence of psychiatric disorders during the second trimester of pregnancy: a population-based study. Am J Obstet Gynecol 2003;189(1):148–54.

21. Larsson C, Sydsjo G, Josefsson A. Health, sociodemographic data, and pregnancy outcome in women with antepartum depressive symptoms. Obstet Gynecol 2004;104(3):459–66.

22. Chung TK, Lau TK, Yip AS, et al. Antepartum depressive symptomatology is associated with adverse obstetric and neonatal outcomes. Psychosom Med 2001;63(5):830–4.

23. Wisner KL, Sit DK, Hanusa BH, et al. Major depression and antidepressant treatment: impact on pregnancy and neonatal outcomes. Am J Psychiatry 2009; 166(5):557–66.

24. Dayan J, Creveuil C, Herlicoviez M, et al. Role of anxiety and depression in the onset of spontaneous preterm labor. Am J Epidemiol 2002;155(4): 293–301.

25. Robertson E, Grace S, Wallington T, et al. Antenatal risk factors for postpartum depression: a synthesis of recent literature. Gen Hosp Psychiatry 2004;26(4): 289–95.

26. Kumar R, Robson KM. A prospective study of emotional disorders in childbearing women. Br J Psychiatry 1984;144:35–47.

27. Kendell RE, McGuire RJ, Connor Y, et al. Mood changes in the first three weeks after childbirth. J Affect Disord 1981;3(4):317–26.

28. Wisner KL, Peindl K, Hanusa BH. Relationship of psychiatric illness to childbearing status: a hospital-based epidemiologic study. J Affect Disord 1993; 28(1):39–50.

29. Vik T, Grote V, Escribano J, et al. Infantile colic, prolonged crying and maternal postnatal depression. Acta Paediatr 2009;98(8):1344–8.

30. McMahon CA, Barnett B, Kowalenko NM, et al. Maternal attachment state of mind moderates the impact of postnatal depression on infant attachment. J Child Psychol Psychiatry 2006;47(7):660–9.

31. Brennan PA, Pargas R, Walker EF, et al. Maternal depression and infant cortisol: influences of timing, comorbidity and treatment. J Child Psychol Psychiatry 2008;49(10):1099–107.
32. Laplante DP, Barr RG, Brunet A, et al. Stress during pregnancy affects general intellectual and language functioning in human toddlers. Pediatr Res 2004; 56(3):400–10.
33. Murray L, Cooper P. Effects of postnatal depression on infant development. Arch Dis Child 1997;77(2):99–101.
34. Dawson GAS. On the origins of a vulnerability to depression: the influence of the early social environment on the development of psychobiological systems related to risk of affective disorder. In: Nelson CA, editor. Minnesota Symposia on Child Psychology: the effects of early adversity on neurobehavioral development, vol. 31. Mahwah (NJ): Lawrence Erlbaum Associates; 2000. p. 245–79.
35. Yonkers KA, Wisner KL, Stewart DE, et al. The management of depression during pregnancy: a report from the American Psychiatric Association and the American College of Obstetricians and Gynecologists. Gen Hosp Psychiatry 2009;31:403–13.
36. Soares CN, Cohen LS. The perimenopause, depressive disorders, and hormonal variability. Sao Paulo Med J 2001;119(2):78–83.
37. Bromberger JT, Assmann SF, Avis NE, et al. Persistent mood symptoms in a multiethnic community cohort of pre- and perimenopausal women. Am J Epidemiol 2003;158(4):347–56.
38. Cohen LS, Soares CN, Vitonis AF, et al. Risk for new onset of depression during the menopausal transition: the Harvard study of moods and cycles. Arch Gen Psychiatry 2006;63(4):385–90.
39. Freeman EW, Sammel MD, Lin H, et al. Associations of hormones and menopausal status with depressed mood in women with no history of depression. Arch Gen Psychiatry 2006;63(4):375–82.
40. Schmidt PJ, Nieman L, Danaceau MA, et al. Estrogen replacement in perimenopause-related depression: a preliminary report. Am J Obstet Gynecol 2000; 183(2):414–20.
41. Carranza-Lira S, Valentino-Figueroa ML. Estrogen therapy for depression in postmenopausal women. Int J Gynaecol Obstet 1999;65(1):35–8.
42. Rossouw JE, Anderson GL, Prentice RL, et al. Risks and benefits of estrogen plus progestin in healthy postmenopausal women: principal results From the Women's Health Initiative randomized controlled trial. JAMA 2002;288(3): 321–33.
43. Hersh AL, Stefanick ML, Stafford RS. National use of postmenopausal hormone therapy: annual trends and response to recent evidence. JAMA 2004;291(1): 47–53.
44. McIntyre RS, Konarski JZ, Grigoriadis S, et al. Hormone replacement therapy and antidepressant prescription patterns: a reciprocal relationship. CMAJ 2005;172(1):57–9.
45. Soares CN. Practical strategies for diagnosing and treating depression in women: menopausal transition. J Clin Psychiatry 2008;69(10):e30.
46. Pirotta MV, Cohen MM, Kotsirilos V, et al. Complementary therapies: have they become accepted in general practice? Med J Aust 2000;172(3):105–9.
47. Barnes PM, Bloom B, Nahin RL. Complementary and alternative medicine use among adults and children: United States, 2007. Natl Health Stat Report 2009;12:1–23.

48. Eisenberg DM, Davis RB, Ettner SL, et al. Trends in alternative medicine use in the United States, 1990–1997: results of a follow-up national survey. JAMA 1998; 280(18):1569–75.

49. Tindle HA, Davis RB, Phillips RS, et al. Trends in use of complementary and alternative medicine by US adults: 1997–2002. Altern Ther Health Med 2005; 11(1):42–9.

50. Mackenzie ER, Taylor L, Bloom BS, et al. Ethnic minority use of complementary and alternative medicine (CAM): a national probability survey of CAM utilizers. Altern Ther Health Med 2003;9(4):50–6.

51. Weissman MM, Leaf PJ, Holzer CE 3rd, et al. The epidemiology of depression. An update on sex differences in rates. J Affect Disord 1984;7(3–4):179–88.

52. Wu P, Fuller C, Liu X, et al. Use of complementary and alternative medicine among women with depression: results of a national survey. Psychiatr Serv 2007;58(3):349–56.

53. Elkins G, Rajab MH, Marcus J. Complementary and alternative medicine use by psychiatric inpatients. Psychol Rep 2005;96(1):163–6.

54. Unutzer J, Klap R, Sturm R, et al. Mental disorders and the use of alternative medicine: results from a national survey. Am J Psychiatry 2000;157(11):1851–7.

55. Mischoulon D, Fava M. Role of S-adenosyl-L-methionine in the treatment of depression: a review of the evidence. Am J Clin Nutr 2002;76(5):1158S–61S.

56. Spillmann M, Fava M. S-adenosyl-methione (ademthionine) in psychiatric disorders. CNS Drugs 1996;6:416–25.

57. Hardy M, Coulter I, Morton SC, et al. S-Adenosyl-L-methionine (SAMe) for depression, osteoarthritis and liver disease. Rockville (MD): Agency for Healthcare Research and Quality; 2002.

58. Delle Chiaie R, Pancheri P, Scapicchio P. Efficacy and tolerability of oral and intramuscular S-adenosyl-L-methionine 1,4-butanedisulfonate (SAMe) in the treatment of major depression: comparison with imipramine in 2 multicenter studies. Am J Clin Nutr 2002;76(5):1172S–6S.

59. Bressa GM. S-Adenosyl-l-methionine (SAMe) as antidepressant: meta-analysis of clinical studies. Acta Neurol Scand Suppl 1994;154:7–14.

60. Pancheri P, Scapicchio P, Chiaie RD. A double-blind, randomized parallel-group, efficacy and safety study of intramuscular S-adenosyl-L-methionine 1,4-butanedisulphonate (SAMe) versus imipramine in patients with major depressive disorder. Int J Neuropsychopharmacol 2002;5(4):287–94.

61. Thachil AF, Mohan R, Bhugra D. The evidence base of complementary and alternative therapies in depression. J Affect Disord 2007;97(1–3):23–35.

62. Alpert JE, Papakostas G, Mischoulon D, et al. S-adenosyl-L-methionine (SAMe) as an adjunct for resistant major depressive disorder: an open trial following partial or nonresponse to selective serotonin reuptake inhibitors or venlafaxine. J Clin Psychopharmacol 2004;24(6):661–4.

63. Goren JL, Stoll AL, Damico KE, et al. Bioavailability and lack of toxicity of S-adenosyl-L-methionine (SAMe) in humans. Pharmacotherapy 2004;24(11): 1501–7.

64. Carney MW, Chary TK, Bottiglieri T, et al. Switch mechanism in affective illness and oral S-adenosylmethionine (SAM). Br J Psychiatry 1987;150:724–5.

65. Cerutti R, Sichel MP, Perin M, et al. Psychological distress during the puerperium: a novel therapeutic approach using S-adenosylmethionine. Curr Ther Res 1993;53(6):701–16.

66. Cozens DO, Barton SJ, Clark R, et al. Reproductive toxicity studies of ademetionine. Arzneimittelforschung 1988;38:1625–9.

67. Salmaggi P, Bressa GM, Nicchia G, et al. Double-blind, placebo-controlled study of S-adenosyl-L-methionine in depressed postmenopausal women. Psychother Psychosom 1993;59(1):34–40.
68. Papakostas GI, Petersen T, Mischoulon D, et al. Serum folate, vitamin B12, and homocysteine in major depressive disorder, Part 1: predictors of clinical response in fluoxetine-resistant depression. J Clin Psychiatry 2004;65(8):1090–5.
69. Bottiglieri T, Laundy M, Crellin R, et al. Homocysteine, folate, methylation, and monoamine metabolism in depression. J Neurol Neurosurg Psychiatry 2000;69(2):228–32.
70. Gilbody S, Lewis S, Lightfoot T. Methylenetetrahydrofolate reductase (MTHFR) genetic polymorphisms and psychiatric disorders: a HuGE review. Am J Epidemiol 2007;165(1):1–13.
71. Lopez-Leon S, Janssens AC, Gonzalez-Zuloeta Ladd AM, et al. Meta-analyses of genetic studies on major depressive disorder. Mol Psychiatry 2008;13(8):772–85.
72. Papakostas GI, Petersen T, Mischoulon D, et al. Serum folate, vitamin B12, and homocysteine in major depressive disorder, Part 2: predictors of relapse during the continuation phase of pharmacotherapy. J Clin Psychiatry 2004;65(8):1096–8.
73. Alpert M, Silva RR, Pouget ER. Prediction of treatment response in geriatric depression from baseline folate level: interaction with an SSRI or a tricyclic antidepressant. J Clin Psychopharmacol 2003;23(3):309–13.
74. Coppen A, Bailey J. Enhancement of the antidepressant action of fluoxetine by folic acid: a randomised, placebo controlled trial. J Affect Disord 2000;60(2):121–30.
75. Miyake Y, Sasaki S, Tanaka K, et al. Dietary folate and vitamins B12, B6, and B2 intake and the risk of postpartum depression in Japan: the Osaka Maternal and Child Health Study. J Affect Disord 2006;96(1–2):133–8.
76. Su KP, Huang SY, Chiu CC, et al. Omega-3 fatty acids in major depressive disorder. A preliminary double-blind, placebo-controlled trial. Eur Neuropsychopharmacol 2003;13(4):267–71.
77. Nemets B, Stahl Z, Belmaker RH. Addition of omega-3 fatty acid to maintenance medication treatment for recurrent unipolar depressive disorder. Am J Psychiatry 2002;159(3):477–9.
78. Marangell LB, Martinez JM, Zboyan HA, et al. A double-blind, placebo-controlled study of the omega-3 fatty acid docosahexaenoic acid in the treatment of major depression. Am J Psychiatry 2003;160(5):996–8.
79. Mischoulon D, Papakostas G, Dording CM, et al. A double-blind randomized controlled trial of ethyl-eicosapentaenoate for major depressive disorder. J Clin Psychiatry 2009;70(12):1636–44.
80. Parker G, Gibson NA, Brotchie H, et al. Omega-3 fatty acids and mood disorders. Am J Psychiatry 2006;163(6):969–78.
81. Kris-Etherton PM, Harris WS, Appel LJ. Omega-3 fatty acids and cardiovascular disease: new recommendations from the American Heart Association. Arterioscler Thromb Vasc Biol 2003;23(2):151–2.
82. Freeman MP, Hibbeln JR, Wisner KL, et al. Randomized dose-ranging pilot trial of omega-3 fatty acids for postpartum depression. Acta Psychiatr Scand 2006;113(1):31–5.
83. McGregor JA, Allen KG, Harris MA, et al. The omega-3 story: nutritional prevention of preterm birth and other adverse pregnancy outcomes. Obstet Gynecol Surv 2001;56(5 Suppl 1):S1–13.

84. Freeman MP. Omega-3 fatty acids and perinatal depression: a review of the literature and recommendations for future research. Prostaglandins Leukot Essent Fatty Acids 2006;75(4–5):291–7.

85. Freeman MP, Hibbeln JR, Wisner KL, et al. Omega-3 fatty acids: evidence basis for treatment and future research in psychiatry. J Clin Psychiatry 2006;67(12): 1954–67.

86. Deutch B. Menstrual pain in Danish women correlated with low n-3 polyunsaturated fatty acid intake. Eur J Clin Nutr 1995;49(7):508–16.

87. Harel Z, Biro FM, Kottenhahn RK, et al. Supplementation with omega-3 polyunsaturated fatty acids in the management of dysmenorrhea in adolescents. Am J Obstet Gynecol 1996;174(4):1335–8.

88. Puolakka J, Makarainen L, Viinikka L, et al. Biochemical and clinical effects of treating the premenstrual syndrome with prostaglandin synthesis precursors. J Reprod Med 1985;30(3):149–53.

89. Callender K, Thomas CS. Treating the premenstrual syndrome. BMJ 1988; 297(6649):684.

90. Collins A, Cerin A, Coleman G, et al. Essential fatty acids in the treatment of premenstrual syndrome. Obstet Gynecol 1993;81(1):93–8.

91. Khoo SK, Munro C, Battistutta D. Evening primrose oil and treatment of premenstrual syndrome. Med J Aust 1990;153(4):189–92.

92. Dunstan JA, Simmer K, Dixon G, et al. Cognitive assessment of children at age 2(1/2) years after maternal fish oil supplementation in pregnancy: a randomised controlled trial. Arch Dis Child Fetal Neonatal Ed 2008;93(1):F45–50.

93. Hibbeln JR, Davis JM, Steer C, et al. Maternal seafood consumption in pregnancy and neurodevelopmental outcomes in childhood (ALSPAC study): an observational cohort study. Lancet 2007;369(9561):578–85.

94. Levant B, Radel JD, Carlson SE. Reduced brain DHA content after a single reproductive cycle in female rats fed a diet deficient in N-3 polyunsaturated fatty acids. Biol Psychiatry 2006;60(9):987–90.

95. Oken E, Kleinman KP, Berland WE, et al. Decline in fish consumption among pregnant women after a national mercury advisory. Obstet Gynecol 2003; 102(2):346–51.

96. Benisek D, Shabert J, Skornick R. Dietary intake of polyunsaturated fatty acids by pregnant or lactating women in the United States. Obstet Gynecol 2000;95: 7778.

97. Hibbeln JR. Seafood consumption, the DHA content of mothers' milk and prevalence rates of postpartum depression: a cross-national, ecological analysis. J Affect Disord 2002;69(1–3):15–29.

98. Golding J, Steer C, Emmett P, et al. High levels of depressive symptoms in pregnancy with low omega-3 fatty acid intake from fish. Epidemiology 2009;20(4): 598–603.

99. Browne JC, Scott KM, Silvers KM. Fish consumption in pregnancy and omega-3 status after birth are not associated with postnatal depression. J Affect Disord 2006;90(2–3):131–9.

100. Miyake Y, Sasaki S, Yokoyama T, et al. Risk of postpartum depression in relation to dietary fish and fat intake in Japan: the Osaka Maternal and Child Health Study. Psychol Med 2006;36(12):1727–35.

101. Strom M, Mortensen EL, Halldorsson TI, et al. Fish and long-chain n-3 polyunsaturated fatty acid intakes during pregnancy and risk of postpartum depression: a prospective study based on a large national birth cohort. Am J Clin Nutr 2009; 90(1):149–55.

102. Rees AM, Austin MP, Owen C, et al. Omega-3 deficiency associated with perinatal depression: case control study. Psychiatry Res 2009;166(2–3): 254–9.

103. Freeman MP, Hibbeln JR, Wisner KL, et al. An open trial of omega-3 fatty acids for depression in pregnancy. Acta Neuropsychiatr 2006;18:21–4.

104. Rees AM, Austin MP, Parker GB. Omega-3 fatty acids as a treatment for perinatal depression: randomized double-blind placebo-controlled trial. Aust N Z J Psychiatry 2008;42(3):199–205.

105. Freeman MP, Davis M, Sinha P, et al. Omega-3 fatty acids and supportive psychotherapy for perinatal depression: a randomized placebo-controlled study. J Affect Disord 2008;110(1–2):142–8.

106. Su KP, Huang SY, Chiu TH, et al. Omega-3 fatty acids for major depressive disorder during pregnancy: results from a randomized, double-blind, placebo-controlled trial. J Clin Psychiatry 2008;69(4):644–51.

107. Freeman MP, Sinha P. Tolerability of omega-3 fatty acid supplements in perinatal women. Prostaglandins Leukot Essent Fatty Acids 2007;77(3–4):203–8.

108. Foran SE, Flood JG, Lewandrowski KB. Measurement of mercury levels in concentrated over-the-counter fish oil preparations: is fish oil healthier than fish? Arch Pathol Lab Med 2003;127(12):1603–5.

109. Newton KM, Reed SD, LaCroix AZ, et al. Treatment of vasomotor symptoms of menopause with black cohosh, multibotanicals, soy, hormone therapy, or placebo: a randomized trial. Ann Intern Med 2006;145(12):869–79.

110. Lucas M, Asselin G, Merette C, et al. Effects of ethyl-eicosapentaenoic acid omega-3 fatty acid supplementation on hot flashes and quality of life among middle-aged women: a double-blind, placebo-controlled, randomized clinical trial. Menopause 2009;16(2):357–66.

111. Terman M, Terman JS, Quitkin FM, et al. Light therapy for seasonal affective disorder. A review of efficacy. Neuropsychopharmacology 1989;2(1):1–22.

112. Eastman CI, Young MA, Fogg LF, et al. Bright light treatment of winter depression: a placebo-controlled trial. Arch Gen Psychiatry 1998;55(10):883–9.

113. Kripke DF, Mullaney DJ, Klauber MR, et al. Controlled trial of bright light for nonseasonal major depressive disorders. Biol Psychiatry 1992;31(2):119–34.

114. Sumaya IC, Rienzi BM, Deegan JF 2nd, et al. Bright light treatment decreases depression in institutionalized older adults: a placebo-controlled crossover study. J Gerontol A Biol Sci Med Sci 2001;56(6):M356–60.

115. Golden RN, Gaynes BN, Ekstrom RD, et al. The efficacy of light therapy in the treatment of mood disorders: a review and meta-analysis of the evidence. Am J Psychiatry 2005;162(4):656–62.

116. Sit D, Wisner KL, Hanusa BH, et al. Light therapy for bipolar disorder: a case series in women. Bipolar Disord 2007;9(8):918–27.

117. Chan PK, Lam RW, Perry KF. Mania precipitated by light therapy for patients with SAD. J Clin Psychiatry 1994;55(10):454.

118. Parry BL, Newton RP. Chronobiological basis of female-specific mood disorders. Neuropsychopharmacology 2001;25(Suppl 5):S102–8.

119. Parry BL, Mahan AM, Mostofi N, et al. Light therapy of late luteal phase dysphoric disorder: an extended study. Am J Psychiatry 1993;150(9):1417–9.

120. Lam RW, Carter D, Misri S, et al. A controlled study of light therapy in women with late luteal phase dysphoric disorder. Psychiatry Res 1999; 86(3):185–92.

121. Oren DA, Wisner KL, Spinelli M, et al. An open trial of morning light therapy for treatment of antepartum depression. Am J Psychiatry 2002;159(4):666–9.

122. Epperson CN, Terman M, Terman JS, et al. Randomized clinical trial of bright light therapy for antepartum depression: preliminary findings. J Clin Psychiatry 2004;65(3):421–5.

123. Corral M, Wardrop AA, Zhang H, et al. Morning light therapy for postpartum depression. Arch Womens Ment Health 2007;10(5):221–4.

124. Trivedi MH, Greer TL, Grannemann BD, et al. Exercise as an augmentation strategy for treatment of major depression. J Psychiatr Pract 2006;12(4): 205–13.

125. Otto MW, Church TS, Craft LL, et al. Exercise for mood and anxiety disorders. J Clin Psychiatry 2007;68(5):669–76.

126. Strawbridge WJ, Deleger S, Roberts RE, et al. Physical activity reduces the risk of subsequent depression for older adults. Am J Epidemiol 2002; 156(4):328–34.

127. Penninx BW, Rejeski WJ, Pandya J, et al. Exercise and depressive symptoms: a comparison of aerobic and resistance exercise effects on emotional and physical function in older persons with high and low depressive symptomatology. J Gerontol B Psychol Sci Soc Sci 2002;57(2):P124–32.

128. Dunn AL, Trivedi MH, Kampert JB, et al. Exercise treatment for depression: efficacy and dose response. Am J Prev Med 2005;28(1):1–8.

129. Prior JC, Vigna Y, Alojada N. Conditioning exercise decreases premenstrual symptoms. A prospective controlled three month trial. Eur J Appl Physiol Occup Physiol 1986;55(4):349–55.

130. Prior JC, Vigna Y, Sciarretta D, et al. Conditioning exercise decreases premenstrual symptoms: a prospective, controlled 6-month trial. Fertil Steril 1987;47(3): 402–8.

131. Steege JF, Blumenthal JA. The effects of aerobic exercise on premenstrual symptoms in middle-aged women: a preliminary study. J Psychosom Res 1993;37(2):127–33.

132. Stoddard JL, Dent CW, Shames L, et al. Exercise training effects on premenstrual distress and ovarian steroid hormones. Eur J Appl Physiol 2007;99(1):27–37.

133. Artal R, O'Toole M. Guidelines of the American College of Obstetricians and Gynecologists for exercise during pregnancy and the postpartum period. Br J Sports Med 2003;37(1):6–12 [discussion: 12].

134. Da Costa D, Rippen N, Dritsa M, et al. Self-reported leisure-time physical activity during pregnancy and relationship to psychological well-being. J Psychosom Obstet Gynaecol 2003;24(2):111–9.

135. Heh SS, Huang LH, Ho SM, et al. Effectiveness of an exercise support program in reducing the severity of postnatal depression in Taiwanese women. Birth 2008;35(1):60–5.

136. Butterweck V. Mechanism of action of St John's wort in depression: what is known? CNS Drugs 2003;17(8):539–62.

137. Simmen U, Burkard W, Berger K, et al. Extracts and constituents of Hypericum perforatum inhibit the binding of various ligands to recombinant receptors expressed with the Semliki Forest virus system. J Recept Signal Transduct Res 1999;19(1–4):59–74.

138. Simmen U, Higelin J, Berger-Buter K, et al. Neurochemical studies with St. John's wort in vitro. Pharmacopsychiatry 2001;34(Suppl 1):S137–42.

139. Gobbi M, Moia M, Pirona L, et al. In vitro binding studies with two Hypericum perforatum extracts–hyperforin, hypericin and biapigenin–on 5-HT6, 5-HT7, GABA(A)/benzodiazepine, sigma, NPY-Y1/Y2 receptors and dopamine transporters. Pharmacopsychiatry 2001;34(Suppl 1):S45–8.

140. Cott JM. In vitro receptor binding and enzyme inhibition by *Hypericum perforatum* extract. Pharmacopsychiatry 1997;30(Suppl 2):108–12.

141. Linde K, Mulrow CD, Berner M, et al. St John's wort for depression. Cochrane Database Syst Rev 2005;(2):CD000448.

142. Roder C, Schaefer M, Leucht S. [Meta-analysis of effectiveness and tolerability of treatment of mild to moderate depression with St. John's Wort]. Fortschr Neurol Psychiatr 2004;72(6):330–43 [in German].

143. Hennessy M, Kelleher D, Spiers JP, et al. St Johns wort increases expression of P-glycoprotein: implications for drug interactions. Br J Clin Pharmacol 2002; 53(1):75–82.

144. Gutmann H, Poller B, Buter KB, et al. *Hypericum perforatum*: which constituents may induce intestinal MDR1 and CYP3A4 mRNA expression? Planta Med 2006; 72(8):685–90.

145. Roby CA, Anderson GD, Kantor E, et al. St John's Wort: effect on CYP3A4 activity. Clin Pharmacol Ther 2000;67(5):451–7.

146. Murphy PA, Kern SE, Stanczyk FZ, et al. Interaction of St. John's Wort with oral contraceptives: effects on the pharmacokinetics of norethindrone and ethinyl estradiol, ovarian activity and breakthrough bleeding. Contraception 2005; 71(6):402–8.

147. Schwarz UI, Buschel B, Kirch W. Unwanted pregnancy on self-medication with St John's wort despite hormonal contraception. Br J Clin Pharmacol 2003;55(1): 112–3.

148. Borges LV, do Carmo Cancino JC, Peters VM, et al. Development of pregnancy in rats treated with *Hypericum perforatum*. Phytother Res 2005;19(10):885–7.

149. Rayburn WF, Christensen HD, Gonzalez CL. Effect of antenatal exposure to Saint John's wort (*Hypericum*) on neurobehavior of developing mice. Am J Obstet Gynecol 2000;183(5):1225–31.

150. Rayburn WF, Gonzalez CL, Christensen HD, et al. Impact of hypericum (St.-John's-wort) given prenatally on cognition of mice offspring. Neurotoxicol Teratol 2001;23(6):629–37.

151. Rayburn WF, Gonzalez CL, Christensen HD, et al. Effect of prenatally administered hypericum (St John's wort) on growth and physical maturation of mouse offspring. Am J Obstet Gynecol 2001;184(2):191–5.

152. Dugoua JJ, Mills E, Perri D, et al. Safety and efficacy of St. John's wort (hypericum) during pregnancy and lactation. Can J Clin Pharmacol 2006;13(3):e268–76.

153. Chan LY, Chiu PY, Lau TK. A study of hypericin-induced teratogenicity during organogenesis using a whole rat embryo culture model. Fertil Steril 2001; 76(5):1073–4.

154. Gregoretti B, Stebel M, Candussio L, et al. Toxicity of *Hypericum perforatum* (St. John's wort) administered during pregnancy and lactation in rats. Toxicol Appl Pharmacol 2004;200(3):201–5.

155. Moretti ME, Maxson A, Hanna F, et al. Evaluating the safety of St. John's Wort in human pregnancy. Reprod Toxicol 2009;28(1):96–9.

156. Klier CM, Schafer MR, Schmid-Siegel B, et al. St. John's wort (*Hypericum perforatum*)–is it safe during breastfeeding? Pharmacopsychiatry 2002; 35(1):29–30.

157. Klier CM, Schmid-Siegel B, Schafer MR, et al. St. John's wort (*Hypericum perforatum*) and breastfeeding: plasma and breast milk concentrations of hyperforin for 5 mothers and 2 infants. J Clin Psychiatry 2006;67(2):305–9.

158. Lee A, Minhas R, Matsuda N, et al. The safety of St. John's wort (*Hypericum perforatum*) during breastfeeding. J Clin Psychiatry 2003;64(8):966–8.

159. van Die MD, Burger HG, Bone KM, et al. *Hypericum perforatum* with *Vitex agnus-castus* in menopausal symptoms: a randomized, controlled trial. Menopause 2009;16(1):156–63.

160. Uebelhack R, Blohmer JU, Graubaum HJ, et al. Black cohosh and St. John's wort for climacteric complaints: a randomized trial. Obstet Gynecol 2006; 107(2 Pt 1):247–55.

161. Allen JJ, Schnyer RN, Chambers AS, et al. Acupuncture for depression: a randomized controlled trial. J Clin Psychiatry 2006;67(11):1665–73.

162. Luo H, Meng F, Jia Y, et al. Clinical research on the therapeutic effect of the electro-acupuncture treatment in patients with depression. Psychiatry Clin Neurosci 1998;52(Suppl):S338–40.

163. Gallagher SM, Allen JJ, Hitt SK, et al. Six-month depression relapse rates among women treated with acupuncture. Complement Ther Med 2001;9(4):216–8.

164. Zhang WJ, Yang XB, Zhong BL. Combination of acupuncture and fluoxetine for depression: a randomized, double-blind, sham-controlled trial. J Altern Complement Med 2009;15(8):837–44.

165. Wang H, Qi H, Wang BS, et al. Is acupuncture beneficial in depression: a meta-analysis of 8 randomized controlled trials? J Affect Disord 2008;111(2–3):125–34.

166. Halbreich U. Systematic reviews of clinical trials of acupuncture as treatment for depression: how systematic and accurate are they? CNS Spectr 2008;13(4): 293–4, 299–300.

167. Streitberger K, Kleinhenz J. Introducing a placebo needle into acupuncture research. Lancet 1998;352(9125):364–5.

168. Rabl M, Ahner R, Bitschnau M, et al. Acupuncture for cervical ripening and induction of labor at term–a randomized controlled trial. Wien Klin Wochenschr 2001;113(23–24):942–6.

169. Motl JM. Acupuncture. In: Shannon S, editor. Handbook of complementary and alternative therapies in mental health. San Francisco (CA): Academic Press; 2002. p. 443–52.

170. Gaudet LM, Dyzak R, Aung SK, et al. Effectiveness of acupuncture for the initiation of labour at term: a pilot randomized controlled trial. J Obstet Gynaecol Can 2008;30(12):1118–23.

171. Manber R, Schnyer RN, Allen JJ, et al. Acupuncture: a promising treatment for depression during pregnancy. J Affect Disord 2004;83(1):89–95.

172. Cho SH, Whang WW. Acupuncture for vasomotor menopausal symptoms: a systematic review. Menopause 2009;16(5):1065–73.

173. Borud EK, Alraek T, White A, et al. The Acupuncture on Hot Flushes Among Menopausal Women (ACUFLASH) study, a randomized controlled trial. Menopause 2009;16(3):484–93.

174. Avis NE, Legault C, Coeytaux RR, et al. A randomized, controlled pilot study of acupuncture treatment for menopausal hot flashes. Menopause 2008;15(6): 1070–8.

175. Nir Y, Huang MI, Schnyer R, et al. Acupuncture for postmenopausal hot flashes. Maturitas 2007;56(4):383–95.

176. Cohen SM, Rousseau ME, Carey BL. Can acupuncture ease the symptoms of menopause? Holist Nurs Pract 2003;17(6):295–9.

177. Huang MI, Nir Y, Chen B, et al. A randomized controlled pilot study of acupuncture for postmenopausal hot flashes: effect on nocturnal hot flashes and sleep quality. Fertil Steril 2006;86(3):700–10.

178. Vincent A, Barton DL, Mandrekar JN, et al. Acupuncture for hot flashes: a randomized, sham-controlled clinical study. Menopause 2007;14(1):45–52.

179. Sandberg M, Wijma K, Wyon Y, et al. Effects of electro-acupuncture on psychological distress in postmenopausal women. Complement Ther Med 2002;10(3): 161–9.
180. Barnes P, Powell-Griner E, McFann K, et al. CDC advance data report #343. Complementary and alternative medicine use among adults: United States, 2002; 2004.
181. Barnes PM, Bloom B, Nahin R. CDC national health statistics report #12. Complementary and alternative medicine use among adults and children: United States, 2007; 2008.

Trauma and Violence: Are Women the Weaker Sex?

Laura C. Pratchett, PsyD[a,b,]*, Michelle R. Pelcovitz, BA[a,b],
Rachel Yehuda, PhD[a,b]

KEYWORDS

• Trauma • Gender • Risk • Prevalence

The defining characteristic of a trauma is that the presented threat of injury or death provokes fear, helplessness, or horror.[1] It has long been recognized that traumatic events can produce pathological stress responses, and in recent years our understanding of these responses has increased. This can be attributed in part to the extremely high rates of exposure to such events. A large body of research indicates that the most the US population will, at some point in their life, be exposed to at least 1 traumatic event, with estimates of prevalence ranging from 58% to 92%.[2–4] Such events might include interpersonal violence (such as rape, assault, and combat), exposure to life threatening accidents (such as motor vehicle accidents), or experiencing a disaster (such as earthquakes, hurricanes, or fire). Recent events have also added the real risk of exposure to terrorism which involves interpersonal violence as well as the mass effect/affect of a disaster.

POSTTRAUMATIC STRESS DISORDER

Psychological sequelae of trauma are varied and include anxiety disorders, substance abuse disorders, and mood disorders.[2] Exposure to childhood trauma, in addition to serving as a risk factor for development of problems following exposure to later trauma, has also been indicated in the etiology of some personality disorders. Post-traumatic stress disorder (PTSD) is unique among psychiatric classifications in that it requires exposure to a traumatic event and a subsequent emotional response of fear, helplessness, or horror.[1] PTSD involves 3 distinct clusters of symptoms consisting of reexperiencing the event, avoidance of reminders of the event, and

[a] Department of Psychiatry, Mount Sinai School of Medicine, One Gustave L. Levy Place, New York, NY, USA
[b] James J. Peters Veterans Affairs Medical Center, 526 OOMH 116/A, 130 West Kingsbridge Road, Bronx, New York, NY 10468, USA
* Corresponding author. James J. Peters Veterans Affairs Medical Center, 526 OOMH 116/A, 130 West Kingsbridge Road, Bronx, New York, NY 10468.
E-mail address: laura.pratchett@va.gov

Psychiatr Clin N Am 33 (2010) 465–474
doi:10.1016/j.psc.2010.01.010
0193-953X/10/$ – see front matter. Published by Elsevier Inc.

psych.theclinics.com

hyperarousal. Reexperiencing may involve unwanted memories in the form of night-mares, intrusive thoughts or images, flashbacks, and either emotional or physiological distress at reminders of the event. Avoidance symptoms include efforts to avoid any people, places, activities, or even thoughts that serve as reminders of the event. Hyperarousal symptoms include difficulty sleeping and concentrating, increased irritability and startle response, and excessive vigilance to threat.

EPIDEMIOLOGICAL ASPECTS

Despite the high rates of exposure to traumatic events, research indicates that PTSD occurs in relatively low numbers of people exposed. Studies examining the prevalence of lifetime history of PTSD in the general US population report rates of 2% to 14%.[2,5,6] Multiple epidemiological studies have found that women are more likely to develop PTSD than men.[2,3,7,8] This is despite the fact that men report significantly more exposure to potentially traumatic events, with the exception of traumatic events during childhood where no sex differences exist for exposure rates.[9] The discrepancy in prevalence of PTSD remains regardless of whether lifetime, current, or conditional (development of PTSD among those who experience trauma) status are studied.[3,10,11] In addition, among those who develop PTSD, women have been found to have more severe symptoms[9] and to experience more reexperiencing symptoms.[12] This apparently greater vulnerability to PTSD among women has been discussed and studied at length and multiple explanatory theories have been developed and explored.

INTERPERSONAL TRAUMA

A common suggestion for this discrepancy focuses on the types of trauma commonly experienced by women versus men. Men are more likely to experience most categories of potentially traumatic event including nonsexual assault, accidents, combat, and witnessing death or injury, and no significant sex differences exist for nonsexual childhood physical abuse and neglect.[9,13] Women, however, are more likely to experience intimate partner violence (IPV) and sexual assault during childhood and adulthood.[9,14]

Intimate Partner Violence

US Department of Justice figures indicate that, annually, 21.5% of nonfatal assaults against women are perpetrated by intimate partners, whereas IPV accounts for only 3.6% of annual assaults against men. Lifetime prevalence rates of IPV by gender are similar with studies suggesting between 3% and 7% of men and 20% and 22% of women experience IPV, meaning women are approximately 3 times more likely to suffer from this kind of violence.[15] Incidences of IPV against women may also have more serious physical consequences than when men are the victim; women who experience IPV are more likely to be injured, receive medical treatment, be hospitalized, and lose time from work.[15] Of those experiencing IPV, 32.6% of women and 26.4% of men received a threat to kill, and 44.7% of women and 19.6% of men reported fearing injury or death. This fear may be somewhat justified. US Department of Justice statistics indicate that 30.1% of female homicide victims are killed by their intimate partner, whereas 5.3% of male homicide victims are killed by their partner. Another difference in severity may be reflected in findings that women were 22.5 times more likely than men to experience rape in the context of IPV, which seems to be the trauma type most associated with PTSD.[2,16] Compounding the experience and significance, assault within the context of IPV is significantly more likely to be part of an abusive pattern that may involve repeated assaults, than assault by a stranger.

Sexual Violence

The statistics for adult sexual assault are equally skewed toward women.[9] Studies suggest that up to 25% of women are victims of sexual assault at some time in their lives.[9,17–19] Although there are considerably fewer studies of male victims of sexual assault, data suggest rates of up to 7%.[13,17,20] These figures are occasionally questioned on the basis that men are more reluctant to report sexual assault. However, prevalence rates of sexual assault are significantly higher among women than men even when study methods address this problem by using anonymous questionnaires rather than individual interviews.[9] Similarly, childhood sexual abuse (CSA) is more common among girls than boys.[13,17,21] A recent meta-analysis of studies representing prevalence rates in 22 countries found that 7.9% of males and 19.7% of females had suffered some form of CSA, making females more than twice as likely to be victimized in this way. This finding is particularly troubling in light of the repeated finding that CSA is a predictor of sexual revictimization.[22] Being female and having a history of CSA are among the strongest identified predictors of adult sexual assault in a community sample, and although a history of CSA does not explain all reported psychological symptoms following adult sexual assault, it is associated with increased distress.[13]

TRAUMA TYPE AND PTSD

It is therefore plausible to speculate that higher rates of PTSD among women could be accounted for by the types of traumas that women are likely to experience, as some types of trauma have been found to lead to PTSD more commonly than others. Specifically, events that involve interpersonal violence precipitate PTSD more often than disasters or motor vehicle accidents. For example, in one study, 55% of rape victims developed PTSD compared with only 7.5% of those involved in a serious accident.[2] A more recent study found that 37.8% of those who had been sexually assaulted and 24.4% of those who had been physically assaulted developed PTSD compared with 4.4% of those who had been in an accident, 2.2% who had experienced a natural disaster, or even 13.3% of those who had been in combat.[16] Therefore, the question has been raised whether the differing prevalence rates reflect female exposure to traumas that more commonly precipitate PTSD.

This question was systematically reviewed in a study that undertook meta-analysis to evaluate whether sex differences in PTSD remain when controlling for trauma type.[9] No sex differences in rates of PTSD were found among individuals who had been sexually assaulted, had experienced childhood sexual or physical abuse or neglect, and women reported more PTSD than men across all other types of traumatic event. Therefore, at first consideration this would seem to disprove the theory that trauma type explains the discrepancy in rates of PTSD. However, before this theory is completely disregarded it is worth noting that the meta-analysis in question was limited by the very small numbers of available studies comparing PTSD rates in male and female victims of sexual assault and CSA (the very types of traumatic experience most likely to lead to PTSD), potentially obscuring differences that may exist. Specifically, the meta-analysis included only 4 studies that compared prevalence rates of PTSD in male and female victims of adult sexual assault, and only 7 did the same for victims of CSA. In addition, no studies used in this meta-analysis compared severity of PTSD for men versus women following adult sexual assault, and only 3 made the comparison following CSA. It is difficult not to speculate that perhaps in the absence of supporting literature on which to base the analysis, these figures represent a very small sampling that does not give sufficient power to identify statistically meaningful differences. For example, 2 studies identified in the preparation of the current article found higher rates of PTSD in men than women following rape: 65% of men versus 46% of women in 1 study, and 67% of men versus 56% of women in another.[2,16] With so few studies included, the question of statistical significance may be relevant; that is, this lack of findings may be a consequence of the limitations of statistical analysis in the evaluation of this question. It seems likely that further investigation of this question is necessary to truly identify and compare rates of PTSD among male and female victims.

With regard to nonsexual assault, the analysis used a general category of assault without examining IPV separately and, as discussed earlier, there are reasons to speculate that IPV may have a different effect than assault by a stranger. In addition, the gender specific significance of specific interpersonal traumas such as assault is not addressed in this type of analysis. It takes little imagination to recognize that being assaulted could have different meaning for a female than a male. For example, the physical consequences of assault on a female are more likely to reflect the differential size and strength of her attacker. Assault on a female by a male is also likely to involve the fear of rape. For men this is not the case.

COGNITIVE MEDIATION AND PTSD

The broad picture of higher rates of PTSD in those who experience interpersonal trauma may indicate a key factor that cannot be examined using even advanced methods of statistical analysis, which cannot take the role of cognitive mediation into account. Given that development of PTSD requires an interpretation of an event as threatening and horrifying and of an inability to control it,[1] there is clearly a role for interpretation. Perhaps, therefore, one missing ingredient in the type of analysis discussed earlier is a way to account for the role of such cognitive mediation and the individual meaning that may be attributed to different types of traumatic events. Specifically, if an event intrinsically threatens an individual's core identity, it may be more likely to produce PTSD. This theory might well provide some explanation for the high rate of PTSD in men and women who have experienced sexual assault, an intrusive act that is beyond comparison and threatens physical safety and identity. This theory would also potentially explain the higher rates of PTSD among women who are physically assaulted, because assault can have implications that are in conflict with the female identity, in a way that perhaps is not the case for men. The term "victim" is used more often in reference to women who have been physically assaulted than men. Sexual assault or rape can also be equally contrary to the male identity, accounting for the high rates of PTSD, as it not only jeopardizes physical integrity but can also be emasculating.

EMOTIONAL REACTIVITY AND PTSD

Another seemingly likely alternative explanation is that socialized gender characteristics influence response to traumatic events such that they contribute not only to risk and resilience but also to specific symptom presentation. At the most basic level, there is a body of research that suggests that men and women tend to differ in terms of emotional reactivity.[23,24] Although this difference is sometimes not substantiated by research, it has been suggested that the absence of findings can be explained by differences in emotion regulation rather than reactivity.[25] The relevance of emotions in the development of PTSD is potentially important because of the role they are believed to play in the development of PTSD. It is theorized that when the emotions experienced in a traumatic situation are overwhelmingly intense, they impede the ability of individuals to fully process the experience at the time and this contributes to a disorganized consolidation of memories that leads to PTSD.[26–28] In fact, among identified risk factors, peritraumatic emotion has been identified as one of the strongest predictors of PTSD.[29] Some support for the theory of emotional differences potentially accounting for discrepant prevalence rates is emerging in recent research. Female police officers, who presumably are socialized by their professional training or earlier life experiences to respond with a more traditionally masculine minimization of emotional reactivity, report less severe PTSD symptoms than civilian women despite exposure to more potentially traumatic experiences. Further, this difference is mediated by intense peritraumatic emotional distress, illustrating that civilian women experienced significantly more emotional distress than female police officers in the face of traumatic events and that this peritraumatic emotion contributed to the development of PTSD.[30] Among female police officers, peritraumatic emotional distress was related to greater levels of somatization, indicating that there is a price connected to the apparent resilience to PTSD. This supports another recent finding that negative affect following trauma predicts somatization in the absence of a diagnosis of PTSD.[31]

GENDER-BIASED PRESENTATIONS

Consideration of these findings raises important questions on the various possible psychological outcomes following trauma. Specifically, it highlights the perspective that the emotional responses to trauma that may be responsible for resilience versus risk to specific posttraumatic sequelae are associated with gender. Other evidence for gender-related differences in emotional responses exist in the literature. For example, it has been shown that immediately following sexual assault, men present with more denial and emotional control.[32] Behavioral responses may also differ somewhat by gender; among adolescents, boys are more likely than girls to report behavioral problems, suicidality, violence, and substance abuse following sexual trauma.[33] In terms of specific symptoms, young girls who are exposed to trauma are more likely to report internalizing symptoms such as depression, anxiety, and hyperarousal,[34,35] whereas boys more often report externalizing symptoms such as aggression and conduct problems.[36,37]

GENDER BIAS IN PERSONALITY DISORDERS

The role of childhood trauma in the development of personality disorders is another area of literature that offers some support for differential responsiveness in males versus females. Although it is a vast oversimplification of etiological factors to view personality disorders as simply trauma spectrum disorders, there is a growing body of literature examining the high prevalence rate of childhood abuse among those who are subsequently diagnosed with certain personality disorders.[38–43] The link with childhood trauma is most commonly made with borderline personality disorder (BPD) and antisocial personality disorder (ASPD).

A personality disorder is diagnosed when an individual presents with an inflexible pervasive pattern of interacting with others and the world that has been present throughout adulthood.[1] In ASPD, this pattern includes deceitfulness, failure to conform to social norms, impulsivity, irritability and aggressiveness, reckless disregard for safety of self or others, pattern of irresponsibility in terms of work or finances, and lack of remorse.[1] BPD is characterized by marked instability in relationships, self-image, and affect as indicated by excessive fear of abandonment, intense and unstable relationships, poor sense of self, recurrent suicidal or self-mutilating behavior, emotional reactivity, chronic feelings of emptiness and, in stressful situations, paranoia or dissociation.[1] In addition, BPD shares some symptoms with

ASPD: impulsivity, irritability and intense expressions of anger. Multiple studies have highlighted that in addition to shared symptoms, there is a high degree of overlap between the 2 disorders with between 10% and 47% of BPD patients also meeting criteria for ASPD[44,45] and up to 70% of ASPD patients meeting criteria for BPD.[46] In the context of a discussion regarding differential expression of symptoms in men versus women, these 2 disorders are particularly relevant; ASPD and BPD have very strong gender specific prevalence. Approximately 80% to 85% of individuals who meet criteria for ASPD are male[47,48] and 70% to 77% of those diagnosed with BPD are female.[1,49]

THE ROLE OF TRAUMA IN ASPD AND BPD

Etiological factors for these 2 disorders are unquestionably complex and involve an interaction with biological and genetic vulnerabilities.[50] However, the literature has consistently found comparatively high rates of childhood abuse among those who are diagnosed with either ASPD or BPD. There is, in particular, a large literature that reports high levels of childhood trauma (particularly relationship trauma) among individuals with BPD. Studies have found rates of CSA in this population ranging from 29% to 71%, with higher estimates for the studies that included participants who are predominantly inpatients and women.[38,51–55] Studies also show that more than 50% of individuals with a diagnosis of BPD report childhood physical abuse.[38,55] Several studies indicate that childhood trauma is significantly more prevalent among individuals with BPD than healthy comparison groups or groups of individuals with other psychiatric diagnoses, including other personality disorders.[51,53,55–59] Although the focus has been on the association of childhood trauma and BPD, several studies have also reported associations with ASPD.[42,60–62] Childhood trauma has been identified as occurring significantly more often in the history of individuals with ASPD than normal controls, or men in the criminal justice system who do not have ASPD.[42,43,61] One prospective study of individuals who were abused or neglected as children found that 17.9% subsequently met criteria for ASPD at some time in their life.[44]

These factors of shared symptoms, comorbidity, and skewed gender prevalence, combined with findings of comparatively high rates of childhood trauma in individuals with either disorder, led to discussion that perhaps these personality disorders are gender specific presentations of the same disorder.[46,54,61] Certainly the symptoms of ASPD can be viewed as externalizing symptoms (aggression, recklessness, failure to conform), whereas many of the symptoms of BPD can be viewed as internalizing (feelings of emptiness, chronic suicidality, fear of abandonment, poor sense of self). Identifying these as either extreme developments of either masculine or feminine responses to childhood trauma is certainly overly simplistic and fails to take into account other etiological considerations. However, the evidence supporting an important role of childhood abuse cannot be ignored, nor can the pronounced gender proportions or the literature that reflects the tendency for males to develop externalizing symptoms in the face of trauma,[36,37] whereas women develop internalizing symptoms.[34,35]

SUMMARY

Although the literature consistently shows that women are significantly more likely than men to develop PTSD, the possible explanations for this are seemingly more complex. Certainly PTSD is most likely to develop following sexual trauma, an event that is much more likely to occur for females than males, and this can unquestionably contribute to some of the skewed gender prevalence in the community. However, it does not seem that the sex difference in PTSD prevalence can be completely attributed to differing exposure to specific types of trauma. Further research on gender prevalence of PTSD following sexual trauma and subcategories of physical assault (such as IPV) is required before the effect of specific trauma types can unequivocally be determined. Regardless, alternative explanations for the difference must also be considered. Rather than considering risk and resilience following trauma as merely a question of development of pathology or not, a more accurate consideration would take a broader perspective: development of specific symptom profiles that are gender biased. Within this paradigm, the role of emotional responsiveness (as a gender-based characteristic that is arguably socially influenced) and cognitive mediation of the traumatic event might influence the specific symptoms that an individual develops. Some support for this perspective can be found in the literature of personality disorders such as ASPD and BPD.

REFERENCES

1. Diagnostic and statistical manual of mental disorders. 4th edition. Text revision: DSM-IV-TR. Washington, DC: American Psychiatric Association; 2000.
2. Kessler RC, Sonnega A, Bromet E, et al. Posttraumatic stress disorder in the national comorbidity survey. Arch Gen Psychiatry 1995;52:1048–60.
3. Breslau N, Kessler RC, Chilcoat Schultz LR, et al. Trauma and posttraumatic stress disorder in the community: the 1996 Detroit Area Survey of Trauma. Arch Gen Psychiatry 1998;55:626–32.
4. Breslau N. The epidemiology of trauma, PTSD, and other posttrauma disorders. Trauma Violence Abuse 2009;10(3):198–210.
5. Shore JH, Vollmer WM, Tatum EI. Community patterns of posttraumatic stress disorders. J Nerv Ment Dis 1989;177:681–5.
6. Resnick HS, Kilpatrick DG, Dansky BS, et al. Prevalence of civilian trauma and posttraumatic stress disorder in a representative national sample of women. J Consult Clin Psychol 1993;61:984–91.
7. Davidson JR, Hughes D, Blazer DG, et al. Post-traumatic stress disorder in the community: an epidemiological study. Psychol Med 1991;21:713–21.
8. Helzer JE, Robins LN, McEvoy L. Post-traumatic stress disorder in the general population: findings of the epidemiologic catchment area survey. N Engl J Med 1987;317:1630–4.
9. Tolin DF, Foa EB. Sex differences in trauma and posttraumatic stress disorder: a quantitative review of 25 years of research. Psychol Trauma 2008;S(1):37–85.
10. Norris FH, Perilla JL, Ibanez GE, et al. Sex differences in symptoms of posttraumatic stress disorder: does culture play a role? J Trauma Stress 2001;14:7–28.
11. Stein MB, Walker JR, Hazen A, et al. Full and partial posttraumatic stress disorder: findings from a community survey. Am J Psychiatry 1997;154:1114–9.
12. Zlotnick C, Zimmerman M, Wolfsdorf BA, et al. Gender differences in patients with posttraumatic stress disorder in a general psychiatric practice. Am J Psychiatry 2001;158:1923–5.
13. Elliott DM, Mok DS, Briere J. Adult sexual assault: prevalence, symptomatology, and sex differences in the general population. J Trauma Stress 2004;17(3):203–11.
14. Norris FH. Epidemiology of trauma: frequency and impact of different potentially traumatic events on different demographic groups. J Consult Clin Psychol 1992;60:409–18.

15. Tjaden P, Thoennes N. Extent, nature, and consequences of intimate partner violence (NMCJ 181867). Washington, DC: US Department of Justice, National Institute on Justice and Centers for Disease Control and Prevention; 2000.

16. Olantunji BO, Babson KA, Smith RC, et al. Gender as a moderator of the relationship between PTSD and disgust: a laboratory test employing individualized script-driven imagery. J Anxiety Disord 2009;23:1091–7.

17. Tjaden P, Thoennes N. Prevalence, incidence, and consequences of violence against women: findings from the National Violence Against Women Survey; 1998.

18. Koss MP, Dinero TE. Discriminant analysis of risk factors for sexual victimization among a national sample of college women. J Consult Clin Psychol 1989;57: 242–50.

19. Sorenson SB, Stein JA, Siegel JM, et al. The prevalence of adult sexual assault: the Los Angeles Epidemiological Catchment Area Project. Am J Epidemiol 1987; 126:1154–65.

20. Martin L, Rosen LN, Durand DB, et al. Prevalence and timing of sexual assaults in a sample of male and female U.S. army soldiers. Mil Med 1998;163:213–6.

21. Pereda N, Guilera G, Forns M, et al. The prevalence of child sexual abuse in community and student samples: a meta-analysis. Clin Psychol Rev 2009;29: 328–38.

22. Roodman AA, Clum GA. Revictimization rates and method variance: a meta-analysis. Clin Psychol Rev 2001;21(2):183–204.

23. Brody LR. Gender and emotion: beyond stereotypes. J Soc Issues 1997;53: 102–50.

24. Bradley MM, Codispoti M, Sabatinelli D, et al. Emotion and motivation II: sex differences in picture processing. Emotion 2001;1:300–19.

25. McRae K, Ochsner KN, Mauss IB, et al. Gender differences in emotion regulation: an fMRI study of cognitive reappraisal. Group Process Intergroup Relat 2008; 11(2):143–62.

26. Brewin CR, Dalgleish T, Joseph S. A dual representation theory of posttraumatic stress disorder. Psychol Rev 1996;103(4):670–86.

27. Ehlers A, Clark DM. A cognitive model of posttraumatic stress disorder. Behav Res Ther 2000;38(4):319–45.

28. Siegel DJ. Memory, trauma, and psychotherapy: a cognitive science view. J Psychother Pract Res 1995;4(2):93–122.

29. Ozer EJ, Best SR, Lipsey TL, et al. Predictors of posttraumatic stress disorder and symptoms in adults. Psychol Bull 2003;129(1):52–73.

30. Lilly MM, Pole N, Best SR, et al. Gender and PTSD: what can we learn from female police officers? J Anxiety Disord 2009;23:767–74.

31. Elklit A, Christiansen DM. Predictive factors for somatization in a trauma sample. Clin Pract Epidemiol Ment Health 2009;5:1.

32. Kaufman A, Divasto P, Jackson R, et al. Male rape victims: noninstitutionalized assault. Am J Psychiatry 1980;137(2):221–3.

33. Darves-Bornoz JM, Choquet M, Ledoux S, et al. Gender differences in symptoms of adolescents reporting sexual assault. Soc Psychiatry Psychiatr Epidemiol 1998;33(3):111–8.

34. Buckner JC, Beardslee WR, Bassuk EL. Exposure to violence and low-income children's mental health: direct, moderated, and mediated relations. Am J Orthop 2004;74(4):413–23.

35. Foster JD, Kuperminc GP, Price AW. Gender differences in posttraumatic stress and related symptoms among inner-city minority youth exposed to community violence. J Youth Adolesc 2004;33(1):59–69.

36. Evans SE, Davies C, DiLillo D. Exposure to domestic violence: a met-analysis of child and adolescent outcomes. Aggress Violent Behav 2008;13(2):131–40.
37. Gustafsson PE, Larsson I, Nelson N, et al. Sociocultural disadvantage, traumatic life events, and psychiatric symptoms in preadolescent children. Am J Orthop 2009;79(3):387–97.
38. Golier J, Yehuda R, Bierer L, et al. The relationship of borderline personality disorder to posttraumatic stress disorder and traumatic events. Am J Psychiatry 2003;160(11):2018–24.
39. Sabo AN. Etiological significance of associations between childhood trauma and borderline personality disorder: conceptual and clinical implications. J Personal Disord 1997;11:50–70.
40. Zanarini MC. Childhood experiences associated with the development of borderline personality disorder. Psychiatr Clin North Am 2000;23:89–101.
41. Paris J, Zweig-Frank H, Guzder J. Psychological risk factors for borderline personality disorder in female patients. Compr Psychiatry 1994;35:301–5.
42. Horwitz AV, Widom CS, McLaughlin J, et al. The impact of childhood abuse and neglect on adult mental health: a prospective study. J Health Soc Behav 2001; 42(2):184–201.
43. Marshall LA, Cooke DJ. The childhood experiences of psychopaths: a retrospective study of familial and societal factors. J Personal Disord 1999;13(3):211–25.
44. Zanari MC, Gunderson JG. Differential diagnoses of antisocial behavior and borderline personality disorder. In: Stoff DM, Breiling J, Maser JD, editors. Handbook of antisocial behavior. New York: Wiley; 1997. p. 83–91.
45. Widiger TA, Trull TJ, Hurt SW, et al. A multidimensional scaling of the DSM-III personality disorders. Arch Gen Psychiatry 1987;44(6):557–63.
46. Widiger TA, Corbitt EM. Comorbidity of antisocial personality disorder with other personality disorders. In: Stoff DM, Breiling J, Maser JD, editors. Handbook of antisocial behavior. New York: Wiley; 1997. p. 75–82.
47. Regier DA, Myers JK, Kramer M, et al. The NIMH epidemiological catchment area program. Arch Gen Psychiatry 1984;41:934–41.
48. Kessler RC, McGonagle KA, Zhao S. Lifetime and twelve month prevalence of DSM-III-R psychiatric disorders in the United States. Results from the National Comorbidity Survey. Arch Gen Psychiatry 1994;51:8–10.
49. Swartz M, Blazer D, George L, et al. Estimating the prevalence of borderline personality disorder in the community. J Personal Disord 1990;4:257–72.
50. Koerner K, Linehan MM. Integrative therapy for borderline personality disorder: dialectical behavior therapy. In: Norcross JC, Goldfried MR, editors. Handbook of psychotherapy integration. New York: Basic Books; 1992. p. 433–59.
51. Herman JL, Perry JC, van der Kolk BA. Childhood trauma in borderline personality disorder. Am J Psychiatry 1989;146:490–5.
52. Zanarini MD, Gunderson JG, Marino MF, et al. Childhood experiences of borderline patients. Compr Psychiatry 1989;30:18–25.
53. Ogata SN, Silk KR, Goodrich S, et al. Childhood sexual and physical abuse in adult patients with borderline personality disorder. Am J Psychiatry 1990;147:1008–13.
54. Hudziak JJ, Boffeli TJ, Kriesman JJ, et al. Clinical study of the relation of borderline personality disorder to Briquet's syndrome (hysteria), somatization disorder, antisocial personality disorder, and substance abuse disorders. Am J Psychiatry 1996;153(12):1598–606.
55. Bandelow B, Krause J, Wedekind D, et al. Early traumatic life events, parental attitudes, family history, and birth risk factors in patients with borderline personality disorder and healthy controls. Psychiatry Res 2005;134:169–79.

56. Zanarini MC, Ruser TF, Frankenburg FR, et al. Risk factors associated with dissociative experiences of borderline patients. J Nerv Ment Dis 2000;188:26–30.
57. Zweig-Frank H, Paris J, Guzder J. Psychological risk factors for dissociation and self-mutilation in female patients with borderline personality disorder. Can J Psychiatry 1994;39:259–64.
58. Ludolph PS, Westen D, Misle B, et al. The borderline diagnosis in adolescents: symptoms and developmental history. Am J Psychiatry 1990;147:470–6.
59. Yen S, Shea MT, Battle CL, et al. Traumatic exposure and posttraumatic stress disorder in borderline, schizotypal, avoidant, and obsessive-compulsive personality disorders: findings from the collaborative longitudinal personality disorders study. J Nerv Ment Dis 2002;190:510–8.
60. Burgess AW, Hartman CR, McCormack A. Abused to abuser: antecedents of socially deviant behaviors. Am J Psychiatry 1987;144(11):1431–6.
61. Lobbestael J, Arntz A, Sieswerda S. Schema modes and childhood abuse in borderline and antisocial personality disorders. J Behav Ther Exp Psychiatry 2005;36:240–53.
62. Wallen J. A comparison of male and female clients in substance abuse treatment. J Subst Abuse Treat 1992;9(3):243–8.

Caring for the Elderly Female Psychiatric Patient

Mudhasir Bashir, MD*, Suzanne Holroyd, MD

KEYWORDS
- Geriatric psychiatry • Female psychiatric patients
- Dementia • Psychiatric disorders

With the growth of the elderly population, and the female elderly population in particular, health providers will be seeing increasing numbers of elderly women with psychiatric disorders. To properly care for this group of patients, better understanding is needed not only of group differences in this patient population but also to understand the differences in each individual, as they age, given their unique life experiences, cohort effects, medical comorbidity, social situation, and personality traits. Understandably, these characteristics will interact with psychiatric disorders in ways that may increase the challenge to correctly diagnose and treat these patients. In addition, understanding late life changes, the prevalence of various mental disorders, and the sometimes unique presentation of mental disorders in this age group are required to better diagnose and treat this population.

As per the Administration on Aging (2002), the numbers of our elderly population will reach 70 million by the year 2030 and will make up 20% of the population. Women will continue to greatly outnumber men despite the fact that the male death rate from heart disease and other causes continues to decline and thus narrow this ratio. The change in death rate between women and men is one example highlighting that differences between men and women are not necessarily genetic, but may be caused by environmental or cohort effects. The latest report from the 2000 US Bureau of Census showed that in the age group of more than 65years of age, men account for 5.1% of the population, whereas women account for 7.3%.

Thus this growing population of elderly women warrants more attention toward their physical and mental well being. Despite some socioeconomic advances by women in recent years, research shows women continue to be at a disadvantage,[1,2] although they still continue to be the primary caregivers as mothers, spouses, and daughters. And because of the increasing life expectancy of the oldest old, their role as caregivers to aging parents, although at high need to receive care themselves, further increases

Department of Psychiatry and Neurobehavioral Sciences, University of Virginia Health System, Box 800623, Charlottesville, VA 22908, USA
* Corresponding author.
E-mail address: mb5qd@virginia.edu

Psychiatr Clin N Am 33 (2010) 475–485
doi:10.1016/j.psc.2010.01.012
0193-953X/10/$ – see front matter © 2010 Elsevier Inc. All rights reserved.

the complexity of their lives. Unfortunately, serious illnesses, such as lung cancer and heart disease, have now reached similar rates for women as men.[3,4] As mental health problems may be intimately linked to physical and socioeconomic health,[5] the previously mentioned problems are indicative of issues facing this growing elderly female population.

Research has revealed that women of older age groups are in a lower socioeconomic status than men.[1] Unfortunately, studies have shown that there are higher rates of most psychiatric disorders among those with lower socioeconomic status.[5] These socioeconomic differences may be in part why women have more anxiety and mood disorders,[5,6] across the life span, whereas men have more substance use.[5,6]

We will now address an approach to the elderly female psychiatric patient and issues specific to psychiatric disorders in this population.

APPROACH TO GERIATRIC FEMALE PSYCHIATRIC PATIENTS

Patients will present for mental health issues to their primary care physician or directly to the psychiatric setting. Frequently, they are brought because of the concerns of others (spouse, children, friends or other physicians) and less frequently because of the legal system or adult protective services, rather than presenting on their own. As such, patients may not want to be evaluated or will deny there are any problems. Thus, in the evaluation of the elderly female patient, outside informants should always be sought. Certainly anyone accompanying patients should be interviewed. If patients come alone, calling relevant outside informants is often the only way to get an accurate history.

Because of the prevalence of cognitive disorders (dementia, mild cognitive impairment, delirium) in the elderly age group, a cognitive assessment should always be done. This assessment is done not only for accurate diagnosis of cognitive disorders but also to assess the potential accuracy of patients' history and the ability of patients to follow through on the treatment plan, be it medication or otherwise. Simple assessments, such as the Folstein Mini Mental State Exam,[7] are adequate for this purpose.

In addition to a routine psychiatric history and examination, special information should be sought for elderly patients. For example, any family history of cognitive impairment or dementia should be sought. A social history should also be sought. Information needed for obtaining a social history includes the current living situation, including any aides or family members who are nearby or help out; current driving status (if still driving, any accidents?); who does the patients' bills/finances; who gets groceries and does the cooking; whether patients are independent regarding bathing, dressing, feeding, and toileting, and gait status (use of a cane/walker/wheelchair). Any care-giving responsibilities of patients should be recorded, because one may be surprised to find patients with dementia still watching grandchildren because the daughter is working, or other such situations. If a spouse or other family is in the home, the relationships of such individuals should be evaluated because abuse may begin for the first time in late life. A simple question regarding how others treat them is often a good starting point in asking about potential abuse.

History of gait instability, or any falls and the circumstances of such falls, should be documented. A detailed medical history, including conditions common in the female elderly population, such as recurrent urinary tract infection (UTI), should be done. History of hormonal therapies and emotional response/side effects to them should be recorded. Any changes of appetite, sleep, and weight loss or gain should be obtained. All patients should have a primary care physician and those that do not should be referred to one because the geriatric psychiatrist will often form a partnership with the primary care doctor in the care of such patients.

DEMENTIA

Dementia is a group of diagnoses that includes memory deficits plus cognitive decline in at least one other cognitive domain to the degree that it effects functioning. Alzheimer's dementia (AD) is the most common type of dementia in the United States followed by vascular dementia and Lewy Body dementia. The prevalence of AD is approximately 5% in people 65 to74 years of age and increases to more than 40% of people older than age 85.[8] As life expectancy for women continues to increase, the number of women with this progressive and devastating illness will likewise increase. There are contradictory studies whether women have a higher incidence of dementia than men, with some showing a higher incidence of AD in women,[9,10] whereas others do not.[9–11]

The association of estrogen to the development or progression of AD has been the subject of speculation and study. The presence of estrogen receptors in multiple areas of the brain has been identified including areas responsible for memory, such as hypothalamus, hippocampus, preoptic area, and basal forebrain.[12] Neuritic growth and synaptogeneses have been shown in animals receiving exogenous estrogen,[13] which may be the direct effect of estrogen or the fact that estrogen serves as a stimulator for neurotrophic factors. Estrogen replacement therapy (ERT) has also been shown to increase cerebral blood flow in women with AD.[13] Some studies have also indicated the modulation of amyloid precursor protein metabolism[14] and inhibition of Apo E levels.[15] Women, especially older thinner women who produce less estrogen, may be more likely to develop AD.[9,10] Animal studies have shown a neuroprotective effect of estrogen and a positive relationship with cholinergic neural function and metabolism.[16,17]

The role of ERT in preventing dementia has been controversial and thus the subject of much study. Early observational studies of long-term estrogen therapy users, although indicating some positive outcome on cognitive function and decreased rates of developing AD and vascular dementia,[18] unfortunately also suggested a higher risk for breast and endometrial cancer and other adverse outcomes.[19–21] Because of these issues, further trials to assess the risk-benefit ratio of ERT have been undertaken. Early results from the Women's Health Initiative Memory study (WHI) revealed that combination therapy of estrogen and progestin increased the risk for dementia in postmenopausal women over 65 years of age.[22] Also ERT was not found to prevent Mild Cognitive Impairment in these women. This study revealed that the risks outweighed the benefits of ERT to the extent that the study was actually stopped early. The Women's International Study of Long Duration Estrogen after Menopause (WISDOM)[23] was a large multicenter study in the United Kingdom that was also terminated early after results from the WHI memory study showed negative outcomes. At present, prevention or treatment of AD with ERT is not supported by current studies, but other researchers are investigating the link of estrogen to dementia using other approaches that leave this area of inquiry still open.[24]

Cognitive enhancers, such as cholinesterase inhibitors or memantine, remain the mainstay of treatment in AD to delay the progression of the illness once diagnosed, and less commonly, to improve cognitive functioning. Psychotic and other behavioral symptoms of dementia are mainly managed with the use of psychotropic medications including antidepressants, mood stabilizers, and antipsychotics, as well as behavioral and environmental approaches. Elderly women with dementia often benefit from behavioral routines consistent with their earlier lives and thus may enjoy appropriate-level tasks, such as folding laundry, holding dolls, and simple cooking. Sudden changes in behavior or mental status is often indicative of delirium caused by medical issues, such as UTIs, and medical workup is appropriate in such cases. For women with recurrent UTIs, prevention through the use of better hygiene, cranberry pill supplement to acidify the urine, or suppressant antibiotic therapy may be crucial in keeping recurrent behaviors under control.

Psychotic Disorders in Older Women

By definition, psychosis is the inability to distinguish reality from fantasy, which may include hallucinations, delusions, or a formal thought disorder. The most common disorders that can cause psychosis in the elderly include delirium, dementia, mood disorders, and primary psychotic disorders. Some forms of psychosis have been observed to be more common in women than men. Delusional disorders have a higher incidence in the elderly female population with persecutory, somatic, and jealous delusions being the most common type.[25] Similarly, typical patients of delusional parasitosis are usually women.[26]

Late onset schizophrenia has been found to be more common in women and has usually been associated with an excellent prognosis, and less negative symptoms.[27,28] However, some studies have found the reverse, with older elderly women having a worse outcome in very late onset (after age 60) cases.[29–31] The possible effect of sex hormones and menopause on psychosis has been proposed. Research has revealed a significantly greater proportion of women (41% in women vs 20% in men) develop late onset schizophrenia, characterized by more positive symptoms and less negative symptoms.[30] A second peak of late onset schizophrenia at menopausal age has been reported, the symptoms of such being more severe in women. Although over-all women have a better prognosis compared with men for this disorder, this may be reversed in the very late onset schizophrenia subgroup.[31] The International Late Onset Schizophrenia Consensus Statement of 2000 achieved a historic consensus on the diagnosis, treatment, and need for further research.[32] They concluded that very late onset schizophrenia (>60 years) has face validity and clinical utility.[32] The report also included a female preponderance in this subgroup with a higher rate of positive symptoms and rare negative symptoms or formal thought disorder.[32] There also seemed to be better premorbid educational, occupational, and psychosocial functioning. The late onset subgroup was also associated with milder cognitive deficits.[32]

Other populations also show an increased association of psychosis in women as compared with men. Data from the National Institute of Mental Health Epidemiological Catchment Area study showed an increase in the rate of visual hallucinations in women more than 80 years of age (40/1000 per year), as compared with women 18- to 80-years old (13/1000 per year). For auditory hallucinations, there was a later peak incidence in women 40- to 50-years old as compared with a male peak at 25- to 30-years old.[33] A study of psychosis in AD revealed that women are more likely than men to have visual hallucinations.[34] There appears to be no difference in prevalence of psychosis in delirium between women and men.[35] Psychosis does not appear to be more common for women with depression.[36,37] In psychotic manic states, women have been found to have a specific pattern of psychosis with more delusions and hallucinations, specifically with more delusions of reference and paranoia.[38]

Although various theories, including differences in reporting, gender specific cultural differences, and hormonal/biological gender differences, have been put forward, it is unclear why elderly women have a higher rate of psychosis than their male counter-parts across different disorders.

When evaluating an elderly woman with new onset psychosis, an organic and medical workup should be undertaken to rule out delirium or other medical process causing such symptoms. Cognitive assessment to help assess for the presence of delirium or dementia must be done. Antipsychotics will typically be used for psychotic symptoms but should be started in low doses in elderly women, observing carefully for effect on gait; alertness/sedation; neurologic side effect, including tremor, dyskinesia or other abnormality, and orthostasis; or effect on cardiac conduction in some cases. The continued need for antipsychotic treatment should be reevaluated on a regular basis, with a trial of reducing the dose attempted where possible.

MOOD DISORDERS

Major depressive disorder (MDD) is estimated to be present in about 5.7% of the residents in the United States, with a much larger percentage (approximately 15%) having subsyndromal depression.[39] Women have a higher rate of depression across the life span,[40,41] although the difference between men and women narrows in late life.[42] The risk for subsyndromal depression increases with age.[39] Bipolar disorder has the same prevalence for men and women across the lifespan.

The presentation of depression may be different between genders. Women may have more anxiety and changes in appetite, sleep, and energy.[43] Mood congruent delusions may also differ, with delusions of paranoia, poverty, or spousal infidelity more common in psychotic depressed women.

It is extremely important that clinicians understand that the diagnosis of depression in the elderly may be a challenge as depressive symptoms may be masked, with depressed mood often denied. Elderly women are more likely to complain of anxiety rather than sadness. New physical complaints or exacerbation of old preexisting ones, such as chronic pain, may be the only presenting complaint. Symptoms, such as weight loss, withdrawal from activity, irritability, and sleep disturbance may be present. Because the elderly are often stoic or view depression as a weakness, using other terms, such as down in the dumps may be more acceptable.

Although age is a risk factor for completed suicide and depression is the most important psychiatric condition associated with completed and attempted suicide in old age,[44] the increase in the elderly suicide rate is mainly caused by the marked increase in rates among elderly men. For women, the age of highest suicide rate is 75 to 79 years (7.9/100,000) dropping to 4.7/100,000 in the 85 and older age group.[45] Among women, white women aged 65 years and older have the higher rate of 6.4/100,000 compared with African Americans at 2.6/100,000. Elderly women are more likely to use lethal means as compared with younger females, with guns[46] and overdose being the most common methods.

To better evaluate mood and suicidal risk, various depression screens have been developed, but most do not take into account the unique presentation of depression in the elderly. The Geriatric Depression Scale (GDS) has proved to be the most valuable tool for this age group.[47] The focus of the GDS is on psychological rather than physical symptoms. Although the GDS may not be helpful in moderately severe to severe dementia, it has been shown to be useful in mild to moderate dementia.[47]

Depression is a major source of morbidity and mortality over and above suicide attempts. Multiple large studies in community-dwelling elderly reveal depression is a powerful and independent risk factor for death in the elderly, and is associated with poorer prognosis of various medical illnesses.[44,48–50]

Treatment of depression in the elderly begins with recognition of the depression, and not just attributing symptoms to age or life stresses. Most classes of antidepressant medications are as effective in the elderly as the young, although there may be a longer time to response and remission. The choice of antidepressants should be based on tolerability and cost. Although selective serotonin reuptake inhibitors (SSRIs), serotonin norepinephrine reuptake inhibitors (SNRIs), and other atypical anti-depressants, such as mirtazapine and bupropion, have not been shown to be superior in efficacy to tricyclics, they generally have a better tolerability profile in the elderly. For selected patients, psychotherapies, including interpersonal, psychodynamic, and cognitive behavioral therapies (CBT) may be useful, although there have been limited studies in the elderly. Electroconvulsive therapy has been shown to have excellent results in geriatric depression, especially psychotic depression where this remains the treatment of choice.[44] First episode depression after 60 years of age has a 70% chance of recurrence within 2 years of remission.[44] Thus, there are differences in opinion regarding the length of maintenance therapy in the elderly. Some recommend that maintenance treatment should be continued for at least 2 years after recovery from a depressive episode, whereas treatment should be continued indefinitely for those with two or more episodes.[44] Clinical judgment comes into play as those with more severe episodes may need lifelong treatment even after the first episode. Left untreated, depression follows a chronic course with high morbidity and mortality in the elderly.

Anxiety Disorders

Although anxiety disorders have a peak age of onset in early adulthood, the elderly still have high rates of anxiety disorders with generalized anxiety disorder and phobias being the most common.[51,52] The most common anxiety disorder in the over 65 age group is simple phobia. Prevalence rates for specific phobias range from 5.9% to 13.1% in the elderly.[53] The rate of comorbid anxiety in the depressed elderly is also high at about 43%,[40] so clinicians should always search for depression in patients pre-senting with anxiety symptoms. Although depression also frequently coexists with phobic disorders, the majority occur in the absence of depression.[54] The National Epidemiologic Survey on Alcohol and Related Conditions (NESARC) study revealed a significant increase in specific phobia among older people with MDD. Despite the high prevalence of anxiety disorders in the elderly, little information is known of how anxiety disorders affect functioning and general well being in the elderly. Social phobia was found to be most strongly associated with specific phobias and it appears that even well-functioning individuals may be at risk for a compromised health-related quality of life. Also using data from NESARC, others have concluded there are signif-icant gender differences in the prevalence, comorbidity pattern, and other clinical correlates of various anxiety disorders.[55] The Health Aging and Body Composition study of persons aged 70 to 79 years reports women were more likely to have anxiety symptoms as compared with men. When anxiety is comorbid with depression in the elderly, time to remission and recovery is longer and risk for relapse stronger.[56]

Anxiety disorders are primarily treated with SSRIs. Unfortunately, many elderly patients will receive initial treatment at their primary care doctors with benzodiaze-pines, which may lead to other problems. Anxiety in the elderly responds as well to SSRIs and SNRIs as the younger population.[57] They are also good candidates for adjuvant psychotherapies, such as CBT or behavioral therapy, which have proved to be very beneficial in anxiety disorders.

ALCOHOL AND OTHER SOURCES OF SUBSTANCE ABUSE IN THE ELDERLY

Use and abuse of alcohol and other drugs in the elderly has been the subject of little research. There are little data available to qualify or quantify this use, especially specific to gender. Because of the physiological changes in the elderly, small amounts of alcohol and other substances can lead to intoxication and functional impairment. The problem of alcohol abuse in the elderly is felt to be largely underestimated and undertreated. Levin and Kruger have described substance abuse as "the silent epidemic," but interest in treatment has been focused mostly toward the young.[58] There is no valid instrument available for screening alcohol abuse and dependence in the elderly. As the present generation of baby boomers ages, predictions are that substance abuse is likely to be a much larger health care problem. An estimated 4.4 million older adults will be in need of substance abuse treatment in 2020 compared with 1.7 million in 2003.[59] Among a group of elderly presenting to the emergency room, the prevalence of alcohol use disorders (abuse and dependence) was 5.3%, with falls and delirium being the main reason for presentation of the elderly to the emergency department.[60]

Although alcohol abuse is a common type of abuse in the elderly, abuse of prescription drugs, primarily benzodiazepines and analgesics, is also common. Abuse of prescription drugs has been reported as high as 11% in elderly women[61] with benzodiazepines making up 17% to 23% of drugs prescribed to the elderly. Social isolation, depression, and history of substance abuse increase the risk.[40] The abuse of prescription drugs by the elderly may at times be unintentional secondary to poor education about these medications, fear of withdrawal symptoms, and trust in prescribing physicians. It has been noted that the elderly are two to three times more likely to be prescribed psychoactive medications, particularly benzodiazepines, for anxiety and insomnia than younger individuals.[62] Unfortunately, such prescribing practices may have serious sequelae, including cognitive impairment, sedation, and falls. Falls are a serious problem in the elderly, with one third of elderly individuals sustaining a fall-related injury each year,[63] with the incidence of falls one and a half times higher in elderly women than men. Falls, of course, are a risk with all substance abuse disorders including alcohol, hypnotics, muscle relaxants, and pain medications.

However, there is also concern that physicians are hesitant to prescribe these medications adequately to treat chronic pain and other symptoms although there are little data to support this in the elderly. Studies have reported there is little evidence to suggest prescription abuse in patients who have no prior history of substance abuse.[64,65] Physical dependence secondary to tolerance may at times be mistaken for abuse.

Clinically, the mix of normal physiologic aging, medical illnesses, and multiple prescription use, when complicated by abuse of alcohol and other substances, can lead to serious problems. If substance use is suspected, information should be obtained from multiple sources, as the elderly frequently minimize their use. Treatment of alcohol abuse should have a multidisciplinary approach and there are multiple treatment strategies. If the traditional 12-step and abstinence model is not acceptable to patients, other approaches, including the Harm reduction model, may be considered (PRISM-E study).[66] Family support is often necessary to have elderly patients gain insight or cooperation for treatment. For benzodiazepine and other prescription abuse and dependence, a slow taper with identification and treatment of comorbid anxiety or mood disorders, reassurance, and support is advisable.

SUMMARY

The population of elderly women will continue to grow, with highly prevalent comorbid psychiatric disorders. Although more research has been done in the last decade studying psychiatric issues in the elderly, less is known about gender specific issues of diagnosis, presentation, treatment, and outcomes. Continued research is urged not only for geriatric psychiatric disorders but for better understanding of differences between women and men.

REFERENCES

1. Moss NE. Gender equity and socioeconomic inequality: a framework for the patterning of women's health. Soc Sci Med 2002;54(5):649–61.
2. Moss N. Socioeconomic disparities in health in the US: an agenda for action. Soc Sci Med 2000;51(11):1627–38.
3. Kiri VA, Soriano J, Visick G, et al. Recent trends in lung cancer and its association with COPD: an analysis using the UK GP research database. Prim Care Respir J 2009. [Epub ahead of print]. PMID: 19756330. DOI:10.4104/pcrj.2009.00048.
4. Lloyd-Jones D, Adams R, Carnethon M, et al. Heart disease and stroke statistics–2009 update: a report from the American heart association statistics committee and stroke statistics subcommittee. Circulation 2009;119(3):480–6.
5. Cross-national comparisons of the prevalences and correlates of mental disorders. WHO international consortium in psychiatric epidemiology. Bull World Health Organ 2000;78(4):413–26.
6. Seedat S, Scott KM, Angermeyer MC, et al. Cross-national associations between gender and mental disorders in the world health organization world mental health surveys. Arch Gen Psychiatry 2009;66(7):785–95.
7. Folstein MF, Folstein SE, McHugh PR. "Mini-mental state". A practical method for grading the cognitive state of patients for the clinician. J Psychiatr Res 1975; 12(3):189–98.
8. Hebert LE, Scherr PA, Bienias JL, et al. Alzheimer disease in the US population: prevalence estimates using the 2000 census. Arch Neurol 2003;60(8):1119–22.
9. Paganini-Hill A, Henderson VW. Estrogen deficiency and risk of Alzheimer's disease in women. Am J Epidemiol 1994;140(3):256–61.
10. Gao S, Hendrie HC, Hall KS, et al. The relationships between age, sex, and the incidence of dementia and Alzheimer disease: a meta-analysis. Arch Gen Psychiatry 1998;55(9):809–15.
11. Ruitenberg A, Ott A, van Swieten JC, et al. Incidence of dementia: does gender make a difference? Neurobiol Aging 2001;22(4):575–80.
12. Stumpf WE, Sar M. Steroid hormone target sites in the brain: the differential distribution of estrogen, progestin, androgen and glucocorticosteroid. J Steroid Biochem 1976;7(11–12):1163–70.
13. Beckmann CR. Alzheimer's disease: an estrogen link? Curr Opin Obstet Gynecol 1997;9(5):295–9.
14. Mani ST, Thakur MK. In the cerebral cortex of female and male mice, amyloid precursor protein (APP) promoter methylation is higher in females and differentially regulated by sex steroids. Brain Res 2006;1067(1):43–7.
15. Struble RG, Cady C, Nathan BP, et al. Apolipoprotein E may be a critical factor in hormone therapy neuroprotection. Front Biosci 2008;13:5387–405.
16. Luine VN, Khylchevskaya RI, McEwen BS. Effect of gonadal steroids on activities of monoamine oxidase and choline acetylase in rat brain. Brain Res 1975;86(2): 293–306.
17. Toran-Allerand CD, Miranda RC, Bentham WD, et al. Estrogen receptors colocalize with low-affinity nerve growth factor receptors in cholinergic neurons of the basal forebrain. Proc Natl Acad Sci U S A 1992;89(10):4668–72.

18. Tang MX, Jacobs D, Stern Y, et al. Effect of estrogen during menopause on risk and age at onset of alzheimer's disease. Lancet 1996;348(9025):429–32.
19. Kawas C, Resnick S, Morrison A, et al. A prospective study of estrogen replacement therapy and the risk of developing Alzheimer's disease: the Baltimore longitudinal study of aging. Neurology 1997;48(6):1517–21.
20. Garton M. Breast cancer and hormone-replacement therapy: the million women study. Lancet 2003;362(9392):1328 [author reply: 1330–1].
21. Grodstein F, Stampfer MJ, Goldhaber SZ, et al. Prospective study of exogenous hormones and risk of pulmonary embolism in women. Lancet 1996;348(9033): 983–7.
22. Craig MC, Maki PM, Murphy DG. The women's health initiative memory study: findings and implications for treatment. Lancet Neurol 2005;4(3):190–4.
23. Vickers MR, Martin J, Meade TW. WISDOM study team. The women's international study of long-duration oestrogen after menopause (WISDOM): a randomised controlled trial. BMC Womens Health 2007;7:2.
24. Maki PM. Hormone therapy and cognitive function: is there a critical period for benefit? Neuroscience 2006;138(3):1027–30.
25. Yamada N, Nakajima S, Noguchi T. Age at onset of delusional disorder is dependent on the delusional theme. Acta Psychiatr Scand 1998;97(2):122–4.
26. Trabert W. 100 years of delusional parasitosis. meta-analysis of 1,223 case reports. Psychopathology 1995;28(5):238–46.
27. Cohen CI, Vahia I, Reyes P, et al. Focus on geriatric psychiatry: Schizophrenia in later life: clinical symptoms and social well-being. Psychiatr Serv 2008;59(3): 232–4.
28. Pearlson GD, Kreger L, Rabins PV, et al. A chart review study of late-onset and early-onset schizophrenia. Am J Psychiatry 1989;146(12):1568–74.
29. Hafner H, Maurer K, Loffler W, et al. Schizophrenia and age. Nervenarzt 1991; 62(9):536–48.
30. Lindamer LA, Lohr JB, Harris MJ, et al. Gender-related clinical differences in older patients with schizophrenia. J Clin Psychiatry 1999;60(1):61–7 [quiz 68–9].
31. Kohler S, van der Werf M, Hart B, et al. Evidence that better outcome of psychosis in women is reversed with increasing age of onset: a population-based 5-year follow-up study. Schizophr Res 2009;113(2–3):226–32.
32. Howard R, Rabins PV, Seeman MV, et al. Late-onset schizophrenia and very-late-onset schizophrenia-like psychosis: an international consensus. the international late-onset schizophrenia group. Am J Psychiatry 2000;157(2):172–8.
33. Tien AY. Distributions of hallucinations in the population. Soc Psychiatry Psychiatr Epidemiol 1991;26(6):287–92.
34. Holroyd S. Visual hallucinations in a geriatric psychiatry clinic: prevalence and associated diagnoses. J Geriatr Psychiatry Neurol 1996;9(4):171–5.
35. Webster R, Holroyd S. Prevalence of psychotic symptoms in delirium. Psychosomatics 2000;41(6):519–22.
36. Fennig S, Bromet E, Jandorf L. Gender differences in clinical characteristics of first-admission psychotic depression. Am J Psychiatry 1993;150(11): 1734–6.
37. Thakur M, Hays J, Krishnan KR. Clinical, demographic and social characteristics of psychotic depression. Psychiatry Res 1999;86(2):99–106.
38. Braunig P, Sarkar R, Effenberger S, et al. Gender differences in psychotic bipolar mania. Gend Med 2009;6(2):356–61.
39. Vanltallie TB. Subsyndromal depression in the elderly: underdiagnosed and undertreated. Metabolism 2005;54(5 Suppl 1):39–44.

40. Mehta KM, Simonsick EM, Penninx BW, et al. Prevalence and correlates of anxiety symptoms in well-functioning older adults: findings from the health aging and body composition study. J Am Geriatr Soc 2003;51(4):499–504.
41. Barry LC, Allore HG, Guo Z, et al. Higher burden of depression among older women: the effect of onset, persistence, and mortality over time. Arch Gen Psychiatry 2008;65(2):172–8.
42. Blazer D, Hughes DC, George LK. The epidemiology of depression in an elderly community population. Gerontologist 1987;27(3):281–7.
43. Silverstein B. Gender differences in the prevalence of somatic versus pure depression: a replication. Am J Psychiatry 2002;159(6):1051–2.
44. Anderson DN. Treating depression in old age: the reasons to be positive. Age Ageing 2001;30(1):13–7.
45. Meehan PJ, Saltzman LE, Sattin RW. Suicides among older united states residents: epidemiologic characteristics and trends. Am J Public Health 1991; 81(9):1198–200.
46. Centers for Disease Control and Prevention (CDC). Suicide among older persons–united states, 1980–1992. MMWR Morb Mortal Wkly Rep 1996;45(1):3–6.
47. Edwards M. Assessing for depression and mood disturbance in later life. Br J Community Nurs 2004;9(11):492–4.
48. Glassman AH, Shapiro PA. Depression and the course of coronary artery disease. Am J Psychiatry 1998;155(1):4–11.
49. Ramasubbu R, Patten SB. Effect of depression on stroke morbidity and mortality. Can J Psychiatry 2003;48(4):250–7.
50. Murphy E, Smith R, Lindesay J, et al. Increased mortality rates in late-life depression. Br J Psychiatry 1988;152:347–53.
51. Flint AJ. Epidemiology and comorbidity of anxiety disorders in the elderly. Am J Psychiatry 1994;151(5):640–9.
52. Lindesay J, Briggs K, Murphy E. The guy's/age concern survey. prevalence rates of cognitive impairment, depression and anxiety in an urban elderly community. Br J Psychiatry 1989;155:317–29.
53. Chou KL. Specific phobia in older adults: evidence from the national epidemiologic survey on alcohol and related conditions. Am J Geriatr Psychiatry 2009; 17(5):376–86.
54. Chou KL. Age at onset of generalized anxiety disorder in older adults. Am J Geriatr Psychiatry 2009;17(6):455–64.
55. Vesga-Lopez O, Schneier FR, Wang S, et al. Gender differences in generalized anxiety disorder: results from the national epidemiologic survey on alcohol and related conditions (NESARC). J Clin Psychiatry 2008;69(10):1606–16.
56. Andreescu C, Lenze EJ, Dew MA, et al. Effect of comorbid anxiety on treatment response and relapse risk in late-life depression: controlled study. Br J Psychiatry 2007;190:344–9.
57. Mancini M, Gianni W, Rossi A, et al. Duloxetine in the management of elderly patients with major depressive disorder: an analysis of published data. Expert Opin Pharmacother 2009;10(5):847–60.
58. Benshoff JJ, Harrawood LK, Koch DS. Substance abuse and the elderly: unique issues and concerns. J Rehabil 2003;69(2):43–8.
59. Gfroerer J, Penne M, Pemberton M, et al. Substance abuse treatment need among older adults in 2020: the impact of the aging baby-boom cohort. Drug Alcohol Depend 2003;69(2):127–35.
60. Onen SH, Onen F, Mangeon JP, et al. Alcohol abuse and dependence in elderly emergency department patients. Arch Gerontol Geriatr 2005;41(2):191–200.

61. Simoni-Wastila L, Yang HK. Psychoactive drug abuse in older adults. Am J Geriatr Pharmacother 2006;4(4):380–94.
62. Ondus KA, Hujer ME, Mann AE, et al. Substance abuse and the hospitalized elderly. Orthop Nurs 1999;18(4):27–34 [quiz 35–6].
63. Finkelstein E, Prabhu M, Chen H. Increased prevalence of falls among elderly individuals with mental health and substance abuse conditions. Am J Geriatr Psychiatry 2007;15(7):611–9.
64. Culberson JW, Ziska M. Prescription drug misuse/abuse in the elderly. Geriatrics 2008;63(9):22–31.
65. Podichetty VK, Mazanec DJ, Biscup RS. Chronic non-malignant musculoskeletal pain in older adults: clinical issues and opioid intervention. Postgrad Med J 2003; 79(937):627–33.
66. Lee HS, Mericle AA, Ayalon L, et al. Harm reduction among at-risk elderly drinkers: a site-specific analysis from the multi-site primary care research in substance abuse and mental health for elderly (PRISM-E) study. Int J Geriatr Psychiatry 2009;24(1):54–60.

Index

Note: Page numbers of article titles are in **boldface** type.

Psychiatr Clin N Am 33 (2010) 487–496
doi:10.1016/S0193-953X(10)00038-9
0193-953X/10/$ – see front matter © 2010 Elsevier Inc. All rights reserved.

psych.theclinics.com

Moving?

Make sure your subscription moves with you!

To notify us of your new address, find your **Clinics Account Number** (located on your mailing label above your name), and contact customer service at:

Email: journalscustomerservice-usa@elsevier.com

800-654-2452 (subscribers in the U.S. & Canada)
314-447-8871 (subscribers outside of the U.S. & Canada)

Fax number: 314-447-8029

Elsevier Health Sciences Division
Subscription Customer Service
3251 Riverport Lane
Maryland Heights, MO 63043

*To ensure uninterrupted delivery of your subscription, please notify us at least 4 weeks in advance of move.